Neurodegeneration in Cognitive Impairment and Mood Disorders for Experimental, Clinical and Translational Neuropsychiatry

Neurodegeneration in Cognitive Impairment and Mood Disorders for Experimental, Clinical and Translational Neuropsychiatry

Editors

Simone Battaglia
Masaru Tanaka

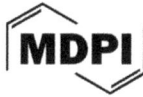

Basel • Beijing • Wuhan • Barcelona • Belgrade • Novi Sad • Cluj • Manchester

Editors

Simone Battaglia
University of Turin
Turin
Italy

Masaru Tanaka
University of Szeged
(HUN-REN-SZTE)
Szeged
Hungary

Editorial Office
MDPI
St. Alban-Anlage 66
4052 Basel, Switzerland

This is a reprint of articles from the Special Issue published online in the open access journal *Biomedicines* (ISSN 2227-9059) (available at: https://www.mdpi.com/journal/biomedicines/special_issues/Neurodegeneration_Neuropsychiatry).

For citation purposes, cite each article independently as indicated on the article page online and as indicated below:

Lastname, A.A.; Lastname, B.B. Article Title. *Journal Name* **Year**, *Volume Number*, Page Range.

ISBN 978-3-7258-0859-5 (Hbk)
ISBN 978-3-7258-0860-1 (PDF)
doi.org/10.3390/books978-3-7258-0860-1

© 2024 by the authors. Articles in this book are Open Access and distributed under the Creative Commons Attribution (CC BY) license. The book as a whole is distributed by MDPI under the terms and conditions of the Creative Commons Attribution-NonCommercial-NoDerivs (CC BY-NC-ND) license.

Contents

About the Editors vii

Preface ix

Simone Battaglia, Alessio Avenanti, László Vécsei and Masaru Tanaka
Neurodegeneration in Cognitive Impairment and Mood Disorders for Experimental, Clinical and Translational Neuropsychiatry
Reprinted from: *Biomedicines* 2024, 12, 574, doi:10.3390/biomedicines12030574 1

Yolanda Cruz-Martínez, Leslie Aguilar-Ponce, Alejandra Romo-Araiza, Almudena Chávez-Guerra, Susana Martiñón, Andrea P. Ibarra-García, et al.
Supplementation with a Symbiotic Induced Neuroprotection and Improved Memory in Rats with Ischemic Stroke
Reprinted from: *Biomedicines* 2024, 12, 209, doi:10.3390/biomedicines12010209 10

Linjing Zhang, Fan Wang, Kailin Xia, Zhou Yu, Yu Fu, Tao Huang and Dongsheng Fan
Unlocking the Medicinal Mysteries: Preventing Lacunar Stroke with Drug Repurposing
Reprinted from: *Biomedicines* 2024, 12, 17, doi:10.3390/biomedicines12010017 22

Deborah E. M. Baliellas, Marcelo P. Barros, Cristina V. Vardaris, Maísa Guariroba, Sandra C. Poppe, Maria F. Martins, et al.
Propentofylline Improves Thiol-Based Antioxidant Defenses and Limits Lipid Peroxidation following Gliotoxic Injury in the Rat Brainstem
Reprinted from: *Biomedicines* 2023, 11, 1652, doi:10.3390/biomedicines11061652 35

Georgi Panov, Silvana Dyulgerova and Presyana Panova
Cognition in Patients with Schizophrenia: Interplay between Working Memory, Disorganized Symptoms, Dissociation, and the Onset and Duration of Psychosis, as Well as Resistance to Treatment
Reprinted from: *Biomedicines* 2023, 11, 3114, doi:10.3390/biomedicines11123114 46

Marcela de Oliveira, Felipe Balistieri Santinelli, Paulo Noronha Lisboa-Filho and Fabio Augusto Barbieri
The Blood Concentration of Metallic Nanoparticles Is Related to Cognitive Performance in People with Multiple Sclerosis: An Exploratory Analysis
Reprinted from: *Biomedicines* 2023, 11, 1819, doi:10.3390/biomedicines11071819 63

Aabid Mustafa Koul, Faisel Ahmad, Abida Bhat, Qurat-ul Aein, Ajaz Ahmad, Aijaz Ahmad Reshi and Rauf-ur-Rashid Kaul
Unraveling Down Syndrome: From Genetic Anomaly to Artificial Intelligence-Enhanced Diagnosis
Reprinted from: *Biomedicines* 2023, 11, 3284, doi:10.3390/biomedicines11123284 74

Khoa Nguyen Tran, Nhi Phuc Khanh Nguyen, Ly Thi Huong Nguyen, Heung-Mook Shin and In-Jun Yang
Screening for Neuroprotective and Rapid Antidepressant-like Effects of 20 Essential Oils
Reprinted from: *Biomedicines* 2023, 11, 1248, doi:10.3390/biomedicines11051248 92

Yangyang Cui, Hankun Zhang, Song Wang, Junzhe Lu, Jinmei He, Lanlan Liu and Weiqiang Liu
Stimulated Parotid Saliva Is a Better Method for Depression Prediction
Reprinted from: *Biomedicines* 2022, 10, 2220, doi:10.3390/biomedicines10092220 122

Ravi Philip Rajkumar
Biomarkers of Neurodegeneration in Post-Traumatic Stress Disorder: An Integrative Review
Reprinted from: *Biomedicines* 2023, 11, 1465, doi:10.3390/biomedicines11051465 . . . . **134**

Catarina Moura, Ana Salomé Correia, Mariana Pereira, Eduarda Ribeiro, Joana Santos and Nuno Vale
Atorvastatin and Nitrofurantoin Repurposed in the Context of Breast Cancer and Neuroblastoma Cells
Reprinted from: *Biomedicines* 2023, 11, 903, doi:10.3390/biomedicines11030903 . . . . **156**

Tosin A. Olasehinde and Oyinlola O. Olaokun
The Beneficial Role of Apigenin against Cognitive and Neurobehavioural Dysfunction: A Systematic Review of Preclinical Investigations
Reprinted from: *Biomedicines* 2024, 12, 178, doi:10.3390/biomedicines12010178 . . . . **176**

Aleksandar Stojsavljević, Novak Lakićević and Sladan Pavlović
Mercury and Autism Spectrum Disorder: Exploring the Link through Comprehensive Review and Meta-Analysis
Reprinted from: *Biomedicines* 2023, 11, 3344, doi:10.3390/biomedicines11123344 . . . . **193**

About the Editors

Simone Battaglia

Simone Battaglia, Ph.D., is an Assistant Professor in Cognitive Neuroscience at the Centre for Studies and Research in Cognitive Neuroscience, Department of Psychology, University of Bologna (Italy), and holds a Research Fellowship at the Department of Psychology, University of Turin (Italy).

His research experience focuses on investigating the intricate functional interplay of different brain areas involved in emotional learning, action control, brain plasticity, decision making, and various cognitive tasks. To this end, his research activities primarily revolve around the utilization of non-invasive brain stimulation techniques, such as transcranial magnetic stimulation (TMS) and transcranial direct current stimulation (tDCS), in addition to employing various neuroscientific techniques to record physiological measures, including EEG, SCR, HRV, and EMG. He has conducted extensive research involving healthy individuals, examining intra/inter-individual differences and patients with acquired brain injuries. He employs a multimodal approach that integrates behavioral assessments, electrophysiological measurements, and neurostimulation techniques in his investigations. His research aims to develop innovative therapeutic protocols, focusing on utilizing the cortico-cortical paired associative stimulation (ccPAS) method to facilitate neuroplasticity and enhance functional recovery.

Masaru Tanaka

Masaru Tanaka, M.D., Ph.D. is a Senior Research Fellow in the Danube Neuroscience Research Laboratory, HUN-REN-SZTE Neuroscience Research Group, Hungarian Research Network, University of Szeged (HUN-REN-SZTE). His scientific interests include depression, anxiety, dementia pain, their comorbid nature, and translational research in neurological diseases and psychiatric disorders. His current research focuses on the antidepressant, anxiolytic, and nootropic effects of neuropeptide, neurohormones, and tryptophan metabolites and their analogs in preclinical neuropsychiatric diseases. He is an Editorial Board Member of Frontiers in Neuroscience, Psychiatry, Anesthesia Research, the Journal of Integrative Neuroscience, Advances in Clinical Experimental Medicine, Biology and Life Sciences, and Biomedicines. He obtained a Ph.D. in Medicine and an MD in General Medicine from the University of Szeged and a bachelor's degree in Biophysics from the University of Illinois, Urbana-Champaign.

Preface

In the quest to understand the complexities of the brain and nervous system, this Reprint shines as a beacon of hope and knowledge. With great pride and a deep sense of purpose, we present a collection of papers exploring the theme of neuroprotection from various perspectives and disciplines. Our journey through the labyrinth of neurological conditions, such as stroke, multiple sclerosis, Down syndrome, major depressive disorder, post-traumatic stress disorder, breast cancer, and neuroblastoma, has been both challenging and rewarding.

We aim to shed light on the potential of various agents and strategies for strengthening the brain's defenses, including symbiotics, pharmaceuticals, essential oils, salivary cortisol, apigenin, and repurposed drugs. The discovery of intricate mechanisms and pathways, such as oxidative stress, inflammation, neurotransmission, neurogenesis, and epigenetics, demonstrates the relentless pursuit of understanding. We emphasize the importance of non-invasive, personalized methods for monitoring and improving neuroprotection, leveraging blood iron concentration, artificial intelligence, and mercury levels.

The introduction of cutting-edge techniques, sophisticated real-time analysis algorithms, machine learning, and physiological biomarkers ushers in a new era in mental healthcare, one that promises to alleviate the societal and economic burdens associated with psychiatric disorders. The contributions on these pages not only advance the field of neuroprotection but also pave the way for new research and treatments.

We sincerely thank all contributors whose tireless efforts have enriched this Special Issue. Their findings emphasize the critical role of neuroprotection in maintaining neurological health and promoting well-being. We sincerely hope this Special Issue will act as a catalyst for further research and discovery in the critical field of neuroprotection.

Simone Battaglia and Masaru Tanaka
Editors

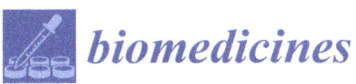 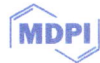

Editorial

Neurodegeneration in Cognitive Impairment and Mood Disorders for Experimental, Clinical and Translational Neuropsychiatry

Simone Battaglia [1,2,*,†], Alessio Avenanti [2,3], László Vécsei [4,5] and Masaru Tanaka [5,*,†]

1. Center for Studies and Research in Cognitive Neuroscience, Department of Psychology "Renzo Canestrari", Cesena Campus, Alma Mater Studiorum Università di Bologna, 47521 Cesena, Italy
2. Department of Psychology, University of Turin, 10124 Turin, Italy; alessio.avenanti@unibo.it
3. Neuropsicology and Cognitive Neuroscience Research Center (CINPSI Neurocog), Universidad Católica del Maule, Talca 3460000, Chile
4. Department of Neurology, Albert Szent-Györgyi Medical School, University of Szeged, Semmelweis u. 6, H-6725 Szeged, Hungary; vecsei.laszlo@med.u-szeged.hu
5. HUN-REN-SZTE Neuroscience Research Group, Hungarian Research Network, University of Szeged (HUN-REN-SZTE), Tisza Lajos krt. 113, H-6725 Szeged, Hungary

* Correspondence: simone.battaglia@unibo.it (S.B.); tanaka.masaru.1@med.u-szeged.hu (M.T.); Tel.: +36-62-342-847 (M.T.)

† These authors contributed equally to this work.

1. Introduction

Neurodegeneration poses a significant challenge for the fields of neuroscience and medicine, as it is the underlying cause of the development and advancement of numerous neurodegenerative and psychiatric disorders [1–3]. It encompasses the progressive decay and loss of neurons across various levels of organization, ranging from molecular to network levels [4–7]. Onset can manifest at various life stages, ranging from early phases, as observed in neurodevelopmental disorders, to later stages, exemplified by conditions like Alzheimer's disease (AD) [8–10]. Neurodegeneration has the potential to impact cognitive, emotional, and behavioral functions, as well as the neural mechanisms associated with consciousness and attention [11–13]. Hence, comprehending the mechanisms and repercussions of neurodegeneration is imperative in order to identify risk factors, biomarkers, and therapeutic targets [14–16]. Nevertheless, the existing therapies for neurodegenerative disorders primarily address alleviate symptoms but are largely inadequate in terms of efficacy. Hence, there is a requirement for new and inventive methods, such as non-invasive brain stimulation, that can regulate neural activity and plasticity in a secure and reversible manner [17–21]. The field is rapidly evolving, with a focus on identifying new avenues of clinical research, elucidating potential mechanisms for the therapeutic effects of non-invasive brain stimulation (NIBS) and exploring the potential synergy between different stimulation protocols and pharmacological interventions [22–27].

The study of neurodegeneration in cognitive impairment and mood disorders is a vast and intricate domain that encounters numerous obstacles in comprehending, diagnosing, and treating these conditions [28–30]. Several existing obstacles include: The diverse and inconsistent nature of neurological and psychiatric disorders, posing challenges for the identification of shared mechanisms, biomarkers, and therapeutic targets across various subtypes, stages, and populations [31–35]. The absence of efficacious disease-altering treatments for the majority of neurodegenerative disorders, which restricts the available choices and results for patients and caregivers; The ethical and practical considerations associated with carrying out clinical trials and translational research in vulnerable and diverse populations, such as the elderly, children, and minority groups [36–38]. The integration and interpretation data derived from various origins and modes, including genetics, epigenetics,

Citation: Battaglia, S.; Avenanti, A.; Vécsei, L.; Tanaka, M. Neurodegeneration in Cognitive Impairment and Mood Disorders for Experimental, Clinical and Translational Neuropsychiatry. *Biomedicines* 2024, 12, 574. https://doi.org/10.3390/biomedicines12030574

Received: 15 February 2024
Accepted: 26 February 2024
Published: 5 March 2024

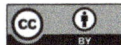

Copyright: © 2024 by the authors. Licensee MDPI, Basel, Switzerland. This article is an open access article distributed under the terms and conditions of the Creative Commons Attribution (CC BY) license (https://creativecommons.org/licenses/by/4.0/).

proteomics, metabolomics, imaging, electrophysiology, and neuropsychology [39–47]. The development and validation of novel methods, such as NIBS, artificial intelligence, and drug repurposing, which necessitate thorough examination and assessment of their safety, effectiveness, and mechanisms [11,48–54]. Addressing these challenges requires collaborative efforts among researchers, clinicians, patients, and policymakers from various fields to enhance our understanding and improve the treatment of neurodegeneration underlying cognitive impairment and mood disorders [55–58]. This special issue focuses on the most recent advancements and hurdles in this area, examining them from experimental, clinical, and translational perspectives.

2. Special Issue Articles

2.1. Stroke and Neuroprotection

Stroke is a critical health issue characterized by the interruption of blood flow to the brain, leading to the death and harm of neurons. Neuroprotection is a key strategy aimed at protecting neurons from damage and preserving their survival and function [59–61]. In this special issue, three articles examined various approaches to promote neuroprotection in animal models of stroke [62–64]. An article by Cruz-Martínez Y et al. investigated the impact of symbiotic supplementation, comprising probiotics and prebiotics, on memory and neuronal survival in rats suffering from ischemic stroke [62]. This study tested the effects of a symbiotic (inulin and Enterococcus faecium). The symbiotic reduced inflammation, protected neurons, and improved memory in subacute phase. This suggests that symbiotics may be useful for stroke treatment and prevention.

To lower the risk of lacunar stroke, a type of stroke that affects the brain's small blood vessels, Zhang L et al. examined the viability of drug repurposing, a strategy that involves using fully approved drugs to treat different medical conditions. The authors used a two-sample Mendelian randomization analysis estimating the genetic variant-exposure and the genetic variant-outcome associations to identify which drugs can prevent lacunar stroke, a type of cerebral infarction [63]. This study found that genetic variants that mimic the effects of calcium channel blockers, statins, ezetimibe, and antisense anti-apoC3 agents can reduce the risk of the condition. The study suggests that these drugs should be repurposed for lacunar stroke prevention to promote healthier brain aging.

The third article by Baliellas et al. examined the impact of propentofylline (PROP), a xanthine derivative, on strengthening antioxidant defenses and decreasing lipid peroxidation in the brainstem of rats with gliotoxic injury, which serves as a model for neurodegeneration [64]. The authors tested the effects of PROP, a drug that reduces inflammation in brain cells in rats exposed to a toxic substance that causes oxidative damage in the brain. The study found that PROP prevented an increase in lipid peroxidation, a marker of oxidative stress, and enhanced the activity of glutathione reductase, an enzyme that recycles antioxidants, in the rat brainstem. This study concluded that PROP could protect the brain from oxidative damage and neurodegeneration. These articles offer a new and valuable understanding of the mechanisms and advantages of neuroprotection against stroke and related disorders.

2.2. Cognitions in Schizophrenia (SCZ), Multiple Sclerosis (MS), and Down Syndrome (DS)

Schizophrenia (SCZ) is a complex mental disorder that affects a range of cognitive capabilities, including memory, attention, reasoning, and language [65–67]. Treatment for this condition generally involves the use of antipsychotic medication, as well as psychotherapy and psychosocial interventions [68–70]. Nevertheless, the outcomes of these treatments can vary depending on several factors [71–73]. This special issue features three articles that explore various aspects of cognition in individuals with SCZ [74–76]. The articles explored how cognition is affected by factors such as the onset and duration of psychosis, severity of symptoms, level of dissociation, and resistance to treatment. Panov et al. examined the relationship between working memory, attention, and SCZ [74]. The study found that most patients with SCZ had problems with working memory and attention and that these problems were worse in patients who did not respond to treatment. The study also found that working memory and attention problems were linked to disorganized behavior, duration of illness, and dissociative symptoms. The study suggests that working memory and attention could be used as indicators of SCZ progression and treatment response.

In another article, de Oliveira et al. investigated the feasibility of utilizing metallic nanoparticles present in the bloodstream as biomarkers for assessing cognitive performance. The research team explored how the blood levels of metallic nanoparticles affect the cognitive abilities of people with multiple sclerosis (MS) [75]. This study measured the blood levels of eight different metals and two cognitive tests in 21 patients with MS. The authors found that higher blood levels of iron, zinc, and total metals were associated with better cognitive performance. This study proposed that blood iron concentration could be a useful indicator of cognitive impairment in people with MS.

Furthermore, they examined the application of artificial intelligence as a means of improving the diagnosis and treatment of SCZ and related conditions. Koul et al. presented a review of Down syndrome (DS), a genetic disorder that causes intellectual and physical impairments [76]. This work discusses how artificial intelligence and machine learning can help diagnose and treat DS by analyzing various data sources. The text highlights the benefits of these technologies in understanding and improving the lives of people with DS. Overall, these articles provide novel knowledge that contributes to our understanding of the cognitive impairments and difficulties experienced by individuals with SCZ and their caregivers.

2.3. Depression and Antidepressants

Major depressive disorder (MDD) is a widespread and debilitating mood disorder that impacts a substantial number of individuals globally [67,77–79]. Characterized by persistent feelings of sadness, reduced interest, diminished self-worth, and various physical and mental symptoms, it often co-occurs with other conditions, such as anxiety, chronic pain, and neurodegenerative diseases [80–83]. In this special issue, three articles explored different approaches for diagnosing and treating depression and its comorbidities [84–86]. The first article assessed the neuroprotective and swiftly acting antidepressant-like properties of 20 essential oils in mice. Tran et al. conducted a study aimed at assessing the potential of essential oils as rapid-acting antidepressants [84]. The study utilized cell and animal models to evaluate the neuroprotective, anti-inflammatory, and behavioral effects of essential oils. The results indicated that certain essential oils and their constituents, possibly operating through glutamate receptors, exhibited positive effects on these parameters. The study recommended additional research on Atractylodes lancea and Chrysanthemum morifolium essential oils.

In the second article, Cui et al. suggests that stimulated parotid saliva is a more accurate indicator of depressive disorder than unstimulated saliva. The authors conducted a study to investigate the influence of various saliva collection methods on cortisol levels, which are thought to be indicative of this emotional state [85]. The results of the study revealed that unstimulated whole-saliva cortisol was most closely related to blood cortisol levels, while stimulated parotid salivary cortisol was the most reliable predictor of the negative emotional condition. Furthermore, the study confirmed that individuals with depression had higher salivary cortisol levels compared to healthy controls, and that salivary cortisol levels demonstrated a positive correlation with the severity of the condition. The study proposed that salivary cortisol could serve as a useful non-invasive method for monitoring MDD.

In the third article, Rajkumar examines biomarkers associated with neurodegeneration in post-traumatic stress disorder (PTSD), a condition that has the potential to initiate or exacerbate depressive symptom. The author conducted a comprehensive review of the relationship between PTSD and neurodegenerative diseases, including AD and Parkinson's disease [86]. According to the review, a range of biomarkers, such as brain structure, genetics, inflammation, metabolism, and sleep, are linked to both PTSD and neurodegenerative disorders. The review also delved into the potential mechanisms and implications of these associations. The review found that PTSD may contribute to an increased risk of developing neurodegenerative diseases and recommended preventive measures.

2.4. Drug Repurposing and Cancer

Cancer is a diverse array of diseases that is distinguished by the uncontrolled expansion and invasion of abnormal cells into neighboring tissues [79,87–89]. The treatment of cancer often involves surgical intervention, chemotherapy, radiation therapy, and immunotherapy; however, these approaches have limitations and may produce adverse effects [90–92]. Therefore, the process of repurposing existing drugs for new applications, referred to as drug repurposing, offers a promising strategy for the development of novel and potent anticancer agents or adjuvants [58,93–95]. In this special issue, three articles were published that explored the potential of drug repurposing in the context of cancer and its associated challenges [96–98]. One article by Moura et al. assessed the anticancer properties of atorvastatin, a medication used to reduce cholesterol levels, and nitrofurantoin, an antibiotic [96]. The authors tested the efficacy of repurposed drugs on breast cancer and neuroblastoma cells to determine their effectiveness, both individually and in combination with doxorubicin. The results indicated that both drugs decreased the viability of both cell lines, and the combination of atorvastatin and nitrofurantoin was more effective in SH-SY5Y cells than in MCF-7 cells. The study underscores the potential use of these drugs in treating breast cancer and neuroblastoma.

In another study, Olasehinde et al. examined the beneficial impact of apigenin, a flavonoid present in plants, on mitigating cognitive and neurobehavioral impairment caused by chemotherapy. The authors conducted a comprehensive review of studies that investigated the effects of apigenin, a plant compound, on various aspects of memory and behavior in animal models of neurological disorders [97]. The review found that apigenin exhibited cognitive and neurobehavioral enhancing effects and modulated several molecular and biochemical pathways related to neuroprotection. However, the review also emphasized the need for further research to establish the optimal dosage and duration of apigenin treatment and to evaluate its efficacy in human subjects.

In the third article, Stojsavljević et al. investigated the correlation between mercury exposure and autism spectrum disorder, a neurodevelopmental condition that may elevate the likelihood of developing cancer [98]. The authors carried out a meta-analysis of studies that investigated mercury levels in various biological samples of children with and without autism. This study revealed that children with autism exhibited higher blood, plasma, and red blood cell mercury levels, but not in their hair and urine. The review proposed that children with autism had impaired mercury detoxification and excretion and that exposure to mercury could exacerbate their condition. Furthermore, the study recommended decreasing Hg^{++} exposure and closely monitoring Hg^{++} levels in children with autism. These articles offer new perspectives on the mechanisms and applications of repurposed drugs in cancer research and therapy.

3. Conclusions

This special issue showcases a series of papers that delve into the theme of neuroprotection from diverse perspectives and disciplines. These papers cover a wide range of conditions that affect the brain and nervous system, such as stroke, MS, DS, MDD, PTSD, breast cancer, and neuroblastoma. Additionally, the studies examine the potential of various agents and strategies to enhance neuroprotection, including symbiotics, drugs, essential oils, salivary cortisol, apigenin, and repurposed drugs. These studies have revealed the intricate and multifaceted mechanisms and pathways that underlie neuroprotection, including oxidative stress, inflammation, neurotransmission, neurogenesis, and epigenetics [99–103]. The papers also emphasize the importance of non-invasive and personalized approaches for monitoring and improving neuroprotection, such as blood iron concentration, artificial intelligence, and mercury levels. The application of these new techniques, advanced real-time analysis algorithms, machine learning, and physiological biomarkers may streamline the mental healthcare process, alleviating the social burden and economic pressures commonly associated with psychiatric disorders [104–107]. These papers make significant contributions to the field of neuroprotection by advancing knowledge and practice, and suggest new avenues for future research and intervention. The special issue highlights the importance and relevance of neuroprotection in preventing and treating various neurological disorders, and promoting brain health and well-being.

Author Contributions: Conceptualization, S.B. and M.T.; writing—original draft preparation, M.T.; writing—review and editing, S.B., A.A., L.V. and M.T.; supervision, S.B. and M.T.; project administration, S.B. and M.T.; funding acquisition, S.B. and M.T. All authors have read and agreed to the published version of the manuscript.

Funding: This work was supported by the National Research, Development, and Innovation Office—NKFIH K138125, SZTE SZAOK-KKA No:2022/5S729, and the HUN-REN Hungarian Research Network to L. Vécsei and M. Tanaka. This work was also supported by #NEXTGENERATIONEU (NGEU) and funded by the Ministry of University and Research (MUR), National Recovery and Resilience Plan (NRRP), project MNESYS (PE0000006)—A Multiscale integrated approach to the study of the nervous system in health and disease (DN. 1553 11.10.2022) to S. Battaglia and A. Avenanti.

Institutional Review Board Statement: Not applicable.

Informed Consent Statement: Not applicable.

Data Availability Statement: Data sharing is not applicable to this article.

Conflicts of Interest: The authors declare no conflict of interest.

Abbreviations

AD	Alzheimer's disease
DS	Down syndrome
MDD	major depressive disorder
MS	multiple sclerosis
NIBS	non-invasive brain stimulation
PROP	propentofylline
PTSD	post-traumatic stress disorder
SCZ	schizophrenia

References

1. Rajkumar, R.P. Comorbid depression and anxiety: Integration of insights from attachment theory and cognitive neuroscience, and their implications for research and treatment. *Front. Behav. Neurosci.* **2022**, *16*, 1104928. [CrossRef]
2. Husain, M. Transdiagnostic neurology: Neuropsychiatric symptoms in neurodegenerative diseases. *Brain* **2017**, *140*, 1535–1536. [CrossRef]
3. Galts, C.P.; Bettio, L.E.; Jewett, D.C.; Yang, C.C.; Brocardo, P.S.; Rodrigues, A.L.S.; Thacker, J.S.; Gil-Mohapel, J. Depression in neurodegenerative diseases: Common mechanisms and current treatment options. *Neurosci. Biobehav. Rev.* **2019**, *102*, 56–84. [CrossRef] [PubMed]
4. Nani, A.; Manuello, J.; Mancuso, L.; Liloia, D.; Costa, T.; Vercelli, A.; Duca, S.; Cauda, F. The pathoconnectivity network analysis of the insular cortex: A morphometric fingerprinting. *NeuroImage* **2021**, *225*, 117481. [CrossRef] [PubMed]
5. Mancuso, L.; Cavuoti-Cabanillas, S.; Liloia, D.; Manuello, J.; Buzi, G.; Duca, S.; Cauda, F.; Costa, T. Default Mode Network spatial configuration varies across task domains. *bioRxiv* **2021**. [CrossRef]
6. Makhlouf, A.T.; Drew, W.; Stubbs, J.L.; Taylor, J.J.; Liloia, D.; Grafman, J.; Silbersweig, D.; Fox, M.D.; Siddiqi, S.H. Heterogenous Patterns of Brain Atrophy in Schizophrenia Localize to A Common Brain Network. 2023. Available online: https://www.researchgate.net/publication/374933868_Heterogenous_Patterns_of_Brain_Atrophy_in_Schizophrenia_Localize_to_A_Common_Brain_Network/fulltext/65385f565d51a8012b6da326/Heterogenous-Patterns-of-Brain-Atrophy-in-Schizophrenia-Localize-to-A-Common-Brain-Network.pdf (accessed on 27 February 2024).
7. Turrini, S.; Wong, B.; Eldaief, M.; Press, D.Z.; Sinclair, D.A.; Koch, G.; Avenanti, A.; Santarnecchi, E. The multifactorial nature of healthy brain ageing: Brain changes, functional decline and protective factors. *Ageing Res. Rev.* **2023**, *88*, 101939. [CrossRef]

8. Du, H.; Yang, B.; Wang, H.; Zeng, Y.; Xin, J.; Li, X. The non-linear correlation between the volume of cerebral white matter lesions and incidence of bipolar disorder: A secondary analysis of data from a cross-sectional study. *Front. Psychiatry* **2023**, *14*, 1149663. [CrossRef] [PubMed]
9. Modgil, S.; Lahiri, D.K.; Sharma, V.L.; Anand, A. Role of early life exposure and environment on neurodegeneration: Implications on brain disorders. *Transl. Neurodegener.* **2014**, *3*, 1–14. [CrossRef] [PubMed]
10. Hickman, R.A.; O'Shea, S.A.; Mehler, M.F.; Chung, W.K. Neurogenetic disorders across the lifespan: From aberrant development to degeneration. *Nat. Rev. Neurol.* **2022**, *18*, 117–124. [CrossRef]
11. Buglio, D.S.; Marton, L.T.; Laurindo, L.F.; Guiguer, E.L.; Araújo, A.C.; Buchaim, R.L.; Goulart, R.d.A.; Rubira, C.J.; Barbalho, S.M. The role of resveratrol in mild cognitive impairment and Alzheimer's disease: A systematic review. *J. Med. Food* **2022**, *25*, 797–806. [CrossRef]
12. Levenson, R.W.; Sturm, V.E.; Haase, C.M. Emotional and behavioral symptoms in neurodegenerative disease: A model for studying the neural bases of psychopathology. *Annu. Rev. Clin. Psychol.* **2014**, *10*, 581–606. [CrossRef] [PubMed]
13. Cieslak, A.; Smith, E.E.; Lysack, J.; Ismail, Z. Case series of mild behavioral impairment: Toward an understanding of the early stages of neurodegenerative diseases affecting behavior and cognition. *Int. Psychogeriatr.* **2018**, *30*, 273–280. [CrossRef] [PubMed]
14. Tanaka, M.; Török, N.; Vécsei, L. Novel pharmaceutical approaches in dementia. In *NeuroPsychopharmacotherapy*; Springer: Berlin/Heidelberg, Germany, 2022; pp. 2803–2820.
15. Polyák, H.; Galla, Z.; Nánási, N.; Cseh, E.K.; Rajda, C.; Veres, G.; Spekker, E.; Szabó, Á.; Klivényi, P.; Tanaka, M. The tryptophan-kynurenine metabolic system is suppressed in cuprizone-induced model of demyelination simulating progressive multiple sclerosis. *Biomedicines* **2023**, *11*, 945. [CrossRef] [PubMed]
16. Hansson, O. Biomarkers for neurodegenerative diseases. *Nat. Med.* **2021**, *27*, 954–963. [CrossRef]
17. Battaglia, S.; Schmidt, A.; Hassel, S.; Tanaka, M. Case reports in neuroimaging and stimulation. *Front. Psychiatry* **2023**, *14*, 1264669. [CrossRef]
18. Tanaka, M.; Diano, M.; Battaglia, S. Insights into structural and functional organization of the brain: Evidence from neuroimaging and non-invasive brain stimulation techniques. *Front. Psychiatry* **2023**, *14*, 1225755. [CrossRef]
19. Turrini, S.; Bevacqua, N.; Cataneo, A.; Chiappini, E.; Fiori, F.; Battaglia, S.; Romei, V.; Avenanti, A. Neurophysiological Markers of Premotor–Motor Network Plasticity Predict Motor Performance in Young and Older Adults. *Biomedicines* **2023**, *11*, 1464. [CrossRef]
20. Turrini, S.; Bevacqua, N.; Cataneo, A.; Chiappini, E.; Fiori, F.; Candidi, M.; Avenanti, A. Transcranial cortico-cortical paired associative stimulation (ccPAS) over ventral premotor-motor pathways enhances action performance and corticomotor excitability in young adults more than in elderly adults. *Front. Aging Neurosci.* **2023**, *15*, 1119508. [CrossRef]
21. Menardi, A.; Rossi, S.; Koch, G.; Hampel, H.; Vergallo, A.; Nitsche, M.A.; Stern, Y.; Borroni, B.; Cappa, S.F.; Cotelli, M.; et al. Toward noninvasive brain stimulation 2.0 in Alzheimer's disease. *Ageing Res. Rev.* **2022**, *75*, 101555. [CrossRef]
22. Battaglia, S.; Di Fazio, C.; Mazzà, M.; Tamietto, M.; Avenanti, A. Targeting Human Glucocorticoid Receptors in Fear Learning: A Multiscale Integrated Approach to Study Functional Connectivity. *Int. J. Mol. Sci.* **2024**, *25*, 864. [CrossRef]
23. Battaglia, M.R.; Di Fazio, C.; Battaglia, S. Activated tryptophan-kynurenine metabolic system in the human brain is associated with learned fear. *Front. Mol. Neurosci.* **2023**, *16*, 1217090. [CrossRef]
24. Battaglia, S.; Di Fazio, C.; Vicario, C.M.; Avenanti, A. Neuropharmacological modulation of N-methyl-D-aspartate, noradrenaline and endocannabinoid receptors in fear extinction learning: Synaptic transmission and plasticity. *Int. J. Mol. Sci.* **2023**, *24*, 5926. [CrossRef]
25. Vila-Merkle, H.; González-Martínez, A.; Campos-Jiménez, R.; Martínez-Ricós, J.; Teruel-Martí, V.; Lloret, A.; Blasco-Serra, A.; Cervera-Ferri, A. Sex differences in amygdalohippocampal oscillations and neuronal activation in a rodent anxiety model and in response to infralimbic deep brain stimulation. *Front. Behav. Neurosci.* **2023**, *17*, 1122163. [CrossRef]
26. Chu, P.-C.; Huang, C.-S.; Chang, P.-K.; Chen, R.-S.; Chen, K.-T.; Hsieh, T.-H.; Liu, H.-L. Weak Ultrasound Contributes to Neuromodulatory Effects in the Rat Motor Cortex. *Int. J. Mol. Sci.* **2023**, *24*, 2578. [CrossRef] [PubMed]
27. Rymaszewska, J.; Wieczorek, T.; Fila-Witecka, K.; Smarzewska, K.; Weiser, A.; Piotrowski, P.; Tabakow, P. Various neuromodulation methods including Deep Brain Stimulation of the medial forebrain bundle combined with psychopharmacotherapy of treatment-resistant depression—Case report. *Front. Psychiatry* **2023**, *13*, 3014. [CrossRef] [PubMed]
28. Deyell, J.S.; Sriparna, M.; Ying, M.; Mao, X. The Interplay between α-Synuclein and Microglia in α-Synucleinopathies. *Int. J. Mol. Sci.* **2023**, *24*, 2477. [CrossRef] [PubMed]
29. Granholm, A.C.; Boger, H.; Emborg, M.E. Mood, memory and movement: An age-related neurodegenerative complex? *Curr. Aging Sci.* **2008**, *1*, 133–139. [CrossRef]
30. Hussain, M.; Kumar, P.; Khan, S.; Gordon, D.K.; Khan, S. Similarities between depression and neurodegenerative diseases: Pathophysiology, challenges in diagnosis and treatment options. *Cureus* **2020**, *12*, e11613. [CrossRef]
31. Battaglia, S.; Nazzi, C.; Thayer, J.F. Genetic differences associated with dopamine and serotonin release mediate fear-induced bradycardia in the human brain. *Transl. Psychiatry* **2024**, *14*, 24. [CrossRef]
32. Battaglia, S.; Nazzi, C.; Thayer, J. Heart's tale of trauma: Fear-conditioned heart rate changes in post-traumatic stress disorder. *Acta Psychiatr. Scand.* **2023**, *148*, 463–466. [CrossRef]
33. Battaglia, S.; Nazzi, C.; Thayer, J. Fear-induced bradycardia in mental disorders: Foundations, current advances, future perspectives. *Neurosci. Biobehav. Rev.* **2023**, *149*, 105163. [CrossRef] [PubMed]
34. Tanaka, M.; Szabó, Á.; Körtési, T.; Szok, D.; Tajti, J.; Vécsei, L. From CGRP to PACAP, VIP, and Beyond: Unraveling the Next Chapters in Migraine Treatment. *Cells* **2023**, *12*, 2649. [CrossRef] [PubMed]

35. Tanaka, M.; Kádár, K.; Tóth, G.; Telegdy, G. Antidepressant-like effects of urocortin 3 fragments. *Brain Res. Bull.* **2011**, *84*, 414–418. [CrossRef] [PubMed]
36. Tanaka, M.; Szabó, Á.; Vécsei, L.; Giménez-Llort, L. Emerging translational research in neurological and psychiatric diseases: From in vitro to in vivo models. *Int. J. Mol. Sci.* **2023**, *24*, 15739. [CrossRef] [PubMed]
37. Guralnik, J.M.; Kritchevsky, S.B. Translating research to promote healthy aging: The complementary role of longitudinal studies and clinical trials. *J. Am. Geriatr. Soc.* **2010**, *58* (Suppl. 2), S337–S342. [CrossRef] [PubMed]
38. Winter, S.S.; Page-Reeves, J.M.; Page, K.A.; Haozous, E.; Solares, A.; Nicole Cordova, C.; Larson, R.S. Inclusion of special populations in clinical research: Important considerations and guidelines. *J. Clin. Transl. Res.* **2018**, *4*, 56–69.
39. Tanaka, M.; Szabó, Á.; Vécsei, L. Preclinical modeling in depression and anxiety: Current challenges and future research directions. *Adv. Clin. Exp. Med.* **2023**, *32*, 505–509. [CrossRef]
40. Gračan, R.; Blažević, S.A.; Brižić, M.; Hranilovic, D. Beyond the Brain: Perinatal Exposure of Rats to Serotonin Enhancers Induces Long-Term Changes in the Jejunum and Liver. *Biomedicines* **2024**, *12*, 357. [CrossRef]
41. Hakamata, Y.; Hori, H.; Mizukami, S.; Izawa, S.; Yoshida, F.; Moriguchi, Y.; Hanakawa, T.; Inoue, Y.; Tagaya, H. Blunted diurnal interleukin-6 rhythm is associated with amygdala emotional hypoactivity and depression: A modulating role of gene-stressor interactions. *Front. Psychiatry* **2023**, *14*, 1196235. [CrossRef]
42. Kim, B.-H.; Kim, S.-H.; Han, C.; Jeong, H.-G.; Lee, M.-S.; Kim, J. Antidepressant-induced mania in panic disorder: A single-case study of clinical and functional connectivity characteristics. *Front. Psychiatry* **2023**, *14*, 1205126. [CrossRef]
43. Adamu, M.J.; Qiang, L.; Nyatega, C.O.; Younis, A.; Kawuwa, H.B.; Jabire, A.H.; Saminu, S. Unraveling the pathophysiology of schizophrenia: Insights from structural magnetic resonance imaging studies. *Front. Psychiatry* **2023**, *14*, 1188603. [CrossRef] [PubMed]
44. Liu, M.; Xie, X.; Xie, J.; Tian, S.; Du, X.; Feng, H.; Zhang, H. Early-onset Alzheimer's disease with depression as the first symptom: A case report with literature review. *Front. Psychiatry* **2023**, *14*, 1192562. [CrossRef] [PubMed]
45. Nyatega, C.O.; Qiang, L.; Adamu, M.J.; Kawuwa, H.B. Gray matter, white matter and cerebrospinal fluid abnormalities in Parkinson's disease: A voxel-based morphometry study. *Front. Psychiatry* **2022**, *13*, 1027907. [CrossRef] [PubMed]
46. Liloia, D.; Cauda, F.; Uddin, L.Q.; Manuello, J.; Mancuso, L.; Keller, R.; Nani, A.; Costa, T. Revealing the selectivity of neuroanatomical alteration in autism spectrum disorder via reverse inference. *Biol. Psychiatry Cogn. Neurosci. Neuroimaging* **2023**, *8*, 1075–1083. [CrossRef]
47. Liloia, D.; Crocetta, A.; Cauda, F.; Duca, S.; Costa, T.; Manuello, J. Seeking Overlapping Neuroanatomical Alterations between Dyslexia and Attention-Deficit/Hyperactivity Disorder: A Meta-Analytic Replication Study. *Brain Sci.* **2022**, *12*, 1367. [CrossRef] [PubMed]
48. Gregorio, F.; Battaglia, S. Advances in EEG-based functional connectivity approaches to the study of the central nervous system in health and disease. *Adv. Clin. Exp. Med.* **2023**, *32*, 607–612. [CrossRef]
49. Di Gregorio, F.; Steinhauser, M.; Maier, M.E.; Thayer, J.F.; Battaglia, S. Error-related cardiac deceleration: Functional interplay between error-related brain activity and autonomic nervous system in performance monitoring. *Neurosci. Biobehav. Rev.* **2024**, *157*, 105542. [CrossRef]
50. Ippolito, G.; Bertaccini, R.; Tarasi, L.; Di Gregorio, F.; Trajkovic, J.; Battaglia, S.; Romei, V. The role of alpha oscillations among the main neuropsychiatric disorders in the adult and developing human brain: Evidence from the last 10 years of research. *Biomedicines* **2022**, *10*, 3189. [CrossRef]
51. Tajti, J.; Szok, D.; Csáti, A.; Szabó, Á.; Tanaka, M.; Vécsei, L. Exploring novel therapeutic targets in the common pathogenic factors in migraine and neuropathic pain. *Int. J. Mol. Sci.* **2023**, *24*, 4114. [CrossRef]
52. Tanaka, M.; Schally, A.; Telegdy, G. Neurotransmission of the antidepressant-like effects of the growth hormone-releasing hormone antagonist MZ-4-71. *Behav. Brain Res.* **2012**, *228*, 388–391. [CrossRef]
53. Tanaka, M.; Szabó, Á.; Vécsei, L. Integrating armchair, bench, and bedside research for behavioral neurology and neuropsychiatry. *Biomedicines* **2022**, *10*, 2999. [CrossRef]
54. Vasiliu, O. Efficacy, Tolerability, and Safety of Toludesvenlafaxine for the Treatment of Major Depressive Disorder—A Narrative Review. *Pharmaceuticals* **2023**, *16*, 411. [CrossRef]
55. Bosso, H.; Barbalho, S.M.; de Alvares Goulart, R.; Otoboni, A.M.M.B. Green coffee: Economic relevance and a systematic review of the effects on human health. *Crit. Rev. Food Sci. Nutr.* **2023**, *63*, 394–410. [CrossRef]
56. Laurindo, L.F.; Barbalho, S.M.; Araújo, A.C.; Guiguer, E.L.; Mondal, A.; Bachtel, G.; Bishayee, A. Açaí (*Euterpe oleracea* Mart.) in health and disease: A critical review. *Nutrients* **2023**, *15*, 989. [CrossRef]
57. Barbalho, S.M.; Direito, R.; Laurindo, L.F.; Marton, L.T.; Guiguer, E.L.; Goulart, R.d.A.; Tofano, R.J.; Carvalho, A.C.; Flato, U.A.P.; Capelluppi Tofano, V.A. Ginkgo biloba in the aging process: A narrative review. *Antioxidants* **2022**, *11*, 525. [CrossRef]
58. de Oliveira Zanuso, B.; Dos Santos, A.R.d.O.; Miola, V.F.B.; Campos, L.M.G.; Spilla, C.S.G.; Barbalho, S.M. Panax ginseng and aging related disorders: A systematic review. *Exp. Gerontol.* **2022**, *161*, 111731. [CrossRef] [PubMed]
59. Huang, Y.; Zhang, X.; Chen, L.; Ren, B.X.; Tang, F.R. Lycium barbarum Ameliorates Neural Damage Induced by Experimental Ischemic Stroke and Radiation Exposure. *Front. Biosci. -Landmark* **2023**, *28*, 38. [CrossRef] [PubMed]
60. Sarkar, S.; Raymick, J.; Imam, S. Neuroprotective and Therapeutic Strategies against Parkinson's Disease: Recent Perspectives. *Int. J. Mol. Sci.* **2016**, *17*, 904. [CrossRef]

61. Teleanu, R.I.; Chircov, C.; Grumezescu, A.M.; Volceanov, A.; Teleanu, D.M. Antioxidant Therapies for Neuroprotection-A Review. *J. Clin. Med.* **2019**, *8*, 1659. [CrossRef] [PubMed]
62. Cruz-Martínez, Y.; Aguilar-Ponce, L.; Romo-Araiza, A.; Chávez-Guerra, A.; Martiñón, S.; Ibarra-García, A.P.; Arias-Santiago, S.; Gálvez-Susano, V.; Ibarra, A. Supplementation with a Symbiotic Induced Neuroprotection and Improved Memory in Rats with Ischemic Stroke. *Biomedicines* **2024**, *12*, 209. [CrossRef] [PubMed]
63. Zhang, L.; Wang, F.; Xia, K.; Yu, Z.; Fu, Y.; Huang, T.; Fan, D. Unlocking the Medicinal Mysteries: Preventing Lacunar Stroke with Drug Repurposing. *Biomedicines* **2023**, *12*, 17. [CrossRef]
64. Baliellas, D.E.; Barros, M.P.; Vardaris, C.V.; Guariroba, M.; Poppe, S.C.; Martins, M.F.; Pereira, Á.A.; Bondan, E.F. Propentofylline Improves Thiol-Based Antioxidant Defenses and Limits Lipid Peroxidation following Gliotoxic Injury in the Rat Brainstem. *Biomedicines* **2023**, *11*, 1652. [CrossRef]
65. Keefe, R.S.; Harvey, P.D. Cognitive impairment in schizophrenia. In *Handbook of Experimental Pharmacology*; Springer: Berlin/Heidelberg, Germany, 2012; pp. 11–37. [CrossRef]
66. Kalkstein, S.; Hurford, I.; Gur, R.C. Neurocognition in schizophrenia. *Curr. Top. Behav. Neurosci.* **2010**, *4*, 373–390. [CrossRef]
67. Reichenberg, A. The assessment of neuropsychological functioning in schizophrenia. *Dialogues Clin. Neurosci.* **2010**, *12*, 383–392. [CrossRef]
68. Ventriglio, A.; Ricci, F.; Magnifico, G.; Chumakov, E.; Torales, J.; Watson, C.; Castaldelli-Maia, J.M.; Petito, A.; Bellomo, A. Psychosocial interventions in schizophrenia: Focus on guidelines. *Int. J. Soc. Psychiatry* **2020**, *66*, 735–747. [CrossRef]
69. De Silva, M.J.; Cooper, S.; Li, H.L.; Lund, C.; Patel, V. Effect of psychosocial interventions on social functioning in depression and schizophrenia: Meta-analysis. *Br. J. Psychiatry* **2013**, *202*, 253–260. [CrossRef] [PubMed]
70. Dickerson, F.B.; Lehman, A.F. Evidence-based psychotherapy for schizophrenia: 2011 update. *J. Nerv. Ment. Dis.* **2011**, *199*, 520–526. [CrossRef] [PubMed]
71. Panov, G.; Panova, P. Obsessive-compulsive symptoms in patient with schizophrenia: The influence of disorganized symptoms, duration of schizophrenia, and drug resistance. *Front. Psychiatry* **2023**, *14*, 1120974. [CrossRef]
72. Lysaker, P.H.; Vohs, J.; Hillis, J.D.; Kukla, M.; Popolo, R.; Salvatore, G.; Dimaggio, G. Poor insight into schizophrenia: Contributing factors, consequences and emerging treatment approaches. *Expert. Rev. Neurother.* **2013**, *13*, 785–793. [CrossRef] [PubMed]
73. Arnold, C.; Farhall, J.; Villagonzalo, K.A.; Sharma, K.; Thomas, N. Engagement with online psychosocial interventions for psychosis: A review and synthesis of relevant factors. *Internet Interv.* **2021**, *25*, 100411. [CrossRef]
74. Panov, G.; Dyulgerova, S.; Panova, P. Cognition in Patients with Schizophrenia: Interplay between Working Memory, Disorganized Symptoms, Dissociation, and the Onset and Duration of Psychosis, as Well as Resistance to Treatment. *Biomedicines* **2023**, *11*, 3114. [CrossRef] [PubMed]
75. de Oliveira, M.; Santinelli, F.B.; Lisboa-Filho, P.N.; Barbieri, F.A. The blood concentration of metallic nanoparticles is related to cognitive performance in people with multiple sclerosis: An exploratory analysis. *Biomedicines* **2023**, *11*, 1819. [CrossRef] [PubMed]
76. Koul, A.M.; Ahmad, F.; Bhat, A.; Aein, Q.-u.; Ahmad, A.; Reshi, A.A.; Kaul, R.-u.-R. Unraveling Down Syndrome: From Genetic Anomaly to Artificial Intelligence-Enhanced Diagnosis. *Biomedicines* **2023**, *11*, 3284. [CrossRef] [PubMed]
77. Kessler, R.C.; Berglund, P.; Demler, O.; Jin, R.; Koretz, D.; Merikangas, K.R.; Rush, A.J.; Walters, E.E.; Wang, P.S. The epidemiology of major depressive disorder: Results from the National Comorbidity Survey Replication (NCS-R). *JAMA* **2003**, *289*, 3095–3105. [CrossRef] [PubMed]
78. Chamberlain, S.R.; Sahakian, B.J. The neuropsychology of mood disorders. *Curr. Psychiatry Rep.* **2006**, *8*, 458–463. [CrossRef] [PubMed]
79. Fernandes, B.S.; Hodge, J.M.; Pasco, J.A.; Berk, M.; Williams, L.J. Effects of Depression and Serotonergic Antidepressants on Bone: Mechanisms and Implications for the Treatment of Depression. *Drugs Aging* **2016**, *33*, 21–25. [CrossRef] [PubMed]
80. Tanaka, M.; Chen, C. Towards a mechanistic understanding of depression, anxiety, and their comorbidity: Perspectives from cognitive neuroscience. *Front. Behav. Neurosci.* **2023**, *17*, 1268156. [CrossRef] [PubMed]
81. Duman, H.; Duman, H.; Puşuroğlu, M.; Yılmaz, A.S. Anxiety disorders and depression are associated with resistant hypertension. *Adv. Clin. Exp. Med.* **2023**, *Online ahead of print*. [CrossRef]
82. Baquero, M.; Martín, N. Depressive symptoms in neurodegenerative diseases. *World J. Clin. Cases* **2015**, *3*, 682–693. [CrossRef]
83. de Tommaso, M.; Arendt-Nielsen, L.; Defrin, R.; Kunz, M.; Pickering, G.; Valeriani, M. Pain in Neurodegenerative Disease: Current Knowledge and Future Perspectives. *Behav. Neurol.* **2016**, *2016*, 7576292. [CrossRef]
84. Tran, K.N.; Nguyen, N.P.K.; Nguyen, L.T.H.; Shin, H.M.; Yang, I.J. Screening for Neuroprotective and Rapid Antidepressant-like Effects of 20 Essential Oils. *Biomedicines* **2023**, *11*, 1248. [CrossRef] [PubMed]
85. Cui, Y.; Zhang, H.; Wang, S.; Lu, J.; He, J.; Liu, L.; Liu, W. Stimulated Parotid Saliva Is a Better Method for Depression Prediction. *Biomedicines* **2022**, *10*, 2220. [CrossRef] [PubMed]
86. Rajkumar, R.P. Biomarkers of Neurodegeneration in Post-Traumatic Stress Disorder: An Integrative Review. *Biomedicines* **2023**, *11*, 1465. [CrossRef] [PubMed]
87. Jinka, R.; Kapoor, R.; Sistla, P.G.; Raj, T.A.; Pande, G. Alterations in Cell-Extracellular Matrix Interactions during Progression of Cancers. *Int. J. Cell Biol.* **2012**, *2012*, 219196. [CrossRef] [PubMed]
88. Mierke, C.T. The fundamental role of mechanical properties in the progression of cancer disease and inflammation. *Rep. Prog. Phys.* **2014**, *77*, 076602. [CrossRef]
89. Brown, J.S.; Amend, S.R.; Austin, R.H.; Gatenby, R.A.; Hammarlund, E.U.; Pienta, K.J. Updating the Definition of Cancer. *Mol. Cancer Res.* **2023**, *21*, 1142–1147. [CrossRef] [PubMed]

90. Wargo, J.A.; Reuben, A.; Cooper, Z.A.; Oh, K.S.; Sullivan, R.J. Immune Effects of Chemotherapy, Radiation, and Targeted Therapy and Opportunities for Combination With Immunotherapy. *Semin. Oncol.* **2015**, *42*, 601–616. [CrossRef]
91. Colaco, R.J.; Martin, P.; Kluger, H.M.; Yu, J.B.; Chiang, V.L. Does immunotherapy increase the rate of radiation necrosis after radiosurgical treatment of brain metastases? *J. Neurosurg.* **2016**, *125*, 17–23. [CrossRef]
92. O'Donnell, J.S.; Hoefsmit, E.P.; Smyth, M.J.; Blank, C.U.; Teng, M.W.L. The Promise of Neoadjuvant Immunotherapy and Surgery for Cancer Treatment. *Clin. Cancer Res.* **2019**, *25*, 5743–5751. [CrossRef]
93. Zhang, M.; Chen, X.; Radacsi, N. New tricks of old drugs: Repurposing non-chemo drugs and dietary phytochemicals as adjuvants in anti-tumor therapies. *J. Control. Release* **2021**, *329*, 96–120. [CrossRef]
94. Augustin, Y.; Staines, H.M.; Krishna, S. Artemisinins as a novel anti-cancer therapy: Targeting a global cancer pandemic through drug repurposing. *Pharmacol. Ther.* **2020**, *216*, 107706. [CrossRef] [PubMed]
95. Ferreira, P.M.P.; Ferreira, J.R.O.; de Sousa, R.W.R.; Bezerra, D.P.; Militão, G.C.G. Aminoquinolines as Translational Models for Drug Repurposing: Anticancer Adjuvant Properties and Toxicokinetic-Related Features. *J. Oncol.* **2021**, *2021*, 3569349. [CrossRef]
96. Moura, C.; Correia, A.S.; Pereira, M.; Ribeiro, E.; Santos, J.; Vale, N. Atorvastatin and Nitrofurantoin Repurposed in the Context of Breast Cancer and Neuroblastoma Cells. *Biomedicines* **2023**, *11*, 903. [CrossRef] [PubMed]
97. Olasehinde, T.A.; Olaokun, O.O. The Beneficial Role of Apigenin against Cognitive and Neurobehavioural Dysfunction: A Systematic Review of Preclinical Investigations. *Biomedicines* **2024**, *12*, 178. [CrossRef] [PubMed]
98. Stojsavljević, A.; Lakićević, N.; Pavlović, S. Mercury and Autism Spectrum Disorder: Exploring the Link through Comprehensive Review and Meta-Analysis. *Biomedicines* **2023**, *11*, 3344. [CrossRef] [PubMed]
99. Jászberényi, M.; Thurzó, B.; Bagosi, Z.; Vécsei, L.; Tanaka, M. The Orexin/Hypocretin System, the Peptidergic Regulator of Vigilance, Orchestrates Adaptation to Stress. *Biomedicines* **2024**, *12*, 448. [CrossRef]
100. Török, N.; Török, R.; Molnár, K.; Szolnoki, Z.; Somogyvári, F.; Boda, K.; Tanaka, M.; Klivényi, P.; Vécsei, L. Single Nucleotide Polymorphisms of Indoleamine 2, 3-Dioxygenase 1 Influenced the Age Onset of Parkinson's Disease. *Front. Biosci. -Landmark* **2022**, *27*, 265.
101. Correia, A.S.; Cardoso, A.; Vale, N. Oxidative Stress in Depression: The Link with the Stress Response, Neuroinflammation, Serotonin, Neurogenesis and Synaptic Plasticity. *Antioxid* **2023**, *12*, 470. [CrossRef]
102. Delgado-Morales, R.; Agís-Balboa, R.C.; Esteller, M.; Berdasco, M. Epigenetic mechanisms during ageing and neurogenesis as novel therapeutic avenues in human brain disorders. *Clin. Epigenetics* **2017**, *9*, 67. [CrossRef]
103. Hwang, J.Y.; Aromolaran, K.A.; Zukin, R.S. The emerging field of epigenetics in neurodegeneration and neuroprotection. *Nat. Rev. Neurosci.* **2017**, *18*, 347–361. [CrossRef]
104. Borgomaneri, S.; Battaglia, S.; Avenanti, A.; di Pellegrino, G. Don't hurt me no more: State-dependent transcranial magnetic stimulation for the treatment of specific phobia. *J. Affect. Disord.* **2021**, *286*, 78–79. [CrossRef] [PubMed]
105. Fan, P.; Miranda, O.; Qi, X.; Kofler, J.; Sweet, R.A.; Wang, L. Unveiling the Enigma: Exploring Risk Factors and Mechanisms for Psychotic Symptoms in Alzheimer's Disease through Electronic Medical Records with Deep Learning Models. *Pharmaceuticals* **2023**, *16*, 911. [CrossRef] [PubMed]
106. Sivananthan, S.; Lee, L.; Anderson, G.; Csanyi, B.; Williams, R.; Gissen, P. Buffy coat score as a biomarker of treatment response in neuronal ceroid lipofuscinosis type 2. *Brain Sci.* **2023**, *13*, 209. [CrossRef]
107. Battaglia, S.; Avenanti, A.; Vécsei, L.; Tanaka, M. Neural Correlates and Molecular Mechanisms of Memory and Learning. *Int. J. Mol. Sci.* **2024**, *25*, 2724. [CrossRef]

Disclaimer/Publisher's Note: The statements, opinions and data contained in all publications are solely those of the individual author(s) and contributor(s) and not of MDPI and/or the editor(s). MDPI and/or the editor(s) disclaim responsibility for any injury to people or property resulting from any ideas, methods, instructions or products referred to in the content.

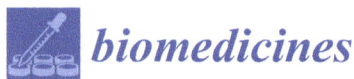 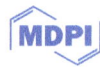

Article

Supplementation with a Symbiotic Induced Neuroprotection and Improved Memory in Rats with Ischemic Stroke

Yolanda Cruz-Martínez [1], Leslie Aguilar-Ponce [1], Alejandra Romo-Araiza [1], Almudena Chávez-Guerra [1], Susana Martiñón [1,2], Andrea P. Ibarra-García [1], Stella Arias-Santiago [1], Vanessa Gálvez-Susano [1] and Antonio Ibarra [1,*]

[1] Centro de Investigación en Ciencias de la Salud (CICSA), Facultad de Ciencias de la Salud, Universidad Anáhuac México Campus Norte, Huixquilucan CP 52786, Edo. de México, Mexico; yolanda.cruz@anahuac.mx (Y.C.-M.); iantonio65@yahoo.com (L.A.-P.); alejandra.romo@anahuac.mx (A.R.-A.); ana.chavezgu@anahuac.mx (A.C.-G.); silvia.martinon@anahuac.mx (S.M.); andrea_ibarra@anahuac.mx (A.P.I.-G.); stella.arias@anahuac.mx (S.A.-S.); jvgs_yaem@hotmail.com (V.G.-S.)

[2] Laboratorio de Inmunología en Adicciones, Subdirección de Investigaciones Clínicas, Instituto Nacional de Psiquiatría Ramón de la Fuente Muñiz, Tlalpan CP 14050, Ciudad de México, Mexico

* Correspondence: jose.ibarra@anahuac.mx

Abstract: After an ischemic stroke, various harmful mechanisms contribute to tissue damage, including the inflammatory response. The increase in pro-inflammatory cytokines has been related to greater damage to the neural tissue and the promotion of neurological alterations, including cognitive impairment. Recent research has shown that the use of prebiotics and/or probiotics counteracts inflammation and improves cognitive function through the production of growth factors, such as brain-derived neurotrophic factor (BDNF), by reducing inflammatory molecules. Therefore, in this study, the effect of the symbiotic inulin and *Enterococcus faecium* on neuroprotection and memory improvement was evaluated in a rat model of transient middle cerebral artery occlusion (tMCAO). In order to accomplish this, the animals were subjected to ischemia; the experimental group was supplemented with the symbiotic and the control group with the vehicle. The neurological deficit as well as spatial and working memory were evaluated using the Zea Longa scale, Morris water maze, and the eight-arm maze tests, respectively. Infarct size, the levels of BDNF, and tumor necrosis factor-alpha (TNF-α) were also assessed. The results show that supplementation with the symbiotic significantly diminished the neurological deficit and infarct size, improved memory and learning, increased BDNF expression, and reduced TNF-α production. These findings provide new evidence about the therapeutic use of symbiotics for ischemic stroke and open up the possibilities for the design of further studies.

Keywords: cognitive impairment; symbiotic; cerebral ischemia; BDNF; TNF-α; tMCAO; *Enterococcus faecium*; cytokines; neuroprotection; memory

Citation: Cruz-Martínez, Y.; Aguilar-Ponce, L.; Romo-Araiza, A.; Chávez-Guerra, A.; Martiñón, S.; Ibarra-García, A.P.; Arias-Santiago, S.; Gálvez-Susano, V.; Ibarra, A. Supplementation with a Symbiotic Induced Neuroprotection and Improved Memory in Rats with Ischemic Stroke. *Biomedicines* **2024**, *12*, 209. https://doi.org/10.3390/biomedicines12010209

Academic Editors: Simone Battaglia and Masaru Tanaka

Received: 9 November 2023
Revised: 14 December 2023
Accepted: 17 December 2023
Published: 17 January 2024

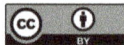

Copyright: © 2024 by the authors. Licensee MDPI, Basel, Switzerland. This article is an open access article distributed under the terms and conditions of the Creative Commons Attribution (CC BY) license (https://creativecommons.org/licenses/by/4.0/).

1. Introduction

Ischemic stroke is caused by a significant reduction in the blood flow to the vessels that supply the brain, causing the activation of several mechanisms such as biochemical dysfunction, an increment of intracellular calcium, excitotoxicity, and activation of lytic enzymes that lead to cell death and, ultimately, a region of damaged neural tissue, or ischemic core [1,2]. Later on, there is a significant increase in free radicals and inflammatory mediators such as IL-6, IL-1β, and TNF-α that contribute to the progression of injured neural tissue [3]. If therapeutic intervention is not carried out, the viable tissue surrounding the infarct area, or ischemic penumbra, dies, and thus the volume of the ischemic core increases.

The cellular changes in neural tissue involve the activation of the microglia and astrocytes, triggering the production of inflammatory mediators even in chronic phases after stroke, especially in areas such as the motor cortex and hippocampus [4]. These events lead to the dysfunction of neurons, resulting in neurological deficits and impairment in memory and learning [2,4,5]. The clinical consequences of stroke will depend on the affected brain region, the intensity of the infarction, and the promptness of medical intervention [6]. The most frequent sequelae are motor alterations and cognitive impairment, mainly in memory, attention, and executive function, including decision-making, working memory, and cognitive flexibility [7].

Recent studies have established that dysbiosis is associated with poor recovery and prognosis after stroke since it increases neuroinflammation and accelerates the progression of cognitive impairment [8,9]. In fact, the composition of the intestinal microbiota could be crucial for the development of stroke. Dysbiosis is associated with a higher risk of stroke since it promotes low-grade inflammation and oxidative stress, contributing to vascular lesions [9,10]. In addition, it has been observed that there is a correlation between the type of pathogenic bacteria in the microbiome and the severity of the neurological dysfunctions caused by stroke [9]. Therefore, restoring the microbiota could become a therapeutic strategy.

In order to restore the microbiome, "a mixture of living microorganisms (probiotics) and substrates (prebiotics) used selectively by microorganisms that confer a beneficial effect on the health of the host" has been proposed [11].

Inulin is a fructan with prebiotic characteristics. In vitro studies have shown that it has anti-inflammatory properties by inhibiting the NF-Kβ pathway [12]. It modulates the composition of microbiota and induces the production of short-chain fatty acids (SCFAs), which also have anti-inflammatory effects [13]. In addition, inulin stimulates the growth of *Enterococcus faecium* [14], a microorganism with the ability to reduce the expression of pro-inflammatory cytokines and increase the production of SCFAs, as well as neurotrophic factors [15].

The use of the symbiotic made with *E. faecium* and agave inulin has shown a reduction in IL-1β and TNF-α expression in aged [15] and obese rats with cognitive impairment. It also increases the expression of BDNF and enhances excitatory synaptic transmissions in the cerebral cortex and hippocampus, improving memory and cognition [16–18]. As a consequence of its anti-inflammatory effects, the symbiotic could also promote neuroprotection after stroke.

In the present study, we evaluated the effect of supplementation with *E. faecium* and agave inulin on neuroprotection and cognition in a murine model of cerebral ischemia.

2. Materials and Methods

2.1. Experimental Design

For this study, 45 male Sprague-Dawley rats, aged three and a half months and weighing an average of 330 ± 20 g, were obtained from the Bioterium of Anáhuac University. The housing conditions of the rats (temperature and humidity) were managed by using automated controlled racks, with food and water available ad libitum, in a 12 h light/dark cycle room, before and after cerebral ischemia was induced using the transient middle cerebral artery occlusion (tMCAO) method.

To explore the effect of the symbiotic on cognitive damage in rats with stroke, we decided to perform a preliminary experiment. Rats were randomly assigned into three groups (15 rats per group) using the GraphPad QuickCals program (https://www.graphpad.com/quickcalcs/randomize1/ accessed on 8 November 2023): (1) tMCAO+ vehicle (control group), (2) tMCAO+ symbiotic (symbiotic-supplemented group), and sham-operated+ vehicle. The control and treated groups were subjected to cerebral ischemia while the sham one was only subjected to the surgical procedure without ischemia. The neurological deficit was evaluated using the Zea Longa scale [19] at 1, 2, 3, 7, and 14 days after ischemia. In order to measure the volume of cerebral infarction, 5 rats were randomly chosen from each group and then euthanized 14 days after ischemia. Three weeks after ischemia, the remaining rats (10 per group) were evaluated for spatial memory and, one week later, their working memory was assessed as well. After clinical evaluations, five weeks after tMCAO, the rats were euthanized in order to measure the hippocampal concentrations of BDNF and TNF-α. Data acquisition was performed using a double-blind design to avoid biases. The experimental design is depicted on the timeline of Figure 1.

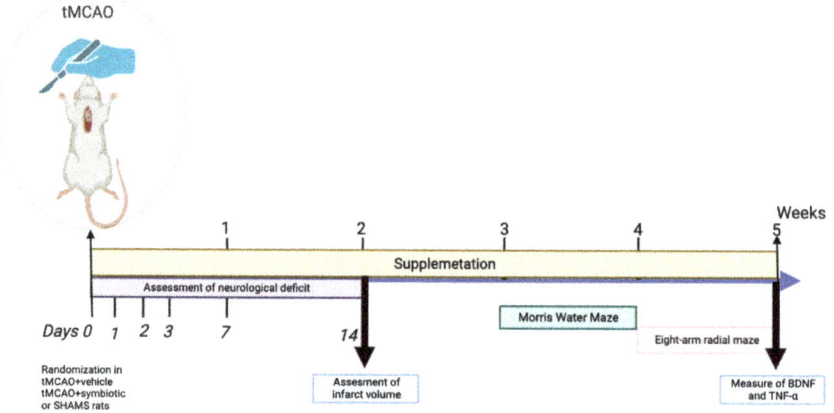

Figure 1. Experimental design.

2.2. Cerebral Ischemia Model

Cerebral ischemia was induced using tMCAO, a procedure that was previously described by Zea Longa in the late 1980s [19]. For this experiment, the rats were anesthetized with a facial mask and 4% isoflurane in oxygen, until a deep anesthetic state was reached; for the rest of the surgery, the concentration of isoflurane was lowered to 1.5%. The body temperature of the rats was maintained at 37 °C using a warm pad until their recovery from the anesthesia. During the procedure, five arteries were identified: the left common carotid (LCC), the internal carotid artery (ICA), the external carotid artery (ECC), and the pterygoid and occipital arteries; the last two were cauterized. A 3-0 nylon monofilament was inserted 18 mm through the ECC until the middle cerebral artery (MCA) was reached. The occlusion was left for 90 min, and afterward, the monofilament was removed, allowing the cerebral blood flow to be restored and the procedure finished with the corresponding stitches. The severity of tMCAO was evaluated by determining the regional cerebral blood flow using a laser Doppler flowmeter (Moor Instruments, Devon, UK). A reduction of around 85% in cerebral perfusion was considered to be focal ischemia. For postoperative care, the animals received acetaminophen 200 mg/kg every 12 h and enrofloxacin 10 mg/kg every 24 h, for 3 days.

2.3. Administration of the Vehicle and Symbiotic

The three groups were supplemented via oral probe; the control and sham groups received one milliliter of water (vehicle of treatment), and the supplemented group received a symbiotic mix of *E. faecium* and agave inulin [4×10^8 CFU and 860 mg/kg, respectively [16]] mixed with the same vehicle. The administration of the vehicle or symbiotic mix was performed daily for 5 weeks. The animals chosen for infarct size evaluation were supplemented for only 14 days.

2.4. Zea Longa Scale

The Zea Longa scale [19] was used to assess the neurological deficit during days 1, 2, 3, 7, and 14 after the tMCAO was performed. This scale provided a score from 0 to 4 points according to the neurological deficit achieved: 0 indicating no neurological deficit, 1 for not being able to lift the right paw, 2 for circling to the left, 3 for decaying to the right, and 4 indicating not being able to walk or referring to a decreased level of consciousness.

2.5. Morris Water Maze

The Morris water maze (MWM) was used to evaluate spatial and associative memory. The rats were placed in a large circular pool (120 cm of diameter) full of water (21–22 °C) and were required to escape to a hidden platform (10 cm of diameter) located 2 cm below the water surface in the south-west quadrant (SWQ) of the pool. The rats were given 3 visual clues shallowly, equidistant from each other, to help them find the location of the platform. The animals underwent a 5-day training protocol consisting of four dives per day, with a maximum duration of 60 s of swimming and 20 s of rest on the platform, for 5 consecutive days. The initial position of the rats was different every day. During the 5-day training protocol, the platform was removed, and the rats were allowed to swim for 60 s to analyze the time they spent in the SWQ versus the time they spent in the remaining quadrants. All trials were recorded using a computerized system (Smart v3.0.02 Panlab Harvard Apparatus, Barcelona, Spain) to determine the latency time taken by each rat to reach the platform below the surface from their initial position, based on the time coordinates of each rat.

2.6. Eight-Arm Radial Maze

An eight-arm radial maze was used to evaluate working and reference memory and provided an indicator of memory deficit. The test consisted of an eight-arm maze in which food was placed on each arm. In 4 of them, food was displayed so that it could not be observed by the rat, but was accessible, whereas in the other 4 arms, access was not provided. This was applied to prevent the animals from be guided by smell. The main objective of this test was to evaluate the working and reference memory simultaneously. The animals have to find the arms with accessible food using extra-maze clues, while avoiding the arms where they already ate the food (working memory), but also avoiding the arms where the food is not accessible to them (reference memory) [20]. The test results were reported as the percentage of correct responses obtained by dividing the number of correct entries in the arms with accessible food by the total number of entries.

2.7. Brain Infarct Volume

Fourteen days after ischemia, five rats (randomly chosen) from each group were euthanized with an overdose of pentobarbital. The brains were extracted without perfusing them and placed at a temperature of -20 Celsius for 15 min, with the purpose of facilitating the slicing process. Each brain was placed in a matrix and 2 mm thick coronal sections were made. The slices were placed in a Petri dish and immersed in 25 mL of 1.5% 2,3,5-triphenyl tetrazolium (TTC) solution (Sigma-Aldrich, St. Louis, MO, USA), for 15 min at 37 °C. The TTC-stained sections were fixed with 4% paraformaldehyde. Afterward, digitized photographs (Canon EOS Rebel SL2; Tokyo, Japan) were obtained. The infarct area was determined using the Image J image analyzer (Image J, National Institutes of Health, Bethesda, MD, USA). The infarct volume was calculated using the Reglodi method, considering edema (EA). The formula used was EA-infarct volume = infarct volume × (contralateral hemisphere/ipsilateral hemisphere) [21].

2.8. Enzyme-Linked Immunosorbent Assay (ELISA)

An ELISA test was performed to measure the levels of brain-derived neurotrophic factor (BDNF) and TNF-α cytokine in 7 rats of each group. The rats were euthanized using a lethal injection of phentobarbital and then decapitated so that the brain could be removed, and the hippocampus dissected: the brain was cut along the longitudinal fissure and the two hemispheres were separated, from both of which the cerebellum and the olfactory bulb were removed. Subsequently, with a spatula, the thalamus and the corpus callosum were removed to expose the entire hippocampus. Once identified, it was separated from the cerebral cortex to be completely removed [22].

The extracted tissue was frozen at a temperature of -80 °C until the study was carried out. The tissue samples were homogenized in a buffer substance at a ratio of 10:1

buffer–tissue weight; the homogenized samples were centrifuged at 14,000× g for half an hour and the supernatant was used to perform an ELISA test. Each sample was run in quintuplicate for each ELISA test, following the instructions provided by the manufacturers (ChemiKineTM from Merck, Darmstadt, Germany, and BioLegend, San Diego, CA, USA).

2.9. Statistical Analysis

Statistical analysis was performed using the Prism 5 software (Prism 5.01, GraphPad Software Inc., San Diego, CA, USA). Data are expressed as mean ± standard deviation and a significance level of $p < 0.05$ was considered. The Shapiro–Wilk normality test was used to analyze the normality of each data set. Neurological deficit was evaluated by using ANOVA for repeated measures. Two-way ANOVA for repeated measures, Student's t-test, and Cohen's d tests were used to assess spatial memory. Working memory, BDNF and TNF-α concentrations, and infarct volume were analyzed using one-way ANOVA and Student's t-test.

3. Results

3.1. Symbiotic Supplementation Reduced the Neurological Deficit Observed after tMCAO

After the rats were subjected to tMCAO, neurological deficit was assessed at 1, 3, 7, and 14 days post-ischemia. The evaluations of the neurological deficit showed that on the first day after ischemia, the control group and the one supplemented with the symbiotic presented a similar neurological deficit (control: 2.8 ± 0.3; symbiotic-supplemented: 3.0 ± 0.02; mean ± SD; $p > 0.05$, Student's t-test, Figure 2). However, at the end of this evaluation (14 days after ischemia), there was a significant improvement in the symbiotic-supplemented group. The neurological deficit was significantly reduced in these animals, (0.57 ± 0.2) in comparison with the control rats (2.57 ± 0.2; $p < 0.0001$, ANOVA for repeated measures). The sham rats did no present any deficit.

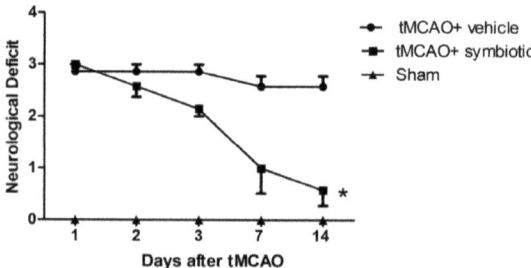

Figure 2. The supplementation with the symbiotic *E. faecium* and agave inulin enhances neurological recovery in rats with tMCAO. Evaluations were performed on days 1, 2, 3, 7, and 14 post-tMCAO. Each point represents mean ± SD of 15 rats per group; * $p < 0.0001$, ANOVA for repeated measures.

3.2. Symbiotic Supplementation Reduced the Infarct Volume after tMCAO

Fourteen days after tMCAO or the sham operation, five rats from each group (randomly chosen) were euthanized for morphological assessment. The 2,3,5-triphenyltetrazolium chloride (TTC) staining method was used to determine the volume of cerebral infarction. Figure 3 shows that the symbiotic-supplemented rats presented a significant reduction in infarct volume (8.84 ± 1.8; mean ± SD) as compared to the control animals (22.15 ± 2.2; $p = 0.003$, Student´s t-test). Animals subjected only to the surgical procedure (sham-operated) did not present infarct signals.

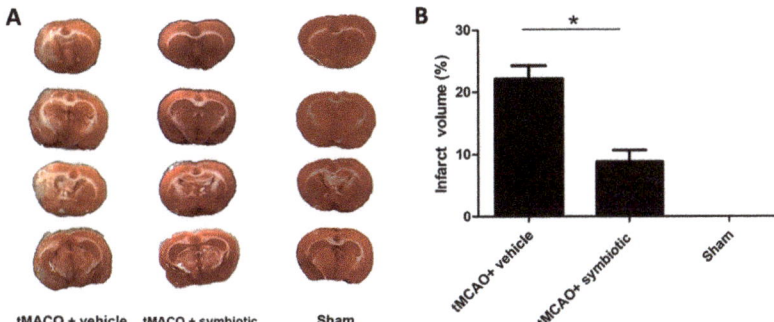

Figure 3. The supplementation with the symbiotic *E. faecium* and agave inulin reduces infarct volume in rats with tMCAO. (**A**) Representative TTC staining of cerebral infarction in comparable coronal sections in rats treated with the symbiotic, vehicle, and sham at 14 days post-tMCAO. (**B**) Quantification of infarct volume based on TTC staining at 14 days post-tMCAO in rats supplemented with the symbiotic, control group, or sham-operated rats. n = 5 mean ± SD (* p = 0.003). Student's *t*-test was employed.

3.3. Supplementation with the Symbiotic Enhances Spatial Memory after tMCAO

In order to evaluate the effect of the symbiotic *E. faecium* and agave inulin on spatial memory three weeks after ischemia, the remaining rats (ten rats per group) were assessed with the Morris water maze test. As expected, the rats subjected to tMCAO showed a significant increase in scape latency time as compared to the sham-operated ones (Figure 4A). However, the time of symbiotic-supplemented rats was lower than that presented by control animals. The interaction between therapy and time was also statistically significant when comparing the symbiotic-supplemented to the control rats (F = 3.37; p = 0.02; ANOVA for repeated measures followed by post hoc Bonferroni test). The last day of acquisition showed a significant difference between the tMCAO-studied groups (symbiotic-supplemented: 19.85 ± 4.66, mean ± SD; control: 43.28 ± 5.89; p = 0.01 Student's *t*-test). In order to know the size of the effect between the groups subjected to tMCAO, we also calculated Cohen's d [23], obtaining a value of 1.14 (large effect) in spatial memory.

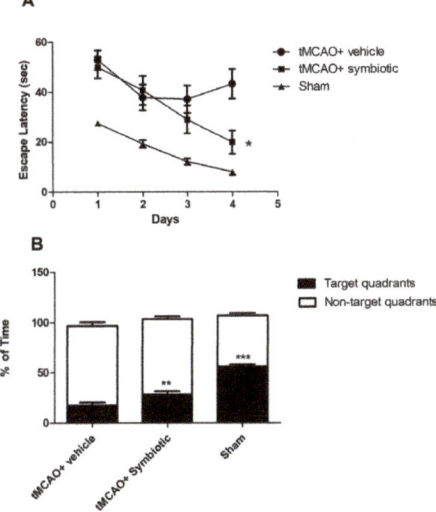

Figure 4. Evaluation of spatial and associative memory in rats with tMCAO supplemented with symbiotic *E. faecium* and agave inulin. (**A**) Escape latency time (seconds) to the platform hidden in

the south-west quadrant (SWQ). (**B**) Time spent (percentage) in the target quadrant compared to the time spent in the non-target quadrants. n = 10 mean ± SD; * p = 0.02; two-way ANOVA for repeated measures followed by post hoc Bonferroni test; ** p = 0.01 vs. control, *** p < 0.001 vs. symbiotic. Student's t-test.

Memory retention was also analyzed on the sixth day by removing the platform and comparing the time spent in the target quadrant to the average time spent in the non-target quadrants (Figure 4B). The sham-operated group spent the longest time in the target quadrant (55.7 ± 2.29). In the case of the tMCAO-subjected rats, the group supplemented with the symbiotic spent more time (28.36 ± 3.14, mean ± SD) when compared to the control one (17.69 ± 2.87; p = 0.01, Student's t-test, Figure 4B).

3.4. Work Memory Was Also Enhanced by Symbiotic Supplementation

With the aim of evaluating the effect of the symbiotic in other domains of memory, the rats were assessed for working memory using an eight-arm radial maze one week after spatial memory evaluation. In this task, working memory was assessed when the rats entered each arm once. In this case, the sham-operated rats performed again the best for this task (95.13 ± 1.44 mean ± SD; Figure 5). In the case of the rats subjected to tMCAO, the symbiotic-supplemented animals showed better performance compared to the control animals (Figure 5). The percentage of correct responses in the symbiotic-supplemented group was significantly higher (72.74 ± 7.02) than that observed in the control one (49.08 ± 3.71; p = 0.003, Student's t-test).

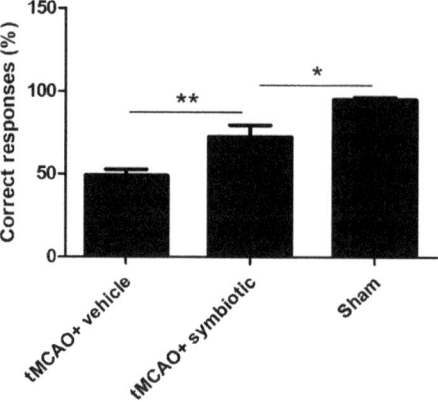

Figure 5. Evaluation of working memory in rats with tMCAO supplemented with symbiotic *E. faecium* and agave inulin. Percentage of correct entries to the eight-armed radial maze. n = 10 mean ± SD; * p < 0.05, ** p = 0.003, Student's t-test.

3.5. Hippocampus of Symbiotic-Supplemented Rats Presented an Increase in BDNF and a Reduction in TNF-α

As the hippocampus is strongly related to memory establishment and this cognitive function depends on BDNF availability [16], we decided to analyze the concentrations of BDNF in this brain region. As shown in Figure 6A, symbiotic supplementation induced an increase in BDNF levels. The concentrations of this molecule were significantly higher in the symbiotic-supplemented rats (5994 ± 124.2; pg/µg of protein, mean ± SD) than those observed in the control (2122 ± 71.94; p < 0.0001) and sham-operated animals (3279 ± 202.7; p < 0.05, one-way ANOVA followed by Tukey's post hoc test). On the other hand, inflammation is one of the phenomena inducing cognitive impairment but also participating in tissue damage after ischemia, especially in the hippocampus. We then evaluated the levels of TNF-α, one of the main cytokines in the inflammatory response observed after stroke (Figure 6B). The concentration of this cytokine was significantly reduced in the symbiotic-supplemented rats (115.2 ± 5.3; pg/μg of protein, mean ± SD) when compared to those observed in the control and sham-operated animals (160.1 ± 11.8; $p = 0.01$ and 132.0 ± 3.3; $p = 0.05$, respectively; one-way ANOVA followed by Tukey´s post hoc test).

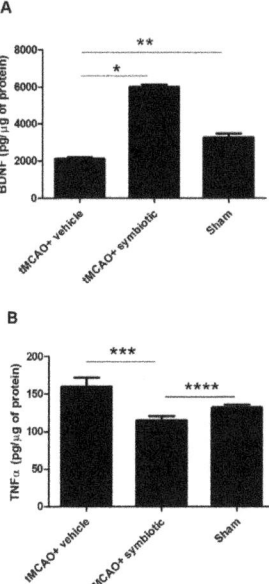

Figure 6. BDNF and TNF-α concentration in rats with tMCAO supplemented with the symbiotic *E. faecium* and agave inulin. (**A**) Concentrations of BDNF. (**B**) Concentrations of TNF-α. n = 7 mean ± SD (* $p \leq 0.0001$); ** $p < 0.05$, *** $p = 0.01$, **** $p = 0.05$. One-way ANOVA followed by Tukey´s post hoc test.

4. Discussion

Recent investigations have proposed the use of symbiotics as therapeutic alternatives for stroke [24,25]. The results of the present investigation show that supplementation with the symbiotic *Enterococcus faecium* and agave inulin as early as 14 days post-stroke improves neurological recovery in a tMCAO model. These results provide significant evidence on the neuroprotective effect that symbiotic supplementation can exert by limiting the size of the infarct, which in turn improves neurological recovery.

In addition, we observed a decrease in TNF-α and an increase in BDNF concentrations in the hippocampus after supplementation with *Enterococcus faecium* and agave inulin. TNF-α is a key cytokine for inducing neuroinflammation [26]. It has been observed that this cytokine contributes to the exacerbation of tissue injury after stroke [27] through different mechanisms, such as mitochondrial dysfunction, leading to apoptosis [28]. It also mediates endothelial necroptosis by increasing the permeability of the blood–brain barrier (BBB) [29] and reducing neurogenesis [30] and neuroplasticity after the ischemic event [31]. On the other hand, BDNF is a growth factor that stimulates cell survival and neural differentiation. The increase in BDNF may mediate the survival of injured neurons through the activation of the PI3K/Akt pathway and MAPK/ERK, inhibiting apoptosis [32]. This molecule also promotes neurotransmission and synaptic plasticity [33]; its deficiency is related to cognitive impairment after an ischemic event [34] and contributes to the prognosis of the neurological outcome.

The changes in the expression of BDNF and TNF-α could be responsible, at least in part, for the neuroprotective effect observed in the supplemented rats. These changes are possible as the symbiotic can selectively increase beneficial bacteria in the intestine as well as levels of short-chain fatty acids [35], such as butyrate, which in turn increases BDNF expression by inhibiting histone deacetylation [12]. Butyrate is obtained as a fermentative product of inulin by *E. faecium* [15]. In addition, *Enterococcus faecium* and agave inulin individually have been shown to possess anti-inflammatory characteristics [11,14]. It has been proven that inulin itself has the ability to reduce the IFN-gamma production by the CD4+ T cells and to increase T reg cells, which express high amounts of IL-10 and a low quantity of IL-6 [36]. Furthermore, inulin also suppresses M1 macrophages and polarizes the M2 phenotype [12], increasing the peripheral blood monocytic myeloid-derived suppressor cells [37]. Moreover, *E. faecium* reduces the IL-8, TNF-α, and IL-6 levels in the macrophages [38], and free radicals overall, and increases the IL-10 and dopamine levels [39].

To corroborate the neuroprotective capacity of *Enterococcus faecium* and agave inulin supplementation, we evaluated the size of the infarct, which was significantly smaller in the treated group. This tissue preservation may be due to the reduction in pro-inflammatory cytokines like TNF-α, one of the main inflammatory mediators that facilitates the infiltration of peripheral leukocytes by increasing permeability and inducing the rupture of the BBB, leading to apoptosis [26]. In the same way, the reduction in leukocyte infiltration could diminish the attack of free radicals. Therefore, a reduction in TNF-α levels contributes to a reduction in infarct volume, leading to greater neurological recovery and preserving neural functions in the hippocampus, such as memory.

Similarly, symbiotic supplementation also enhanced spatial and working memory recovery. These data are very similar to the results obtained by the group of Lee et al., who performed a fecal transplant from young mice with a healthy intestinal microbiome to aged mice subjected to tMCAO. This study showed improvement in behavior and memory two weeks after the intervention. Furthermore, 11 days after the transplant, the microbiome of the mice with tMCAO was very similar to that of the donors [40].

After stroke, inflammation causes alterations in the microenvironment of the hypothalamus that directly affect the functioning of the hypothalamic neurons, mainly affecting memory. The process of neuroinflammation has been observed persisting into the chronic stages. Radenovic et al. reported the presence of activated microglial cells and astrocytes up to two years post-ischemia, particularly notable in the CA1 and CA3 regions of the hippocampus. These findings are associated with progressive neurodegeneration and suggest a potential link to the development of dementia [4]. Previous studies have shown that the symbiotic inulin and *E. faecium* can reduce inflammation in this area of the brain and induce the expression of neurotrophic factors [15]. The results of our present work are consistent with these findings.

Furthermore, BDNF is capable of inducing neuroplasticity and is involved in long-term potentiation (LTP) processes during memory recall and learning [15]. These effects indicate the possible mechanisms that may be involved in cognitive recovery after an ischemic event, since BDNF is a key molecule for memory establishment.

The findings of this study represent the first approach analyzing the effect of supplementation with *E. faecium* and agave inulin after cerebral ischemia. These promising results provide some bases to contemplate the potential impact of this therapeutic strategy on the chronic phase of ischemia [4]. In line with this, it will be necessary to plan the assessment of diverse parameters including both local and systemic inflammation and morphological alteration, among others.

5. Conclusions

Supplementation with the symbiotic *E. faecium* and agave inulin can induce neuroprotection (infarct size reduction) in a model of cerebral ischemia. This could be the result of reducing the TNF-α concentrations and increasing BDNF expression. This neuroprotective effect promoted better neurological recovery. In the same way, symbiotic supplementation induced a significant recovery of spatial and working memory. Therefore, symbiotic supplementation could work as an adjuvant therapy to improve neurological recovery in stroke patients. Further research is needed to provide more evidence supporting the usefulness of this therapeutic strategy.

Author Contributions: Y.C.-M.: conception and design of the study, data collection, and analysis and interpretation of the data; performed research; A.R.-A.: data collection, and analysis and interpretation of the data; performed research; A.C.-G.: data collection, and analysis and interpretation of the data; performed research; L.A.-P.: performed research; data collection; S.M.: writing the manuscript or providing critical revision of the manuscript for intellectual content; analyzed data; A.P.I.-G.: writing the manuscript or providing critical revision of the manuscript for intellectual content; analyzed data; S.A.-S.: data collection, and analysis and interpretation of the data; V.G.-S.: data collection, and analysis and interpretation of the data; A.I.: conception and design of the study; writing the manuscript or providing critical revision of the manuscript for intellectual content; obtaining funding; administrative operation. All authors have read and agreed to the published version of the manuscript.

Funding: This research was funded by la Universidad Anáhuac, México, grant number 201859. The APC was funded by la Universidad Anáhuac, México.

Institutional Review Board Statement: All the experiments were performed according to the guidelines of the National Institute of Health (NIH) [41] and the Official Mexican Standard NOM-062-ZOO-1999 [42]. Under the review of the Research Committee of la Universidad Anáhuac and the Internal Committee for the Care and Use of Laboratory Animals (CICUAL), this work was accepted on 23 November 2018 and registered under number 201859.

Data Availability Statement: The data presented in this study are available on request from the corresponding author.

Acknowledgments: We acknowledge Lisset Navarro for the manuscript language supervision.

Conflicts of Interest: The authors declare no conflicts of interest. The funders had no role in the design of the study; in the collection, analyses, or interpretation of data; in the writing of the manuscript; or in the decision to publish the results.

References

1. Feigin, V.L.; Brainin, M.; Norrving, B.; Martins, S.; Sacco, R.L.; Hacke, W.; Fisher, M.; Pandian, J.; Lindsay, P. World Stroke Organization (WSO): Global Stroke Fact Sheet 2022. *Int. J. Stroke* **2022**, *17*, 18–29. [CrossRef] [PubMed]
2. Zhang, Q.; Jia, M.; Wang, Y.; Wang, Q.; Wu, J. Cell Death Mechanisms in Cerebral Ischemia-Reperfusion Injury. *Neurochem. Res.* **2022**, *47*, 3525–3542. [CrossRef] [PubMed]
3. Jurcau, A.; Simion, A. Neuroinflammation in Cerebral Ischemia and Ischemia/Reperfusion Injuries: From Pathophysiology to Therapeutic Strategies. *Int. J. Mol. Sci.* **2021**, *23*, 14. [CrossRef] [PubMed]
4. Radenovic, L.; Nenadic, M.; Ułamek-Kozioł, M.; Januszewski, S.; Czuczwar, S.J.; Andjus, P.R.; Pluta, R. Heterogeneity in brain distribution of activated microglia and astrocytes in a rat ischemic model of Alzheimer's disease after 2 years of survival. *Aging* **2020**, *12*, 12251–12267. [CrossRef] [PubMed]
5. Hoffmann, T.; Bennett, S.; Koh, C.L.; McKenna, K.T. Occupational therapy for cognitive impairment in stroke patients. *Cochrane Database Syst. Rev.* **2010**, *2010*, CD006430. [CrossRef] [PubMed]
6. Zhao, L.; Biesbroek, J.M.; Shi, L.; Liu, W.; Kuijf, H.J.; Chu, W.W.; Abrigo, J.M.; Lee, R.K.; Leung, T.W.; Lau, A.Y.; et al. Strategic infarct location for post-stroke cognitive impairment: A multivariate lesion-symptom mapping study. *J. Cereb. Blood Flow Metab.* **2018**, *38*, 1299–1311. [CrossRef]
7. Lugtmeijer, S.; Lammers, N.A.; de Haan, E.H.F.; de Leeuw, F.E.; Kessels, R.P.C. Post-Stroke Working Memory Dysfunction: A Meta-Analysis and Systematic Review. *Neuropsychol. Rev.* **2021**, *31*, 202–219. [CrossRef]
8. Morrison, H.W.; White, M.M.; Rothers, J.L.; Taylor-Piliae, R.E. Examining the Associations between Post-Stroke Cognitive Function and Common Comorbid Conditions among Stroke Survivors. *Int. J. Environ. Res. Public Health* **2022**, *19*, 13445. [CrossRef]
9. Li, N.; Wang, X.; Sun, C.; Wu, X.; Lu, M.; Si, Y.; Ye, X.; Wang, T.; Yu, X.; Zhao, X.; et al. Change of intestinal microbiota in cerebral ischemic stroke patients. *BMC Microbiol.* **2019**, *19*, 191. [CrossRef]
10. Yamashiro, K.; Kurita, N.; Urabe, T.; Hattori, N. Role of the Gut Microbiota in Stroke Pathogenesis and Potential Therapeutic Implications. *Ann. Nutr. Metab.* **2021**, *77*, 36–44. [CrossRef]
11. Swanson, K.S.; Gibson, G.R.; Hutkins, R.; Reimer, R.A.; Reid, G.; Verbeke, K.; Scott, K.P.; Holscher, H.D.; Azad, M.B.; Delzenne, N.M.; et al. The International Scientific Association for Probiotics and Prebiotics (ISAPP) consensus statement on the definition and scope of synbiotics. *Nat. Rev. Gastroenterol. Hepatol.* **2020**, *17*, 687–701. [CrossRef] [PubMed]

12. Farabegoli, F.; Santaclara, F.J.; Costas, D.; Alonso, M.; Abril, A.G.; Espiñeira, M.; Ortea, I.; Costas, C. Exploring the Anti-Inflammatory Effect of Inulin by Integrating Transcriptomic and Proteomic Analyses in a Murine Macrophage Cell Model. *Nutrients* **2023**, *15*, 859. [CrossRef] [PubMed]
13. Wang, Z.; Zhang, X.; Zhu, L.; Yang, X.; He, F.; Wang, T.; Bao, T.; Lu, H.; Wang, H.; Yang, S. Inulin alleviates inflammation of alcoholic liver disease via SCFAs-inducing suppression of M1 and facilitation of M2 macrophages in mice. *Int. Immunopharmacol.* **2020**, *78*, 106062. [CrossRef] [PubMed]
14. Ayala Monter, M.A.; Pinto Ruiz, R.; González Muñoz, S.S.; Bárcena Gama, J.R.; Hernández Mendo, O.; Torres Salado, N. Efecto prebiótico de dos fuentes de inulina en el crecimiento in vitro de *Lactobacillus salivarius* y *Enterococcus faecium*. *Rev. Mex. Cienc. Pecu.* **2018**, *9*, 346–361. [CrossRef]
15. Yang, Q.; He, Y.; Tian, L.L.; Zhang, Z.; Qiu, L.; Tao, X.Y.; Wei, H. Anti-tumor effect of infant-derived *Enterococcus* via the inhibition of proliferation and inflammation as well as the promotion of apoptosis. *Food Funct.* **2023**, *14*, 2223–2238. [CrossRef] [PubMed]
16. Romo-Araiza, A.; Gutiérrez-Salmeán, G.; Galván, E.J.; Hernández-Frausto, M.; Herrera-López, G.; Romo-Parra, H.; García-Contreras, V.; Fernández-Presas, A.M.; Jasso-Chávez, R.; Borlongan, C.V.; et al. Probiotics and Prebiotics as a Therapeutic Strategy to Improve Memory in a Model of Middle-Aged Rats. *Front. Aging Neurosci.* **2018**, *10*, 416. [CrossRef] [PubMed]
17. Servín-Casas, G.A.; Romo-Araiza, A.; Gutierrez-Salmean, G.; Martinez-Solis, E.; Ibarra-García, A.P.; Cruz-Martinez, Y.; Rodriguez-Barrera, R.; García, E.; Incontri-Abraham, D.; Ibarra, A. Memory improvement in senile rats after prebiotic and probiotic supplementation is not induced by GLP-1. *CNS Neurosci. Ther.* **2022**, *28*, 1986–1992. [CrossRef]
18. Romo-Araiza, A.; Picazo-Aguilar, R.I.; Griego, E.; Márquez, L.A.; Galván, E.J.; Cruz, Y.; Fernández-Presas, A.M.; Chávez-Guerra, A.; Rodríguez-Barrera, R.; Azpiri-Cardós, A.P.; et al. Symbiotic Supplementation (*E. faecium* and Agave Inulin) Improves Spatial Memory and Increases Plasticity in the Hippocampus of Obese Rats: A Proof-of-Concept Study. *Cell Transplant.* **2023**, *32*, 9636897231177357. [CrossRef]
19. Longa, E.Z.; Weinstein, P.R.; Carlson, S.; Cummins, R. Reversible middle cerebral artery occlusion without craniectomy in rats. *Stroke* **1989**, *20*, 84–91. [CrossRef]
20. Penley, S.C.; Gaudet, C.M.; Threlkeld, S.W. Use of an eight-arm radial water maze to assess working and reference memory following neonatal brain injury. *J. Vis. Exp.* **2013**, *82*, 50940.
21. Nouraee, C.; Fisher, M.; Di Napoli, M.; Salazar, P.; Farr, T.D.; Jafarli, A.; Divani, A.A. A Brief Review of Edema-Adjusted Infarct Volume Measurement Techniques for Rodent Focal Cerebral Ischemia Models with Practical Recommendations. *J. Vasc. Interv. Neurol.* **2019**, *10*, 38–45.
22. Chiu, K.; Lau, W.M.; Lau, H.T.; So, K.F.; Chang, R.C. Micro-dissection of rat brain for RNA or protein extraction from specific brain region. *J. Vis. Exp.* **2007**, *7*, 269.
23. Dominguez-Lara, S. Magnitud del efecto, una guía rápida. *Educ. Méd.* **2018**, *19*, 251–254. [CrossRef]
24. Honarpisheh, P.; Bryan, R.M.; McCullough, L.D. Aging Microbiota-Gut-Brain Axis in Stroke Risk and Outcome. *Circ. Res.* **2022**, *130*, 1112–1144. [CrossRef] [PubMed]
25. Pluta, R.; Januszewski, S.; Czuczwar, S.J. The Role of Gut Microbiota in an Ischemic Stroke. *Int. J. Mol. Sci.* **2021**, *22*, 915. [CrossRef] [PubMed]
26. Zhao, Y.; Zhu, Q.; Bi, C.; Yuan, J.; Chen, Y.; Hu, X. Bibliometric analysis of tumor necrosis factor in post-stroke neuroinflammation from 2003 to 2021. *Front. Immunol.* **2022**, *13*, 1040686. [CrossRef] [PubMed]
27. Lin, S.-Y.; Wang, Y.-Y.; Chang, C.-Y.; Wu, C.-C.; Chen, W.-Y.; Liao, S.-L.; Chen, C.-J. TNF-α Receptor Inhibitor Alleviates Metabolic and Inflammatory Changes in a Rat Model of Ischemic Stroke. *Antioxidants* **2021**, *10*, 851. [CrossRef] [PubMed]
28. Wilkins, H.M.; Swerdlow, R.H. TNF-α in cerebral ischemia: Another stroke against you? *J. Neurochem.* **2015**, *132*, 369–372. [CrossRef]
29. Chen, A.Q.; Fang, Z.; Chen, X.L.; Yang, S.; Zhou, Y.F.; Mao, L.; Xia, Y.P.; Jin, H.J.; Li, Y.N.; You, M.F.; et al. Microglia-derived TNF-α mediates endothelial necroptosis aggravating blood brain–barrier disruption after ischemic stroke. *Cell Death Dis.* **2019**, *10*, 487. [CrossRef]
30. Iosif, R.E.; Ahlenius, H.; Ekdahl, C.T.; Darsalia, V.; Thored, P.; Jovinge, S.; Kokaia, Z.; Lindvall, O. Suppression of stroke-induced progenitor proliferation in adult subventricular zone by tumor necrosis factor receptor 1. *J. Cereb. Blood Flow Metab.* **2008**, *28*, 1574–1587. [CrossRef]
31. Liguz-Lecznar, M.; Zakrzewska, R.; Kossut, M. Inhibition of TNF-α R1 signaling can rescue functional cortical plasticity impaired in early post-stroke period. *Neurobiol. Aging* **2015**, *36*, 2877–2884. [CrossRef] [PubMed]
32. Sayyah, M.; Seydyousefi, M.; Moghanlou, A.E.; Metz, G.A.S.; Shamsaei, N.; Faghfoori, M.H.; Faghfoori, Z. Activation of BDNF- and VEGF-mediated Neuroprotection by Treadmill Exercise Training in Experimental Stroke. *Metab. Brain Dis.* **2022**, *37*, 1843–1853. [CrossRef] [PubMed]
33. Eyileten, C.; Sharif, L.; Wicik, Z.; Jakubik, D.; Jarosz-Popek, J.; Soplinska, A.; Postula, M.; Czlonkowska, A.; Kaplon-Cieslicka, A.; Mirowska-Guzel, D. The Relation of the Brain-Derived Neurotrophic Factor with MicroRNAs in Neurodegenerative Diseases and Ischemic Stroke. *Mol. Neurobiol.* **2021**, *58*, 329–347. [CrossRef] [PubMed]
34. Havlovska, Y.Y.; Lytvynenko, N.V.; Shkodina, A.D. Serum Level of Brain-Derived Neurotrophic Factor and Thrombotic Type Are Predictive of Cognitive Impairment in the Acute Period of Ischemic Strokes Patients. *Neurol. Res. Int.* **2023**, *2023*, 5578850. [CrossRef]

35. Guo, J.; Zhang, M.; Wang, H.; Li, N.; Lu, Z.; Li, L.; Hui, S.; Xu, H. Gut microbiota and short chain fatty acids partially mediate the beneficial effects of inulin on metabolic disorders in obese ob/ob mice. *J. Food Biochem.* **2022**, *46*, e14063. [CrossRef] [PubMed]
36. Li, K.; Zhang, L.; Xue, J.; Yang, X.; Dong, X.; Sha, L.; Lei, H.; Zhang, X.; Zhu, L.; Wang, Z.; et al. Dietary inulin alleviates diverse stages of type 2 diabetes mellitus via anti-inflammation and modulating gut microbiota in db/db mice. *Food Funct.* **2019**, *10*, 1915–1927. [CrossRef] [PubMed]
37. Bao, T.; Wang, Z.; Zhu, L.; Lu, H.; Wang, T.; Zhang, Y.; Zhang, X.; Wang, H.; Yang, S. Inulin increases the proportion of monocytic myeloid-derived suppressor cells in peripheral blood, liver, spleen and regulates the secretion of plasma inflammatory cytokines in mice with non-alcoholic fatty liver disease. *Xi Bao Yu Fen Zi Mian Yi Xue Za Zhi* **2020**, *36*, 228–235. [PubMed]
38. Ondee, T.; Pongpirul, K.; Janchot, K.; Kanacharoen, S.; Lertmongkolaksorn, T.; Wongsaroj, L.; Somboonna, N.; Ngamwongsatit, N.; Leelahavanichkul, A. *Lactiplantibacillus plantarum* dfa1 Outperforms *Enterococcus faecium* dfa1 on Anti-Obesity in High Fat-Induced Obesity Mice Possibly through the Differences in Gut Dysbiosis Attenuation, despite the Similar Anti-Inflammatory Properties. *Nutrients* **2021**, *14*, 80. [CrossRef]
39. Divyashri, G.; Krishna, G.; Muralidhara; Prapulla, S.G. Probiotic attributes, antioxidant, anti-inflammatory and neuromodulatory effects of Enterococcus faecium CFR 3003: In vitro and in vivo evidence. *J. Med. Microbiol.* **2015**, *64*, 1527–1540. [CrossRef]
40. Lee, J.; D'aigle, J.; Atadja, L.; Quaicoe, V.; Honarpisheh, P.; Ganesh, B.P.; Hassan, A.; Graf, J.; Petrosino, J.F.; Putluri, N.; et al. Gut Microbiota-Derived Short-Chain Fatty Acids Promote Poststroke Recovery in Aged Mice. *Circ. Res.* **2020**, *127*, 453–465. [CrossRef]
41. National Research Council. *Guía Para el Cuidado y Uso de Animales de Laboratorio*; Ediciones UC: Santiago, Chile, 2017; ISBN-13: 978-9561421080.
42. Diario Oficial de la Federación. *Norma Oficial Mexicana NOM-062-ZOO-1999. Especificaciones Técnicas para la Producción, Cuidado y uso de los Animales de Laboratorio*. México. 2001. Available online: chrome-extension://efaidnbmnnnibpcajpcglclefindmkaj/https://www.gob.mx/cms/uploads/attachment/file/203498/NOM-062-ZOO-1999_220801.pdf (accessed on 8 November 2023).

Disclaimer/Publisher's Note: The statements, opinions and data contained in all publications are solely those of the individual author(s) and contributor(s) and not of MDPI and/or the editor(s). MDPI and/or the editor(s) disclaim responsibility for any injury to people or property resulting from any ideas, methods, instructions or products referred to in the content.

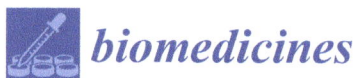 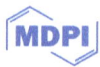

Article

Unlocking the Medicinal Mysteries: Preventing Lacunar Stroke with Drug Repurposing

Linjing Zhang [1,†], Fan Wang [1,†], Kailin Xia [1], Zhou Yu [1], Yu Fu [1], Tao Huang [1,2,3,*] and Dongsheng Fan [1,4,5,*]

1. Department of Neurology, Peking University Third Hospital, Beijing 100191, China; zhanglinjing@bjmu.edu.cn (L.Z.); yifan.1103@163.com (F.W.); kllook@pku.edu.cn (K.X.); yuzhou_1995@126.com (Z.Y.); lilac_fu@126.com (Y.F.)
2. Department of Epidemiology and Biostatistics, School of Public Health, Peking University, Beijing 100871, China
3. Center for Intelligent Public Health, Institute for Artificial Intelligence, Peking University, Beijing 100871, China
4. Beijing Key Laboratory of Biomarker and Translational Research in Neurodegenerative Diseases, Beijing 100191, China
5. Key Laboratory for Neuroscience, National Health Commission/Ministry of Education, Peking University, Beijing 100871, China

* Correspondence: huangtao@bjmu.edu.cn (T.H.); dsfan2010@aliyun.com (D.F.); Tel.: +86-13488745828 (T.H.); +86-13701023871 (D.F.); Fax: +86-010-82266250 (D.F.)

† These authors contributed equally to this work.

Citation: Zhang, L.; Wang, F.; Xia, K.; Yu, Z.; Fu, Y.; Huang, T.; Fan, D. Unlocking the Medicinal Mysteries: Preventing Lacunar Stroke with Drug Repurposing. *Biomedicines* **2024**, *12*, 17. https://doi.org/10.3390/biomedicines12010017

Academic Editors: Masaru Tanaka and Kuen-Jer Tsai

Received: 26 October 2023
Revised: 10 December 2023
Accepted: 11 December 2023
Published: 20 December 2023

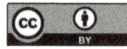

Copyright: © 2023 by the authors. Licensee MDPI, Basel, Switzerland. This article is an open access article distributed under the terms and conditions of the Creative Commons Attribution (CC BY) license (https://creativecommons.org/licenses/by/4.0/).

Abstract: Currently, only the general control of the risk factors is known to prevent lacunar cerebral infarction, but it is unknown which type of medication for controlling the risk factors has a causal relationship with reducing the risk of lacunar infarction. To unlock this medical mystery, drug-target Mendelian randomization analysis was applied to estimate the effect of common antihypertensive agents, hypolipidemic agents, and hypoglycemic agents on lacunar stroke. Lacunar stroke data for the transethnic analysis were derived from meta-analyses comprising 7338 cases and 254,798 controls. We have confirmed that genetic variants mimicking calcium channel blockers were found to most stably prevent lacunar stroke. The genetic variants at or near *HMGCR*, *NPC1L1*, and *APOC3* were predicted to decrease lacunar stroke incidence in drug-target MR analysis. These variants mimic the effects of statins, ezetimibe, and antisense anti-*apoC3* agents, respectively. Genetically proxied *GLP1R* agonism had a marginal effect on lacunar stroke, while a genetically proxied improvement in overall glycemic control was associated with reduced lacunar stroke risk. Here, we show that certain categories of drugs currently used in clinical practice can more effectively reduce the risk of stroke. Repurposing several drugs with well-established safety and low costs for lacunar stroke prevention should be given high priority when doctors are making decisions in clinical practice. This may contribute to healthier brain aging.

Keywords: stroke; lacunar; mendelian randomization analysis; drug repurposing; antihypertensive agent; hypolipidemic agents; hypoglycemic agents; aging; healthy; precision medicine; genetic association studies; preventive medicine

1. Introduction

Lacunar stroke is a small subcortical infarct that arises from ischemia in the territory of the deep perforating arteries of the brain [1]. These arteries, also known as lenticulostriate arteries, supply blood to the brain's deep structures, including the basal ganglia, thalamus, internal capsule, and white matter. Lacunar stroke accounts for one-quarter of the overall number of ischemic strokes. Despite their small size, they can have significant impacts on a person's health and quality of life. They can lead to long-term intellectual and physical disabilities, including difficulties with movement, speech, and cognitive functions. The exact cause of lacunar strokes is not fully understood, but they are often associated with conditions that affect the health of blood vessels, such as hypertension, diabetes, and high cholesterol.

These conditions can lead to the hardening and narrowing of the small blood vessels in the brain, reducing blood flow and increasing the risk of a lacunar stroke. Preventive treatments are generally aimed at controlling these three risk factors. However, it is not yet known which specific medication for controlling these three risk factors can have a causal relationship with reducing the risk of lacunar infarction. In other words, the exact relationship between specific medications for these risk factors and the reduction of lacunar infarction risk is still under investigation. This is an area where further research is needed.

Recently, Matthew Traylor et al. made substantial progress in identifying the genetic mechanisms underlying lacunar stroke by genome-wide association studies (GWAS) [2]. Their research has shed light on novel mechanisms underlying lacunar stroke pathogenesis, pointing to pathways that could potentially be targeted by more precision therapeutics [3].

The Mendelian randomization (MR) approach is a popular genetic epidemiological method that uses genetic variants as instrumental variables (*IVs*) for exposure to assess causal associations between risk factors and disease [4]. This method exploits the random allocation of genetic variants at conception to minimize any bias due to confounding and reverse causation that can restrict causal inference in observational research [5]. Genetic variation in drug-target proteins, such as *HMGCR*, can be leveraged to extend the application of Mendelian randomization (MR) to investigate drug effects [5,6]. Specifically, single-nucleotide polymorphisms (SNPs) in or near the *HMGCR* gene were used as proxies for *HMGCR* inhibition by statins [7]. Drug repurposing, otherwise known as drug repositioning, is a strategy that seeks to identify new indications and targets for approved drugs that are beyond the scope of their original medical indications [8]. Drug repurposing can be a time- and cost-effective way to discover novel therapeutics. Therefore, drug repurposing can be a useful strategy for lacunar stroke by exploring the potential of existing drugs that have already been proven safe and effective in humans [9].

Thus, to estimate which class of medication for antihypertensive, lipid-lowering, and antidiabetic drugs can exert a causal relationship with reducing the risk of lacunar infarction, we conducted this comprehensive MR analysis. We first exploited a two-sample MR approach to examine the causal associations of modifiable risk factors with lacunar stroke. Second, multivariable MR was conducted to estimate the direct causal effect of blood pressure and lipids on lacunar stroke. Third, drug-targeted MR was applied to evaluate several commonly used classes of antihypertensive, lipid-lowering agents and *GLP1R* agonism for hypoglycemic drugs likely to have efficacy in preventing lacunar stroke. The study design is presented in Figure 1.

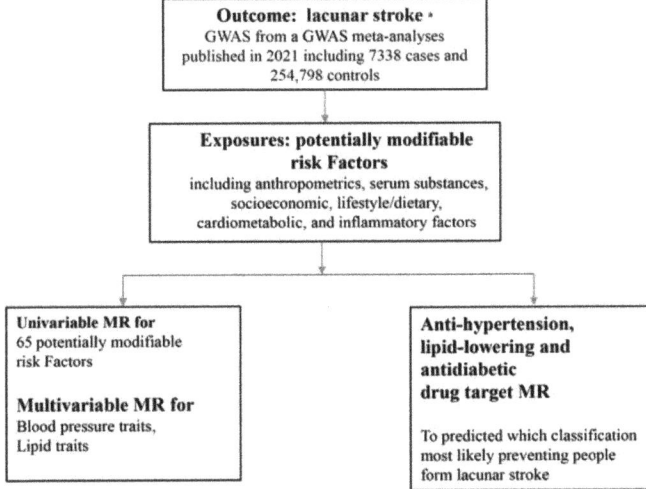

Figure 1. Overall study design. ᵃ: [2]. GWAS: genome-wide association study; MR: Mendelian randomization.

The purpose of this drug-target MR study was to determine whether some pre-existing drugs had a causal effect on lacunar stroke, with the ultimate goal of repurposing these drugs for new therapeutic applications. The study proposed that certain categories of medication could be identified and prioritized for use in the prevention of lacunar stroke.

2. Materials and Methods

We utilize a method known as Mendelian randomization (MR), which uses genetic variants as instrumental variables to estimate the causal effect of an exposure on an outcome. Our data sources include published genome-wide association studies (GWASs) and summary data from the MR base. Through this rigorous approach, we aim to shed light on the complex interplay of genetic and modifiable risk factors in the development of lacunar stroke, ultimately contributing to improved prevention and treatment strategies.

2.1. Potential Risk Factors

We considered potential risk factors that can be grouped under the following categories: anthropometry (waist-to-hip ratio, body fat, height, body mass index, bone mineral density, childhood BMI, birth weight), socioeconomic (education, intelligence), lifestyle/dietary (diphenylamine, smoking (number), eicosapntemacnioc acid, linoleic acid (LA; 18:2,n6), coffee, morning person, subjective well-being, adrenic acid (22:4,n6), arachidonic acid (AA; 20:4,n6), sedentary, carbohydrate, gamma linolenic acid (GLA; 18:3,n6)), cardiometabolic (common carotid intima-media thickness, coronary heart disease, HDL cholesterol ‖ id:ieu-b-109, total cholesterol, homocysteine (Hcy), C-reaction protein (CRP), type 2 diabetes, lipoprotein(a), fasting glucose, heart rate, fasting proinsulin, fasting insulin, pulse pressure, apolipoprotein A-I ‖ id:ieu-b-107, diastolic blood pressure (DBP), triglycerides ‖ id:ieu-b-111, hypertension, fibrinogen, adiponectin, atrial fibrillation, leptin), LDL cholesterol ‖ id:ieu-b-110, *HbA1C*, 2h glucose, systolic blood pressure (SBP), apolipoprotein B ‖ id: ieu-b-108), endogenous substances (serum creatinine, vitamin E, uric acid, eGFRcrea, blood urea nitrogen, vitamin b12, protein, vitamin D), neuropsychiatric disorders (anorexia nervosa, schizophrenia, neuroticism, major depression, Parkinson's disease) and other system diseases (chronic obstructive pulmonary disease, rheumatoid arthritis, osteoporotic fracture, Crohn's disease, asthma). These 65 risk factors are listed in Table S1. The eligible risk factors had the most solid evidence from previous observational studies, indicating that they may predispose an individual to lacunar stroke.

2.2. Data Sources

We searched PubMed for published genome-wide association studies to obtain the summary data (effect size estimates and standard errors) of risk factors. We also derived data from the MR base https://gwas.mrcieu.ac.uk/ (accessed on 29 August 2023) [10]. Details on the risk factors (including traits, number of IVs in the study ($p < 5 \times 10^{-8}$), the GWASs that the traits were interested, number of samples that the GWASs included, and units of the traits) that showed significant effects on lacunar stroke from which we obtained summary data for the current analyses are presented in Table S2.

Lacunar stroke data were obtained from meta-analyses conducted in Europe, the USA, and Australia [2]. The meta-analyses included previous genome-wide association studies (GWASs) and additional cases and controls from the U.K. DNA lacunar stroke studies and the International Stroke Genetics Consortium. The study comprised a total of 6030 cases and 248,929 controls of European ancestry. In addition, the transethnic analysis included 7338 cases and 254,798 controls [11–14]. These lacunar stroke cases were MRI-confirmed cases, as MRI confirmation of lacunar stroke is more reliable than standard phenotyping. Genotyping arrays, quality control filters, and imputation reference panels could be found in the study [2]. Summary-level GWAS data could be derived from https://cd.hugeamp.org/downloads.html (accessed on 23 August 2023).

2.3. Genetic Variants

For univariable MR analyses, SNPs with genome-wide significance ($p < 5 \times 10^{-8}$) for each risk factor and their effect size estimates and standard errors were also collected. Only independent variants are not in linkage disequilibrium (defined as $r^2 < 0.001$) with other genetic variants for the same risk factor. The IVs (F statistic > 10) for all the exposures were sufficiently informative [15]. F-statistics were calculated for each variant using the formula $F = beta^2 / SE^2$ [16].

For blood pressure (BP)-related (SBP: systolic blood pressure; DBP: diastolic blood pressure; PP: pulse pressure) or lipid-related (ApoB: apolipoprotein B; LDL-C: low-density lipoprotein; TG: triglyceride; ApoA1: apolipoprotein A-I; HDL-C: high-density lipoprotein) traits, one exposure is genetically correlated with other exposures. Thus, we employed multivariable MR (MVMR) analysis to estimate the independent causal effect of each exposure [17,18]. As an extension of univariable MR, MVMR concatenating a set of IVs for each exposure estimates the direct effect of exposures on lacunar stroke risk, whereas univariable MR calculates the total effect. SNPs for the BP traits were obtained from summary statistics of a large GWAS of BP traits with over 1 million people of European ancestry [19]. All SNPs with genome-wide significance ($n = 255$, LD_$r^2 < 0.1$) that were associated with any of the BP traits were included in the set of IVs. For the lipid multivariable MR analyses, in Model 1, we pooled all SNPs with genome-wide significance that were associated with any of the traits, including ApoB, LDL-C, and TG. In Model 2, the traits included ApoA1 and HDL-C [20]. The IVs were derived from the MR base with a threshold clump_$r^2 = 0.001$ and clump_kb = 1000. In all, 384 and 435 IVs were concatenated for Model 1 and Model 2.

For antihypertensive drug-MR, MR analyses were performed to estimate the effect of a 10 mmHg reduction in blood pressure by antihypertensive drugs. Genetic instruments were selected based on their association with each blood pressure (BP) trait at genome-wide significance ($p < 5 \times 10^{-8}$) and their proximity to genes (near (+/−200 kb) or within encoding protein targets of 12 antihypertensive medication classes. Effect estimates for each genetic variant were derived for each BP trait from the trans-ancestry BP GWAS [21–23] (Table S3). The primary analysis focused on the SBP-lowering effect, with sensitivity analyses considering the remaining BP traits (DBP, PP).

To investigate the effects of lipid-lowering drugs, the Mendelian randomization (MR) approach used *HMG*-CoA reductase as a proxy for statins. Five single-nucleotide polymorphisms (SNPs) associated with low-density lipoprotein (LDL) cholesterol at the genome-wide significant level ($p < 5.0 \times 10^{-8}$) and located within ±100 kb windows from the gene region of HMGCR were obtained (Figure 2). Variants located in the HMGCR, PCSK9, and NPC1L1 regions were selected using the method described by B. A. Ference [24]. The method proposed by Do et al. was used to select variants located in or near the APOC3 regions [25]. Variants were selected based on their associations with either low-density lipoprotein cholesterol (LDL-C) or triglycerides (TG), and they were not highly correlated ($r^2 < 0.4$ or $r^2 < 0.3$) (Table S3).

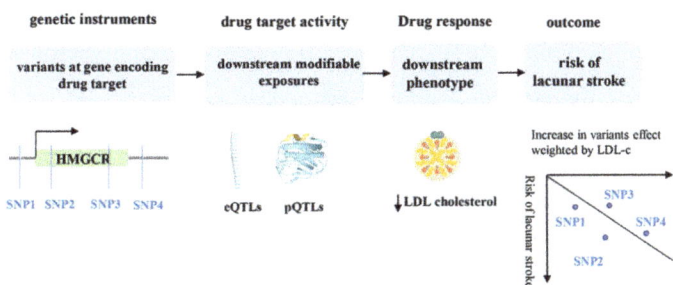

Figure 2. Principles of drug-target MR analysis framework. MR: Mendelian randomization. SNP: single-nucleotide polymorphism; HMGCR: 3-Hydroxy-3-Methylglutaryl-CoA reductase; eQTLs: expression quantitative trait loci; pQTLs: protein quantitative trait loci; LDL: low-density lipoprotein.

For antidiabetic drugs, genetic proxies for glucagon-like peptide 1 receptor (GLP1R) agonism and glycemic control by any mechanism estimated to be associated with glycated hemoglobin (mmol/mol) were derived from 337,000 samples in the U.K. Biobank [26,27]. The linkage disequilibrium r^2 values for variants used as proxies for GLP1R agonism and glycemic control were $r^2 < 0.1$ and 0.001, respectively (Table S3).

2.4. Mendelian Randomization Analysis

The principle and main analyses were described in our previous study [20,28,29]. Inverse-variance weighted (*IVW*) was the primary MR approach in the study. MR–Egger [30,31], the weighted median [32], and the simple median were calculated, and the MR–Egger intercept test was used to assess horizontal pleiotropy. We also used the Cochran Q statistic to test for heterogeneity and pleiotropy [33]. For instruments with only 1 variant, Wald-ratio MR was performed.

Next, the multivariable IVW method was used as the primary approach in conducting multivariable MR [33–35]. Univariable MR results reflect the total effect of each exposure on the outcome, including both direct and indirect effects through interactions with other exposures. Multivariable MR is often used in lipid analysis to estimate the direct causal effect of each exposure on an outcome [17]. Mendelian randomization (MR) can also provide valuable information about drugs, such as predicting their efficacy and revealing target-mediated adverse effects, which is also known as drug-target MR [5]. Drug-target MR can demonstrate the effect of modifying biomarkers through specific therapeutic targets on long-term health outcomes [36]. To account for both measured and unmeasured pleiotropy, we also used the multivariable MR-Egger [34] and the MR-Lasso method [37]. To test for heterogeneity and pleiotropy, we performed the Cochran Q statistic and multivariable MR-Egger test (intercept) [17,37].

The analyses were performed with R version 4.1.1 (R Core Team, Vienna, Austria) and the "Two Sample MR" (version 0.5.6) and "Mendelian Randomization" (version 0.5.1) packages [38]. Given that there was only one outcome under investigation (lacunar stroke), we used a 2-tailed p-value < 0.05 to denote evidence against the null hypothesis (i.e., $p < 0.05$ provided evidence in favor of an association between the exposure and outcome).

3. Results

Among all 65 risk factors (i.e., anthropometric, serum substances, socioeconomic, lifestyle/dietary, cardiometabolic, and inflammatory factors), not surprisingly, genetically predicted hypertension, hyperlipidemia, and type 2 diabetes were identified as the predominant high-risk factors for the development of lacunar stroke (Figure 3). Greater height, higher educational level, fibrinogen, and atrial fibrillation have also been found to be associated with the incidence of lacunar stroke (Figure 3).

The odds ratio for lacunar stroke estimated for a 1-SD increase in predisposition to elevated SBP was 1.06, and the effect was also validated and similar with SBP through analysis estimated for DBP and PP.

For lipids, genetically predicted 1-SD increases in triglyceride and apolipoprotein B levels showed a causal detrimental effect on lacunar stroke, respectively.

The analysis showed a decreased risk of lacunar stroke with genetically predicted high levels of apolipoprotein A-I and HDL. A genetic predisposition to type 2 diabetes significantly increases the risk of lacunar stroke. In addition, a high level of fasting proinsulin had a detrimental influence on the risk of lacunar stroke. The main results of significant risk factors in univariable MR are presented in Table S4.

In blood pressure MVMR analysis, we found little evidence for the direct effects of any blood pressure factor on the risk of lacunar stroke. Specifically, the ORs of lacunar stroke per 1-SD increase in SBP, DBP, and PP were 0.97, 1.08, and 1.07, respectively. For lipid MVMR, when ApoB, LDL-C, and TG were assessed together in Model 1 using the multivariable *IVW* method, elevated TG levels remained significantly associated with a higher risk of lacunar stroke. In Model 2, neither apolipoprotein A-I nor HDL levels showed direct effects on lacunar stroke risk. The MVMR results are listed in Table S5, and the MR–Egger intercept and Q test results in the study are listed in Table S6.

Furthermore, the antihypertensive drug MR demonstrated that genetic variants mimicking the effect of calcium channel blockers (CCBs) showed the most potent effects in preventing lacunar stroke for each 1 SD decrease in genetically predicted SBP. The protective effects remained stable in the sensitivity analyses when variants mimicking CCB effects were estimated using DBP and PP (Figure 4). We also found that loop diuretics may prevent lacunar stroke, as estimated by SBP and DBP (Figure 4). Genetically predicted alpha-adrenoceptor blockers may have marginally protective effects on lacunar stroke, but only when estimated with SBP (Figure 4). No evidence of efficacy was identified for other antihypertensive drug classes in the analysis.

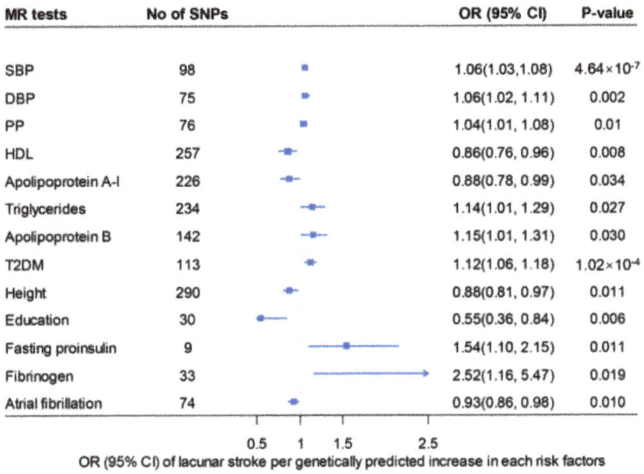

MR tests	No of SNPs	OR (95% CI)	P-value
SBP	98	1.06(1.03,1.08)	4.64×10^{-7}
DBP	75	1.06(1.02, 1.11)	0.002
PP	76	1.04(1.01, 1.08)	0.01
HDL	257	0.86(0.76, 0.96)	0.008
Apolipoprotein A-I	226	0.88(0.78, 0.99)	0.034
Triglycerides	234	1.14(1.01, 1.29)	0.027
Apolipoprotein B	142	1.15(1.01, 1.31)	0.030
T2DM	113	1.12(1.06, 1.18)	1.02×10^{-4}
Height	290	0.88(0.81, 0.97)	0.011
Education	30	0.55(0.36, 0.84)	0.006
Fasting proinsulin	9	1.54(1.10, 2.15)	0.011
Fibrinogen	33	2.52(1.16, 5.47)	0.019
Atrial fibrillation	74	0.93(0.86, 0.98)	0.010

OR (95% CI) of lacunar stroke per genetically predicted increase in each risk factors

Figure 3. Odds ratios for associations between genetically predicted significant factors and lacunar stroke conduct by univariable MR. MR: mendelian randomization. DBP: diastolic blood pressure; PP: pulse pressure; SBP: systolic blood pressure; HDL: high-density lipoprotein; T2DM: diabetes mellitus type 2; OR: odds ratio. 95% CI: 95% confidence interval. HDL, apolipoprotein A-I, triglycerides, apolipoprotein B, height used the multiplicative random effects model due to instrumental heterogeneity (Cochran Q test $p < 0.05$).

In the LDL-lowering target MR, the LDL-lowering effect predicted by the genetic variants at or near the *HMGCR* gene (i.e., mimicking the effect of statins), *NPC1L1* (mimicking the effects of ezetimibe), and *APOC3* (mimicking antisense anti-apoC3 agents) may decrease the risk of lacunar stroke (Figure 5). Genetic proxies for *HMGCR* agonism were associated with a reduced risk of lacunar stroke, and genetic proxies for *NPC1L1* inhibition were associated with a reduced risk of lacunar stroke. Significant protective associations of genetically proxied *APOC3* inhibition estimated either by LDL or triglyceride lowering with lacunar stroke risk were also observed (Figure 5).

We found little evidence for genetic proxies for *GLP1R* agonism effects on lacunar stroke; genetically proxied *GLP1R* agonism showed a marginal effect on lacunar stroke, while a genetically proxied improvement in overall glycemic control was associated with a reduced risk of lacunar stroke.

There were causal associations between genetically predicted greater height, higher education level, and lower odds of lacunar stroke, respectively. We also found that a high level of fibrinogen was associated with an increased risk of lacunar stroke, and a high risk of atrial fibrillation was associated with a decreased risk of lacunar stroke. No other causal evidence of lacunar stroke risk was found in the analysis. The main results of significant risk factors in univariable MR are presented in Table S4.

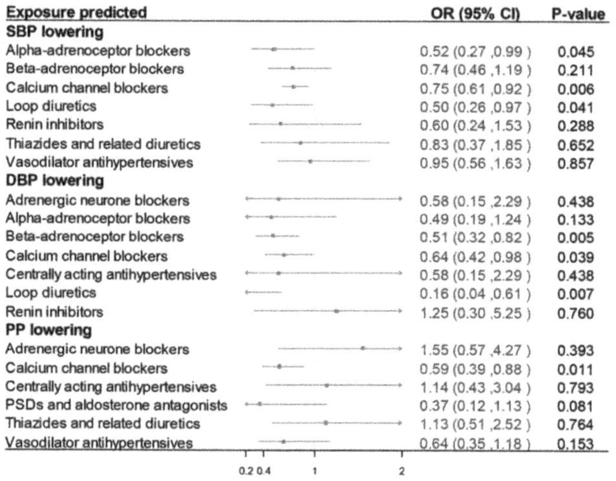

Exposure predicted	OR (95% CI)	P-value
SBP lowering		
Alpha-adrenoceptor blockers	0.52 (0.27 ,0.99)	0.045
Beta-adrenoceptor blockers	0.74 (0.46 ,1.19)	0.211
Calcium channel blockers	0.75 (0.61 ,0.92)	0.006
Loop diuretics	0.50 (0.26 ,0.97)	0.041
Renin inhibitors	0.60 (0.24 ,1.53)	0.288
Thiazides and related diuretics	0.83 (0.37 ,1.85)	0.652
Vasodilator antihypertensives	0.95 (0.56 ,1.63)	0.857
DBP lowering		
Adrenergic neurone blockers	0.58 (0.15 ,2.29)	0.438
Alpha-adrenoceptor blockers	0.49 (0.19 ,1.24)	0.133
Beta-adrenoceptor blockers	0.51 (0.32 ,0.82)	0.005
Calcium channel blockers	0.64 (0.42 ,0.98)	0.039
Centrally acting antihypertensives	0.58 (0.15 ,2.29)	0.438
Loop diuretics	0.16 (0.04 ,0.61)	0.007
Renin inhibitors	1.25 (0.30 ,5.25)	0.760
PP lowering		
Adrenergic neurone blockers	1.55 (0.57 ,4.27)	0.393
Calcium channel blockers	0.59 (0.39 ,0.88)	0.011
Centrally acting antihypertensives	1.14 (0.43 ,3.04)	0.793
PSDs and aldosterone antagonists	0.37 (0.12 ,1.13)	0.081
Thiazides and related diuretics	1.13 (0.51 ,2.52)	0.764
Vasodilator antihypertensives	0.64 (0.35 ,1.18)	0.153

Figure 4. Results of blood pressure-lowering drug-target MR analysis. Estimated for SBP-lowering target weighted by SBP, DBP-lowering target weighted by DBP, and PP-lowering target weighted by PP. On the left of x-axis = 1 presented drug use protective, and on the right of x-axis = 1 presented drug use detrimental. MR: Mendelian randomization; DBP: diastolic blood pressure; PP: pulse pressure; SBP: systolic blood pressure. OR: odds ratio. 95% CI: 95% confidence interval.

Exposure predicted	OR (95% CI)	P-value
LDL-lowering targets		
HMGCR inhibition	0.53(0.38,0.73)	8.42×10^{-5}
PCSK9 inhibition	1.12(0.91, 1.37)	0.289
NPC1L1 blockade	0.33(0.18, 0.59)	2.36×10^{-4}
APOC3 inhibition	0.68(0.51, 0.91)	8.56×10^{-3}
Triglyceride-lowering targets		
APOA5/APOC3 modulation	1.13(0.90, 1.44)	0.276
LPL activation	1.23(0.86, 1.79)	0.250
ANGPTL3 inhibition	0.61(0.36, 1.08)	0.089
APOB inhibition	0.50(0.27, 0.92)	0.027

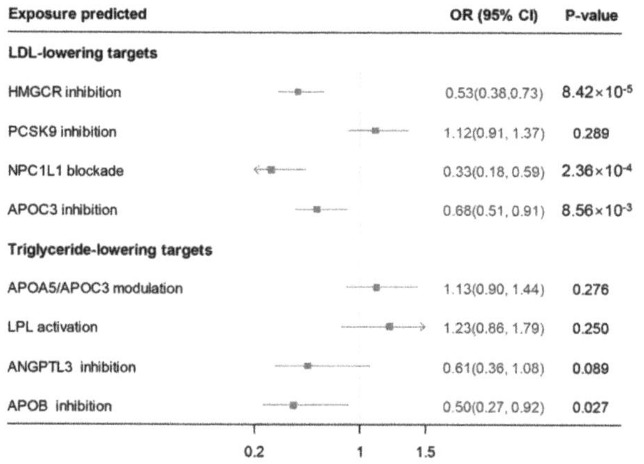

Figure 5. Results of lipid-lowering drug-target MR analysis. Estimated for LDL-lowering target weighted by LDL, triglyceride-lowering target weighted by triglyceride. On the left of x-axis = 1 presented drug use protective, and on the right of x-axis = 1 presented drug use detrimental. MR: Mendelian randomization; LDL: low-density lipoprotein; HMGCR: 3-Hydroxy-3-Methylglutaryl-CoA reductase; PCSK9: proprotein convertase subtilisin kexin type 9; NPC1L1: NPC1-like intracellular cholesterol transporter 1; APOC3: apolipoprotein C3; APOA5: apolipoprotein A5; LPL: lipoprotein lipase; ANGPTL3: angiopoietin-like 3; APOB: apolipoprotein B; OR: odds ratio. 95% CI: 95% confidence interval.

Our MR analysis provided strong genetic evidence that hypertension, hyperlipidemia, and type 2 diabetes were the predominant risk factors for the development of lacunar stroke. Moreover, our MVMR analysis documented that genetically predicted elevated TG levels were still associated with a higher risk of lacunar stroke. Importantly, the comprehensive drug-target MR approach identified the protective effects of common antihypertensive, lipid-lowering medications on lacunar stroke. CCBs, statins, ezetimibe, and anti-*apoC3* agents were most likely to have potential effects of preventing lacunar stroke. *GLP1R* agonism did not show such effects, but improvement in overall glycemic control was associated with a reduced risk of lacunar stroke.

4. Discussion

In conclusion, this study provides valuable insights into the genetic and modifiable risk factors for lacunar stroke. The findings could potentially guide the development of preventive strategies and treatments for this condition [39]. This study indicated that old drugs could be repurposed to prevent lacunar stroke more precisely with substantially lower overall development costs and shorter development timelines [40]. Such drugs should be given high priority when doctors are making decisions and may contribute to a healthier brain during aging.

Antihypertensive, lipid-lowering agents have been explored with stroke in a previous study. Georgakis MK et al. found that genetic proxies for CCBs showed an inverse association with the risk of ischemic stroke compared with proxies for β-blockade, which was particularly strong for small vessel stroke [41]. Our study showed that among the 12 antihypertensive drug classes, CCBs had the most potent effects in preventing lacunar stroke and that loop diuretics may prevent the development of lacunar stroke, as estimated by SBP. β-Blockade did not show protective effects against the risk of lacunar stroke estimated by SBP. Large-scale meta-analyses of clinical trials have shown that calcium channel blockers have a stronger effect on reducing the risk of stroke than β blockers [42,43]. However, the association between lipid-lowering variants mimicking statin use and a lower risk of ischemic stroke was statistically significant only for large artery stroke [44]. The possible explanation was that the data we used as outcomes made substantial progress in identifying the genetic mechanisms underlying lacunar stroke. We also found little evidence for the effect of *PCSK9* inhibitors in preventing lacunar stroke. Our findings agree with the results by Hopewell JC et al. in that *PCSK9* inhibitors are unlikely to have an effect on lacunar stroke risk. Notably, genetic proxies for *HMGCR* agonism, *NPC1L1* (mimicking the effects of ezetimibe) and *APOC3*, were predicted to decrease the risk of lacunar stroke; they do affect the risk of lacunar stroke, but they may not do so via LDL. We found little evidence to suggest that LDL itself affects the risk of developing lacunar stroke. The underlying mechanism needs to be explored in the future.

Blood pressure showed a significant association with lacunar stroke risk in univariable MR but not in MVMR. A possible explanation for this is that MVMR analysis is used to estimate the independent causal effect of each exposure, whereas univariable MR is used to calculate the total effect. Elevated TG levels were found to be associated with a higher risk of lacunar stroke conditional on ApoB and LDL-C levels in multivariable MR, which was consistent with the results from univariable MR. This result suggests that compared with ApoB or LDL-C, TG may be more likely to have a detrimental causal effect on lacunar stroke. Thus, in drug-targeted MR, we applied proxies for lipid-lowering agents estimated by TG-lowering targets.

In this screening Mendelian randomization analysis, we also found that higher height and education levels are associated with a reduced risk of lacunar stroke. Currently, it is well understood that higher education levels often indicate that individuals are more likely to have access to healthy diets, appropriate physical exercise, and harmless work environments and are more concerned about their health status. These characteristics are all favorable factors in reducing the risk of lacunar stroke. However, the biological mechanism behind the association between higher height and reduced risk of lacunar stroke is currently unclear. For both of these results, further mediation analysis would be helpful in uncovering their underlying biological mechanisms.

The relationship between fibrinogen and lacunar stroke can be explained by the fact that high levels of fibrinogen can lead to the formation of blood clots, which can block small arteries in the brain and cause a lacunar stroke [45]. Further research is needed to understand the underlying biological mechanisms behind this association. However, this finding suggests that monitoring fibrinogen levels may be an important factor in reducing the risk of lacunar stroke [46].

Additionally, this result may imply that atrial fibrillation patients are less likely to develop lacunar stroke. However, more research is needed to confirm this hypothesis and to determine the underlying biological mechanisms. One possible explanation for this association is that atrial fibrillation may lead to changes in blood flow and pressure within the brain, which could reduce the risk of lacunar stroke. Another possibility is that the medications used to treat atrial fibrillation may also have a protective effect against lacunar stroke. Future studies could investigate the effects of different types of medications on the risk of lacunar stroke in individuals with atrial fibrillation, as well as the potential role of lifestyle factors such as diet and exercise.

The term lipohyalinosis refers to a concentric accumulation of hyaline material in the walls of small cerebral vessels, which causes narrowing and blockage of the penetrating arteries [47]. This is among the first and most frequent mechanisms of lacunar stroke that have been documented and confirmed by pathology. High blood pressure may cause the vessel walls to thicken and degenerate, as well as foam cells to fill up the lumen of small arteries that penetrate the brain, leading to lipohyalinosis. Diabetes is a condition that affects the metabolism of blood glucose (or blood sugar) and blood lipids, causing chronic inflammation [48]. These factors harm the vessel wall, leading to the accumulation of lipid, fibrous tissue, and calcification and the formation of atherosclerotic plaques. Our study suggests that CCBs, statins, ezetimibe, and anti-*apoC3* agents may prevent lacunar stroke by lowering blood pressure and lipid levels. Additionally, the potential role of statins in improving lacunar stroke might be due to the anti-inflammatory effect of statins [49]. The antihyperglycemic effect alone is able to reduce oxidative stress, with improvement in endothelial function, which is one of the triggers for the Virchow triad [50]. Future studies should investigate whether other mechanisms are also involved, which may help identify new targets for interventions or therapies. A strength of our study was the use of two-sample MR, which allowed us to utilize the latest GWASs for lacunar stroke outcomes, which included 7338 cases and 254,798 controls [2]. MR is a more effective approach than traditional pharmacoepidemiological methods in addressing certain types of confounding. This includes confounding by indication, as well as confounding by environmental and lifestyle factors that cannot be fully adjusted for using observational data. Residual confounding is an inevitable consequence of measurement error and incomplete capture of all potential confounding factors. Importantly, drug repurposing, being a less expensive and time-consuming approach, brings effective therapies to patients compared with the cumbersome traditional processes of discovery and development. Repurposing candidates have already undergone several stages of clinical development and have well-established safety and pharmacological profiles. This translates to lower development costs, faster development times, and ultimately lower out-of-pocket costs for patients, reducing the actual cost of therapy [51].

Several limitations merit consideration. Our study was constrained by the fact that MR estimates the effect of lifelong exposure, while drugs typically have much shorter periods of exposure [52]. Additionally, systolic blood pressure may have age-dependent effects. As a result, the effect sizes we estimated may not directly reflect what is observed in trials or clinical practice and may not be able to identify critical periods of exposure. Nevertheless, our study assumed a linear relationship between exposures and lacunar stroke and did not investigate the nonlinear effects of the exposures [30,32]. The populations of exposures and outcomes we explored in the study were not all from subjects of European ancestry; the lacunar stroke GWAS data were derived from transethnic studies, and the underlying populations were primarily composed of individuals of European ancestry [53]. Thus, bias from population stratification is deemed likely [54]. In this analysis, we only analyzed *GLP1R* agonism for hypoglycemic drugs and did not analyze other commonly used hypoglycemic drugs in clinical practice, such as metformin and *DPP4* inhibitors, which may result in missing information. Metformin is a multi-target drug that is not suitable for MR analysis [55], and there are not enough available instrumental variables to proxy DPP4 inhibitors as far as we know. Finally, completely ruling out pleiotropy or an alternative direct causal pathway is a challenge for all MR analyses because there are probably some unknown confounders that could influence lacunar stroke [56]. These limitations highlight the importance of cautious interpretation of findings [54]. Further research is needed to validate these findings and to explore their clinical implications.

Precision medicine technology is continuously developing, and we believe that it will play an increasingly important role in the diagnosis and treatment of lacunar stroke [57]. To foster the potential of MR analysis, it is crucial to acquire large datasets that comprise subject-level information on hundreds to thousands of patients [58]. This will enable the development of more accurate and reliable predictive models for lacunar stroke, which can help clinicians identify high-risk patients and provide them with timely and effective interventions [59]. In conclusion, precision medicine, particularly using drug-target MR, is a promising approach for the prevention and treatment of lacunar stroke and an area that deserves further research and development [9,39,60].

5. Conclusions

Using an MR design to comprehensively repurpose approved drugs to precisely prevent lacunar stroke with well-established safety and low costs. CCBs, statins, ezetimibe, and anti-*apoC3* agents were most likely to have potential effects of preventing lacunar stroke. This study provided solid evidence for doctors to consider when making decisions in clinical practice and may contribute to a healthier brain during aging.

Supplementary Materials: The following supporting information can be downloaded at: https://www.mdpi.com/article/10.3390/biomedicines12010017/s1, Table S1. All potential modifaiable risk factors classification groups; Table S2. Summarised GWAS data for potentially modifiable risk factors that shown significant effects on lacunar stroke in univariable MR; Table S3. Genetic variants included in drug-target analyses for each region; Table S4. the main results of significant risk factors in univariable MR; Table S5. Multivariable MR estimates for blood pressure and lipids; Table S6. MR-Egger intercept and Q test result in the study.

Author Contributions: L.Z.: conceptualization, data curation, formal analysis, writing—original draft; F.W.: methodology, software, validation; K.X.: methodology, software, validation; Z.Y.: methodology, software, validation; Y.F.: writing—conceptualization, writing—review and editing; T.H.: conceptualization, writing—review and editing; D.F.: conceptualization, writing—review and editing. All authors have read and agreed to the published version of the manuscript.

Funding: This study was supported by the National Natural Science Foundation of China (grant numbers 82101490, 81030019, and 81873784) and the Beijing Key Laboratory of Biomarker and Translational Research in Neurodegenerative Disorders.

Institutional Review Board Statement: All human research was approved by the relevant institutional review boards and conducted according to the Declaration of Helsinki. Ethical approval was obtained from relevant Research Ethics Committees and from the review boards of Peking University Third Hospital.

Data Availability Statement: All data collected for the study and code used in the analysis will be made available to others.

Conflicts of Interest: The authors report no conflict of interest.

References

1. Pantoni, L. Cerebral small vessel disease: From pathogenesis and clinical characteristics to therapeutic challenges. *Lancet Neurol.* **2010**, *9*, 689–701. [CrossRef]
2. Traylor, M.; Persyn, E.; Tomppo, L.; Klasson, S.; Abedi, V.; Bakker, M.K.; Torres, N.; Li, L.; Bell, S.; Rutten-Jacobs, L.; et al. Genetic basis of lacunar stroke: A pooled analysis of individual patient data and genome-wide association studies. *Lancet Neurol.* **2021**, *20*, 351–361. [CrossRef]
3. Nelson, M.R.; Tipney, H.; Painter, J.L.; Shen, J.; Nicoletti, P.; Shen, Y.; Floratos, A.; Sham, P.C.; Li, M.J.; Wang, J.; et al. The support of human genetic evidence for approved drug indications. *Nat. Genet.* **2015**, *47*, 856–860. [CrossRef]

4. Davey Smith, G.; Hemani, G. Mendelian randomization: Genetic anchors for causal inference in epidemiological studies. *Human. Mol. Genet.* **2014**, *23*, R89–R98. [CrossRef]
5. Schmidt, A.F.; Finan, C.; Gordillo-Marañón, M.; Asselbergs, F.W.; Freitag, D.F.; Patel, R.S.; Tyl, B.; Chopade, S.; Faraway, R.; Zwierzyna, M.; et al. Genetic drug target validation using Mendelian randomisation. *Nat. Commun.* **2020**, *11*, 3255. [CrossRef]
6. Swerdlow, D.I.; Holmes, M.V.; Kuchenbaecker, K.B.; Engmann, J.E.; Shah, T.; Sofat, R.; Guo, Y.; Chung, C.; Peasey, A.; Pfister, R.; et al. The interleukin-6 receptor as a target for prevention of coronary heart disease: A mendelian randomisation analysis. *Lancet* **2012**, *379*, 1214–1224. [CrossRef]
7. Swerdlow, D.I.; Preiss, D.; Kuchenbaecker, K.B.; Holmes, M.V.; Engmann, J.E.; Shah, T.; Sofat, R.; Stender, S.; Johnson, P.C.; Scott, R.A.; et al. HMG-coenzyme A reductase inhibition, type 2 diabetes, and bodyweight: Evidence from genetic analysis and randomised trials. *Lancet* **2015**, *385*, 351–361. [CrossRef]
8. Ashburn, T.T.; Thor, K.B. Drug repositioning: Identifying and developing new uses for existing drugs. *Nat. Rev. Drug Discov.* **2004**, *3*, 673–683. [CrossRef]
9. Acosta, J.N.; Szejko, N.; Falcone, G.J. Mendelian Randomization in Stroke: A Powerful Approach to Causal Inference and Drug Target Validation. *Front. Genet.* **2021**, *12*, 683082. [CrossRef]
10. Hemani, G.; Zheng, J.; Elsworth, B.; Wade, K.H.; Haberland, V.; Baird, D.; Laurin, C.; Burgess, S.; Bowden, J.; Langdon, R.; et al. The MR-Base platform supports systematic causal inference across the human phenome. *eLife* **2018**, *7*, e34408. [CrossRef]
11. Kilarski, L.L.; Rutten-Jacobs, L.C.; Bevan, S.; Baker, R.; Hassan, A.; Hughes, D.A.; Markus, H.S. Prevalence of CADASIL and Fabry Disease in a Cohort of MRI Defined Younger Onset Lacunar Stroke. *PLoS ONE* **2015**, *10*, e0136352. [CrossRef]
12. Adams, H.P., Jr.; Bendixen, B.H.; Kappelle, L.J.; Biller, J.; Love, B.B.; Gordon, D.L.; Marsh, E.E., 3rd. Classification of subtype of acute ischemic stroke. Definitions for use in a multicenter clinical trial. TOAST. Trial of Org 10172 in Acute Stroke Treatment. *Stroke* **1993**, *24*, 35–41. [CrossRef]
13. Bellenguez, C.; Bevan, S.; Gschwendtner, A.; Spencer, C.C.; Burgess, A.I.; Pirinen, M.; Jackson, C.A.; Traylor, M.; Strange, A.; Su, Z.; et al. Genome-wide association study identifies a variant in HDAC9 associated with large vessel ischemic stroke. *Nat. Genet.* **2012**, *44*, 328–333. [CrossRef]
14. NINDS Stroke Genetics Network (SiGN); International Stroke Genetics Consortium (ISGC). Loci associated with ischaemic stroke and its subtypes (SiGN): A genome-wide association study. *Lancet Neurol.* **2016**, *15*, 174–184. [CrossRef]
15. Pierce, B.L.; Ahsan, H.; Vanderweele, T.J. Power and instrument strength requirements for Mendelian randomization studies using multiple genetic variants. *Int. J. Epidemiol.* **2011**, *40*, 740–752. [CrossRef]
16. Bowden, J.; Del Greco, M.F.; Minelli, C.; Davey Smith, G.; Sheehan, N.A.; Thompson, J.R. Assessing the suitability of summary data for two-sample Mendelian randomization analyses using MR-Egger regression: The role of the I2 statistic. *Int. J. Epidemiol.* **2016**, *45*, 1961–1974. [CrossRef]
17. Sanderson, E.; Davey Smith, G.; Windmeijer, F.; Bowden, J. An examination of multivariable Mendelian randomization in the single-sample and two-sample summary data settings. *Int. J. Epidemiol.* **2019**, *48*, 713–727. [CrossRef]
18. Sanderson, E. Multivariable Mendelian Randomization and Mediation. *Cold Spring Harb. Perspect. Med.* **2021**, *11*, a038984. [CrossRef]
19. Evangelou, E.; Warren, H.R.; Mosen-Ansorena, D.; Mifsud, B.; Pazoki, R.; Gao, H.; Ntritsos, G.; Dimou, N.; Cabrera, C.P.; Karaman, I.; et al. Genetic analysis of over 1 million people identifies 535 new loci associated with blood pressure traits. *Nat. Genet.* **2018**, *50*, 1412–1425. [CrossRef]
20. Yu, Z.; Zhang, L.; Zhang, G.; Xia, K.; Yang, Q.; Huang, T.; Fan, D. Lipids, Apolipoproteins, Statins and ICH: A Mendelian Randomization Study. *Ann. Neurol.* **2022**, *92*, 390–399. [CrossRef]
21. Gill, D.; Georgakis, M.K.; Koskeridis, F.; Jiang, L.; Feng, Q.; Wei, W.Q.; Theodoratou, E.; Elliott, P.; Denny, J.C.; Malik, R.; et al. Use of Genetic Variants Related to Antihypertensive Drugs to Inform on Efficacy and Side Effects. *Circulation* **2019**, *140*, 270–279. [CrossRef]
22. Walker, V.M.; Kehoe, P.G.; Martin, R.M.; Davies, N.M. Repurposing antihypertensive drugs for the prevention of Alzheimer's disease: A Mendelian randomization study. *Int. J. Epidemiol.* **2020**, *49*, 1132–1140. [CrossRef]
23. Levin, M.G.; Klarin, D.; Walker, V.M.; Gill, D.; Lynch, J.; Hellwege, J.N.; Keaton, J.M.; Lee, K.M.; Assimes, T.L.; Natarajan, P.; et al. Association Between Genetic Variation in Blood Pressure and Increased Lifetime Risk of Peripheral Artery Disease. *Arterioscler. Thromb. Vasc. Biol.* **2021**, *41*, 2027–2034. [CrossRef]
24. Ference, B.A.; Ray, K.K.; Catapano, A.L.; Ference, T.B.; Burgess, S.; Neff, D.R.; Oliver-Williams, C.; Wood, A.M.; Butterworth, A.S.; Di Angelantonio, E.; et al. Mendelian Randomization Study of ACLY and Cardiovascular Disease. *N. Engl. J. Med.* **2019**, *380*, 1033–1042. [CrossRef]
25. Do, R.; Willer, C.J.; Schmidt, E.M.; Sengupta, S.; Gao, C.; Peloso, G.M.; Gustafsson, S.; Kanoni, S.; Ganna, A.; Chen, J.; et al. Common variants associated with plasma triglycerides and risk for coronary artery disease. *Nat. Genet.* **2013**, *45*, 1345–1352. [CrossRef]
26. Daghlas, I.; Karhunen, V.; Ray, D.; Zuber, V.; Burgess, S.; Tsao, P.S.; Lynch, J.A.; Lee, K.M.; Voight, B.F.; Chang, K.M.; et al. Genetic Evidence for Repurposing of GLP1R (Glucagon-Like Peptide-1 Receptor) Agonists to Prevent Heart Failure. *J. Am. Heart Assoc.* **2021**, *10*, e020331. [CrossRef]

27. Vujkovic, M.; Keaton, J.M.; Lynch, J.A.; Miller, D.R.; Zhou, J.; Tcheandjieu, C.; Huffman, J.E.; Assimes, T.L.; Lorenz, K.; Zhu, X.; et al. Discovery of 318 new risk loci for type 2 diabetes and related vascular outcomes among 1.4 million participants in a multi-ancestry meta-analysis. *Nat. Genet.* **2020**, *52*, 680–691. [CrossRef]
28. Burgess, S.; Davey Smith, G.; Davies, N.M.; Dudbridge, F.; Gill, D.; Glymour, M.M.; Hartwig, F.P.; Kutalik, Z.; Holmes, M.V.; Minelli, C.; et al. Guidelines for performing Mendelian randomization investigations: Update for summer 2023. *Wellcome Open. Res.* **2019**, *4*, 186. [CrossRef]
29. Bowden, J.; Spiller, W.; Del Greco, M.F.; Sheehan, N.; Thompson, J.; Minelli, C.; Davey Smith, G. Improving the visualization, interpretation and analysis of two-sample summary data Mendelian randomization via the Radial plot and Radial regression. *Int. J. Epidemiol.* **2018**, *47*, 1264–1278. [CrossRef]
30. Burgess, S.; Bowden, J.; Fall, T.; Ingelsson, E.; Thompson, S.G. Sensitivity Analyses for Robust Causal Inference from Mendelian Randomization Analyses with Multiple Genetic Variants. *Epidemiology* **2017**, *28*, 30–42. [CrossRef]
31. Bowden, J.; Davey Smith, G.; Burgess, S. Mendelian randomization with invalid instruments: Effect estimation and bias detection through Egger regression. *Int. J. Epidemiol.* **2015**, *44*, 512–525. [CrossRef]
32. Bowden, J.; Davey Smith, G.; Haycock, P.C.; Burgess, S. Consistent Estimation in Mendelian Randomization with Some Invalid Instruments Using a Weighted Median Estimator. *Genet. Epidemiol.* **2016**, *40*, 304–314. [CrossRef]
33. Sanderson, E.; Spiller, W.; Bowden, J. Testing and correcting for weak and pleiotropic instruments in two-sample multivariable Mendelian randomization. *Stat. Med.* **2021**, *40*, 5434–5452. [CrossRef]
34. Rees, J.M.B.; Wood, A.M.; Burgess, S. Extending the MR-Egger method for multivariable Mendelian randomization to correct for both measured and unmeasured pleiotropy. *Stat. Med.* **2017**, *36*, 4705–4718. [CrossRef]
35. Zheng, J.; Brion, M.J.; Kemp, J.P.; Warrington, N.M.; Borges, M.C.; Hemani, G.; Richardson, T.G.; Rasheed, H.; Qiao, Z.; Haycock, P.; et al. The Effect of Plasma Lipids and Lipid-Lowering Interventions on Bone Mineral Density: A Mendelian Randomization Study. *J. Bone Miner. Res.* **2020**, *35*, 1224–1235. [CrossRef]
36. Williams, D.M.; Finan, C.; Schmidt, A.F.; Burgess, S.; Hingorani, A.D. Lipid lowering and Alzheimer disease risk: A mendelian randomization study. *Ann. Neurol.* **2020**, *87*, 30–39. [CrossRef]
37. Grant, A.J.; Burgess, S. Pleiotropy robust methods for multivariable Mendelian randomization. *Stat. Med.* **2021**, *40*, 5813–5830. [CrossRef]
38. Rasooly, D.; Patel, C.J. Conducting a Reproducible Mendelian Randomization Analysis Using the R Analytic Statistical Environment. *Curr. Protoc. Hum. Genet.* **2019**, *101*, e82. [CrossRef]
39. Daghlas, I.; Gill, D. Mendelian randomization as a tool to inform drug development using human genetics. *Camb. Prism. Precis. Med.* **2023**, *1*, e16. [CrossRef]
40. Pushpakom, S.; Iorio, F.; Eyers, P.A.; Escott, K.J.; Hopper, S.; Wells, A.; Doig, A.; Guilliams, T.; Latimer, J.; McNamee, C.; et al. Drug repurposing: Progress, challenges and recommendations. *Nat. Rev. Drug. Discov.* **2019**, *18*, 41–58. [CrossRef]
41. Georgakis, M.K.; Gill, D.; Webb, A.J.S.; Evangelou, E.; Elliott, P.; Sudlow, C.L.M.; Dehghan, A.; Malik, R.; Tzoulaki, I.; Dichgans, M. Genetically determined blood pressure, antihypertensive drug classes, and risk of stroke subtypes. *Neurology* **2020**, *95*, e353–e361. [CrossRef] [PubMed]
42. Rothwell, P.M.; Howard, S.C.; Dolan, E.; O'Brien, E.; Dobson, J.E.; Dahlöf, B.; Poulter, N.R.; Sever, P.S. Effects of beta blockers and calcium-channel blockers on within-individual variability in blood pressure and risk of stroke. *Lancet. Neurol.* **2010**, *9*, 469–480. [CrossRef] [PubMed]
43. Webb, A.J.; Fischer, U.; Mehta, Z.; Rothwell, P.M. Effects of antihypertensive-drug class on interindividual variation in blood pressure and risk of stroke: A systematic review and meta-analysis. *Lancet* **2010**, *375*, 906–915. [CrossRef] [PubMed]
44. Hindy, G.; Engström, G.; Larsson, S.C.; Traylor, M.; Markus, H.S.; Melander, O.; Orho-Melander, M. Role of Blood Lipids in the Development of Ischemic Stroke and its Subtypes. *Stroke* **2018**, *49*, 820–827. [CrossRef]
45. Rothwell, P.M.; Howard, S.C.; Power, D.A.; Gutnikov, S.A.; Algra, A.; van Gijn, J.; Clark, T.G.; Murphy, M.F.; Warlow, C.P. Fibrinogen concentration and risk of ischemic stroke and acute coronary events in 5113 patients with transient ischemic attack and minor ischemic stroke. *Stroke* **2004**, *35*, 2300–2305. [CrossRef]
46. Martiskainen, M.; Pohjasvaara, T.; Mikkelsson, J.; Mäntylä, R.; Kunnas, T.; Laippala, P.; Ilveskoski, E.; Kaste, M.; Karhunen, P.J.; Erkinjuntti, T. Fibrinogen gene promoter -455 A allele as a risk factor for lacunar stroke. *Stroke* **2003**, *34*, 886–891. [CrossRef]
47. Onodera, O.; Uemura, M.; Ando, S.; Hayashi, H.; Kanazawa, M. Rethinking Lacunar Stroke: Beyond Fisher's Curse. *Brain Nerve* **2021**, *73*, 991–998. [CrossRef]
48. Palmer, A.K.; Tchkonia, T.; LeBrasseur, N.K.; Chini, E.N.; Xu, M.; Kirkland, J.L. Cellular Senescence in Type 2 Diabetes: A Therapeutic Opportunity. *Diabetes* **2015**, *64*, 2289–2298. [CrossRef]
49. Satny, M.; Hubacek, J.A.; Vrablik, M. Statins and Inflammation. *Curr. Atheroscler. Rep.* **2021**, *23*, 80. [CrossRef]
50. Caturano, A.; D'Angelo, M.; Mormone, A.; Russo, V.; Mollica, M.P.; Salvatore, T.; Galiero, R.; Rinaldi, L.; Vetrano, E.; Marfella, R.; et al. Oxidative Stress in Type 2 Diabetes: Impacts from Pathogenesis to Lifestyle Modifications. *Curr. Issues Mol. Biol.* **2023**, *45*, 6651–6666. [CrossRef]
51. Ng, Y.L.; Salim, C.K.; Chu, J.J.H. Drug repurposing for COVID-19: Approaches, challenges and promising candidates. *Pharmacol. Ther.* **2021**, *228*, 107930. [CrossRef]
52. Smith, G.D.; Ebrahim, S. Mendelian randomization: Prospects, potentials, and limitations. *Int. J. Epidemiol.* **2004**, *33*, 30–42. [CrossRef] [PubMed]

53. Pierce, B.L.; Burgess, S. Efficient design for Mendelian randomization studies: Subsample and 2-sample instrumental variable estimators. *Am. J. Epidemiol.* **2013**, *178*, 1177–1184. [CrossRef] [PubMed]
54. VanderWeele, T.J.; Tchetgen Tchetgen, E.J.; Cornelis, M.; Kraft, P. Methodological challenges in mendelian randomization. *Epidemiology* **2014**, *25*, 427–435. [CrossRef] [PubMed]
55. Ma, T.; Tian, X.; Zhang, B.; Li, M.; Wang, Y.; Yang, C.; Wu, J.; Wei, X.; Qu, Q.; Yu, Y.; et al. Low-dose metformin targets the lysosomal AMPK pathway through PEN2. *Nature* **2022**, *603*, 159–165. [CrossRef] [PubMed]
56. Hemani, G.; Bowden, J.; Davey Smith, G. Evaluating the potential role of pleiotropy in Mendelian randomization studies. *Hum. Mol. Genet.* **2018**, *27*, R195–R208. [CrossRef] [PubMed]
57. Bonkhoff, A.K.; Grefkes, C. Precision medicine in stroke: Towards personalized outcome predictions using artificial intelligence. *Brain* **2021**, *145*, 457–475. [CrossRef]
58. Emdin, C.A.; Khera, A.V.; Kathiresan, S. Mendelian Randomization. *JAMA* **2017**, *318*, 1925–1926. [CrossRef]
59. Gill, D.; Vujkovic, M. The Potential of Genetic Data for Prioritizing Drug Repurposing Efforts. *Neurology* **2022**, *99*, 267–268. [CrossRef]
60. Georgakis, M.K.; Malik, R.; Gill, D.; Franceschini, N.; Sudlow, C.L.M.; Dichgans, M. Interleukin-6 Signaling Effects on Ischemic Stroke and Other Cardiovascular Outcomes: A Mendelian Randomization Study. *Circ. Genom. Precis. Med.* **2020**, *13*, e002872. [CrossRef]

Disclaimer/Publisher's Note: The statements, opinions and data contained in all publications are solely those of the individual author(s) and contributor(s) and not of MDPI and/or the editor(s). MDPI and/or the editor(s) disclaim responsibility for any injury to people or property resulting from any ideas, methods, instructions or products referred to in the content.

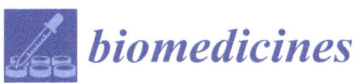

Article

Propentofylline Improves Thiol-Based Antioxidant Defenses and Limits Lipid Peroxidation following Gliotoxic Injury in the Rat Brainstem

Deborah E. M. Baliellas [1], Marcelo P. Barros [2,*], Cristina V. Vardaris [2], Maísa Guariroba [1,2], Sandra C. Poppe [1], Maria F. Martins [1,3], Álvaro A. F. Pereira [1,†] and Eduardo F. Bondan [3,*]

[1] Department of Veterinary Medicine, Cruzeiro do Sul University, São Paulo 08060070, Brazil; dbaliellas@gmail.com (D.E.M.B.); maisa_bizie@hotmail.com (M.G.); sandra.poppe@cruzeirodosul.edu.br (S.C.P.); fa3m@terra.com.br (M.F.M.)

[2] Interdisciplinary Programs in Health Sciences, Institute of Physical Activity and Sport Sciences (ICAFE), Cruzeiro do Sul University, São Paulo 01506000, Brazil; crisvardaris@gmail.com

[3] Graduate Program in Environmental and Experimental Pathology, University Paulista (UNIP), São Paulo 04057000, Brazil

* Correspondence: marcelo.barros@cruzeirodosul.edu.br (M.P.B.); eduardo.bondan@docente.unip.br (E.F.B.); Tel.: +55-11-33853103 (M.P.B.); +55-11-55864171 (E.F.B.)

† in memoriam.

Abstract: Propentofylline (PROP) is a methylated xanthine compound that diminishes the activation of microglial cells and astrocytes, which are neuronal cells strongly associated with many neurodegenerative diseases. Based on previously observed remyelination and neuroprotective effects, PROP has also been proposed to increment antioxidant defenses and to prevent oxidative damage in neural tissues. Since most neurodegenerative processes have free radicals as molecular pathological agents, the aim of this study was to evaluate the antioxidant effects of 12.5 mg·kg^{-1}·day^{-1} PROP in plasma and the brainstem of Wistar rats exposed to the gliotoxic agent 0.1% ethidium bromide (EB) for 7–31 days. The bulk of the data here demonstrates that, after 7 days of EB treatment, TBARS levels were 2-fold higher in the rat CNS than in control, reaching a maximum of 2.4-fold within 15 days. After 31 days of EB treatment, lipoperoxidation in CNS was still 65% higher than that in the control. Clearly, PROP treatment limited the progression of lipoperoxidation in EB-oxidized CNS: it was, for example, 76% lower than in the EB-treated group after 15 days. Most of these effects were associated with PROP-induced activity of glutathione reductase in the brainstem: the EB + PROP group showed 59% higher GR activity than that of the EB or control groups within 7 days. In summary, aligning with previous studies from our group and with literature about MTXs, we observed that propentofylline (PROP) improved the thiol-based antioxidant defenses in the rat brainstem by the induction of the enzymatic activity of glutathione reductase (GR), which diminished lipid oxidation progression and rebalanced the redox status in the CNS.

Keywords: astrocyte; glial cells; xanthine; oxidative stress; free radicals; neurodegenerative; caffeine

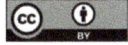

1. Introduction

Methylxanthines (MTXs) are purine-based alkaloids that are frequently found in highly consumed foods and beverages such as coffee, cacao, chocolate, and tea [1,2]. After uptake by the human body, MTXs are freely distributed in the bloodstream to different tissues, where they are absorbed at different rates. Among all absorbing tissues/organs, MTXs easily cross the blood–brain barrier to accumulate in several segments of the central nervous system (CNS) [3].

Many MTXs display substantial neuro-boosting properties, similar to that of caffeine, which were associated with important antioxidant and neuroprotective effects that significantly diminish oxidative stress in brain portions and neuronal circuits [4]. Moreover,

MTXs were shown to modulate inflammatory immune responses, usually by controlling the release of pro-inflammatory cytokines and the attenuation of microglial activation [5]. On the molecular level, MTXs and their phosphate-derivatives are potential chelating agents of redox-active metals, such as ferrous and cupreous ions (Fe^{2+} and Cu^+, respectively), which are catalysts for the formation of more aggressive reactive oxygen/nitrogen species (ROS/RNS) in biological systems [6]. Moreover, MTXs treatment was shown to affect major thiol-dependent antioxidant defenses, mainly glutathione (GSH), probably via redox-signaling cascades, such as the Keap1-Nrf2 and NF-kB pathways [7]. Thiol-dependent antioxidants, such as GSH, peroxiredoxin, and glutaredoxin, are direct scavengers of ROS/RNS, as well as substrates for major antioxidant enzymes, such as glutathione peroxidase (GPx), glutathione reductase (GR), and glutathione-S-transferase (GST) [8]. Figure 1 shows natural and synthetic MTXs.

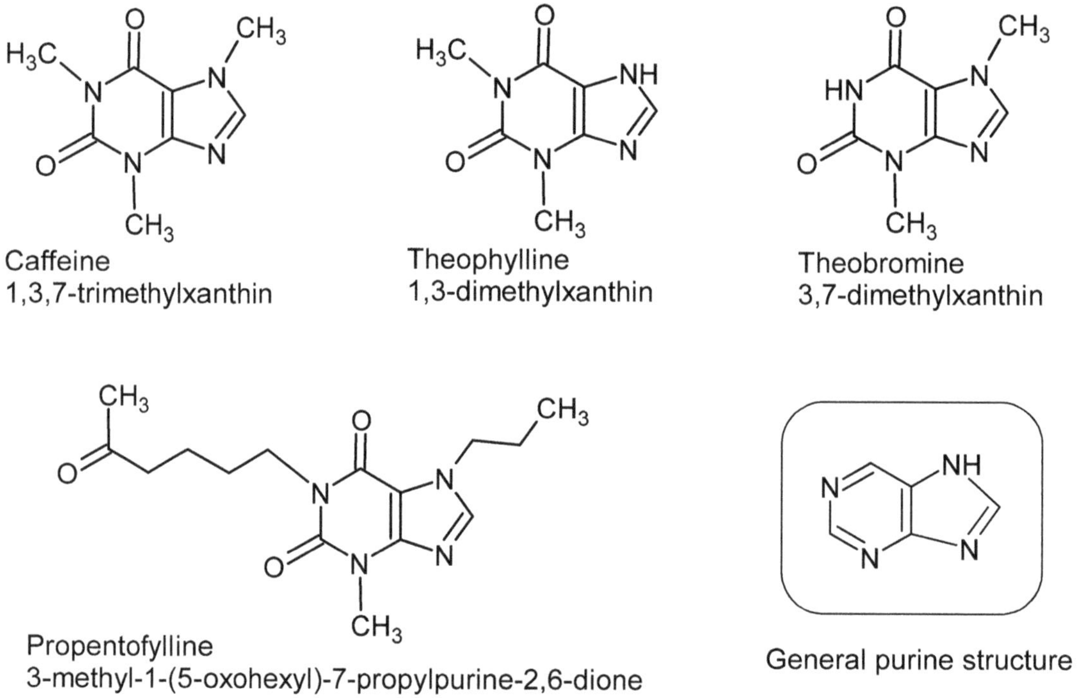

Caffeine
1,3,7-trimethylxanthin

Theophylline
1,3-dimethylxanthin

Theobromine
3,7-dimethylxanthin

Propentofylline
3-methyl-1-(5-oxohexyl)-7-propylpurine-2,6-dione

General purine structure

Figure 1. Chemical structures of common purines, caffeine, theophylline, theobromine, and the synthetic methylxanthine, propentofylline.

The CNS, all brain regions included, is particularly sensitive to oxidative stress [8]. The animal brain is a highly (ATP) energy-demanding organ, normally supplied with an enormous amount of molecular oxygen (O_2), engaged with intense mitochondrial activity, and it is particularly rich in polyunsaturated fatty acids, which, altogether, constantly expose this organ to harmful oxidative/nitrative conditions [9]. In an even worse scenario, the brain accumulates prooxidant iron ions for proper cognitive functions (although with distinguished distribution between brain regions) and surprisingly limited antioxidant capacities, especially in terms of the H_2O_2-removing enzyme catalase [10]. Therefore, ROS/RNS accumulation in brain regions (acute or chronic) is a cellular threat that, if not properly counteracted by local and systemic antioxidants, can cause significant neuronal damage [8]. From all subcellular sources of ROS/RNS, mitochondria are unquestionably the main organelles associated with oxidative/nitrative injuries to biomolecules during aging and neurodegenerative processes [11].

Ethidium bromide (EB) has been applied as a gliotoxin to impose oxidative conditions within brain regions, causing oligodendroglial and astrocytic death, severe demyelination (although "naked" axons remain preserved), blood–brain barrier impairments, and Schwann cell invasion, especially when injected in the white matter of the CNS [12]. Previous studies from our group have shown that propentofylline (PROP), a synthetic MTX, acts to (i) decrease astrocytic activation, thus reducing glial scar development following injury [12], (ii) increase both oligodendroglial and Schwann cell remyelination after 31 days, compared to untreated animals [13], and (iii) even reverse the neuronal dysfunction caused by demyelination induced by the diabetic state in Wistar rats [14]. Considering that most of the PROP-mediated healing processes involve redox (free radical) chemistry, we aimed here to investigate the effect of 12.5 mg·kg^{-1}·day^{-1} PROP on biomarkers of oxidative stress in plasma and the brainstem regions (pons and mesencephalon) of Wistar rats treated with 0.1% EB (as a gliotoxin) after 7, 15, and 31 days. Based on previous behavioral and morphological data, we expected to observe significant antioxidant activity of PROP, both in plasma and the brain regions, in EB-injured animals.

2. Materials and Methods

2.1. Animals

Adult (4–5 months old) male Wistar rats were obtained from the Laboratory of Animal Resources, Paulista University (UNIP), São Paulo, Brazil, and were randomly distributed in a four-arm parallel group experiment [15]. Three sets of 24 animals each were initially used in experimental treatments, from which 21 samples were collected after 7 days of treatment; 23 samples were collected after the 15-day intervention; and 22 samples were collected after the 31-day intervention. The animals were kept under controlled light conditions (12 h light-dark cycle) and water and standard laboratory animal feed (52% carbohydrate, 21% protein, and 4% lipid; Nuvilab CR1, Nuvital, Curitiba, PR, Brazil) were provided ad libitum during the experimental period. All animal procedures were performed in accordance with the guidelines of the Committee on Care and Use of Laboratory Animal Resources and Brazilian Institutional Ethics Committee, Paulista University (protocol number 182/13, CEUA/ICS/UNIP).

This study presents four experimental groups: (i) control; (ii) treated with 0.1% ethidium bromide (EB); (iii) treated with 12.5 mg·kg^{-1}·day^{-1} of propentofylline (PROP); and (iv) both EB and PROP treatments, in the same doses. All rats were anaesthetized with 2.5% thiopental (50 mg·kg^{-1}) by an intraperitoneal route. After that, a burr-hole was made on the right side of the skull, 8 mm behind the frontoparietal suture for drug administration. Injections of 10 µL of 0.1% EB were performed into the cisterna pontis (an enlarged subarachnoid space below the ventral surface of the pons). The pons is a connective structure that links the base of the brain to animal spinal cord and is associated with unvoluntary tasks, such as the sleep–wake cycle and breathing [16]. Injections were performed freehand using a Hamilton syringe, fitted with a 35° angled polished 26-gauge needle into the cisterna pontis. Rats treated with propentofylline (PROP) received 12.5 mg·kg^{-1}·day^{-1} of PROP (Agener União Química, São Paulo, SP, 20 mg·mL^{-1} solution) by an intraperitoneal route daily during the experimental period.

2.2. Plasma and Tissue Samples

The choice of the appropriate sampling method is known to be crucial for accurate haematological and clinico-biochemical measurements [17]. Blood samples were collected in EDTA-containing Vacutainer® flasks for plasma isolation (after centrifugation for 5 min, at 4× g, RT). Heparin-coated tubes were avoided here, as the study aimed to measure indices involving iron metabolism or iron-chelating capacities. For biochemical analysis in the nervous tissue, all rats from experimental groups were euthanized and whole brains were collected at each of the sampling periods: 7, 15, and 31 days post-EB injection (p.i.). Pons and mesencephalon portions of the brainstem were cautiously removed, immediately frozen in liquid nitrogen, and stored in a −80 °C freezer for further analyses. Figure 2 sketches the experimental design of our study.

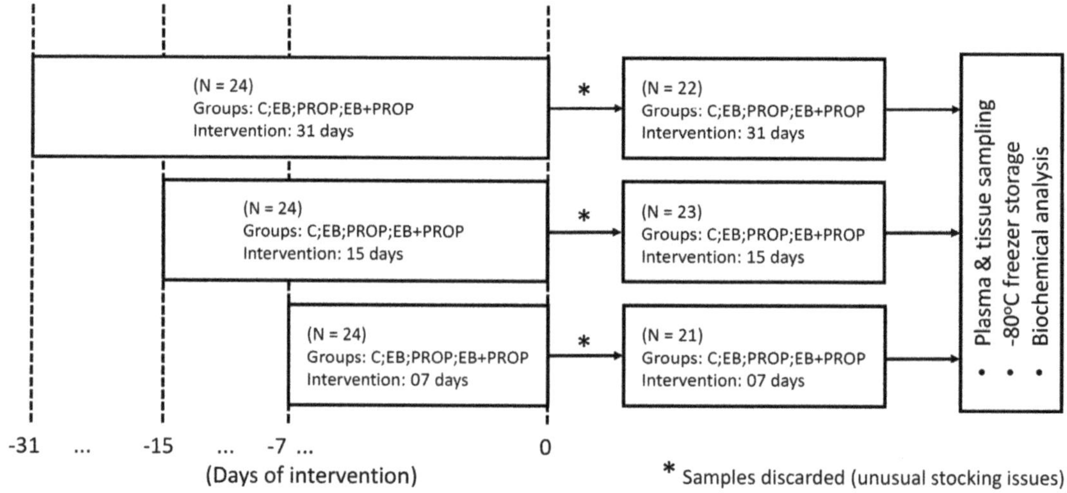

Figure 2. Experimental design of the study.

2.3. Biochemical Analyses

The brainstem (including pons and mesencephalon) of the animals was rapidly thawed and homogenized using a pestle (or a Potter apparatus) in 1–2 mL of 50 mM phosphate buffer, pH 7.4, then centrifuged for 10 min at $10,000 \times g$ and 4 °C. Tissue/cellular debris was discarded and homogenates were kept in an ice-water bath for immediate enzyme and other biochemical determinations.

Catalase activity was determined by H_2O_2 consumption for 5 min at 25 °C. In each assay, 10 μL of sample were added to the reaction system composed by 10 mM H_2O_2 in 50 mM KPO (potassium phosphate) buffer, pH 7.4, and absorbance was monitored at 240 nm ($\varepsilon_{240nm} = 0.071$ mM^{-1}·cm^{-1}). Catalase activity was expressed in mU$_{CAT}$·mg protein^{-1} [18].

Glutathione reductase (GR) activities were measured based on the oxidation of β-NADPH (at 340 nm; $\varepsilon = 6.2 \times 10^3$ M^{-1}·cm^{-1}). In the presence of 0.25 mM NaN$_3$ (for catalase inhibition), a 10 μL sample was mixed with 1 mM of oxidized glutathione (GSSG) and 0.12 mM β-NADPH in reaction buffer (143 mM sodium phosphate and 6.3 mM EDTA, pH 7.4), at 25 °C. GR activity was expressed in mU$_{GR}$·mg protein^{-1} [19]. All protein analyses were performed using the Coomassie-blue method described by Bradford, 1976 [20].

The total antioxidant capacity of the nervous tissue was measured by the ferric-reducing activity method (FRAP) [21]. The FRAP method quantifies metal ligands in samples that form [Fe(L)]$^{n+}$ complexes that restrain Fenton-type reactions and the formation of more aggressive radicals, such as the hydroxyl radical (HO$^\bullet$). We adapted the method by replacing the classic ferrous-chelating agent 2,4,6-tripyridyl-S-triazine (TPTZ) by its analog 2,3-bis(2-pyridyl)-pyrazine (DPP) [22]. Briefly, 10–20 μL of samples were mixed with 10 mM DPP (from a stock solution in 40 mM HCl) and 20 mM of FeCl$_3$ in a 0.30 M acetate buffer (pH 3.6). Absorbance at 593 nm was recorded for 4 min to determine the rate of Fe^{2+}-DPP complex formation and was compared to a standard curve. Total iron content in brain tissue was estimated by the modified colorimetric method based on the formation of a Fe^{2+}: bipyridyl complexes [23].

Measurements of reduced (GSH) and oxidized glutathione contents (GSSG) applied the stoichiometric reaction of reduced thiol groups (-SH) with 5,5′-dithio-2-nitrobenzoic acid (DTNB) to form TNB, which was monitored spectrophotometrically at 412 nm in 5 mM phosphate buffer, with 5 mM EDTA, pH 7.5. For GSSG determination, the current GSH forms in samples were prevented from oxidation by adding 0.2 mM 2-vinylpyridine (2VP) and its excess was eliminated by the further addition of 2 mM triethylamine (TEA). Then, the reaction system was added to 4 mM DTNB, 1 mM β-NADPH, and 0.25 U.mL^{-1} of enzyme GR for (i) full reduction of GSSG forms to GSH (total glutathione content) and (ii) reaction of total GSH with DTNB for TNB formation and detection at 412 nm [24]. The GSH and GSSG contents in the brainstem samples were expressed in mmol.mg protein^{-1}. Finally, the ratio between GSH and GSSG contents was calculated and presented here as the "reducing power" in samples (dimensionless), as shown in Equation (1).

$$\text{Reducing power (RP)} = [\text{GSH}]/[\text{GSSG}], \qquad (1)$$

where [GSH] is the reduced glutathione concentration in the samples and [GSSG] is the oxidized glutathione concentration in the samples.

Lipid oxidation was estimated by the method of thiobarbituric acid-reactive substances (TBARS). Briefly, 250 µL of samples reacted with 0.35% thiobarbituric acid, with 1% Triton X-100, in 0.25 mM HCl to produce a pinkish chromophore that was detected by absorbance at 535 nm. A standard curve with 1,1′,3,3′-tetraethoxypropane was used for TBARS determination. The formation of TBARS occurred in plastic microtubes in a boiling bath (100 °C), for 10 min [25]. All spectrophotometric determinations were performed in a microplate reader SpectraMax M2 (Silicon Valley, CA, USA).

2.4. Statistical Analyses

The software Jamovi version 1.1.5 was used to perform the normality tests—Shapiro–Wilk, skewness and kurtosis, generalized linear model (GLM), and post-hoc with correction of the error rate to the significance level by Fisher method.

Outliers were determined using the interquartile range method (IQR × 2.2) [26] and, when necessary, the data were winsorized [27]. The boxplot graphics were made using the following site: http://shiny.chemgrid.org/boxplotr/. The results were analyzed for the significance level and the effect size for each experiment performed. The significance level adopted was $p \leq 0.05$ and the differences reported in the comparison of groups, times, and interactions were reported by the difference (diff.) between group means, considering the type of distribution presented.

3. Results

For 31 days, lipoperoxidation was monitored in plasma and the brainstem tissue of experimental animals, with similar variation patterns in both matrices, depending on the treatment applied (Table 1). Higher levels of lipoperoxidation were especially found in the CNS following EB treatment. After 7 days, the TBARS levels were 2-fold higher in the rat CNS than in saline administered rats (control), reaching a maximum of 2.4-fold within 15 days. After 31 days of EB treatment, lipoperoxidation was still 65% higher than that of the control in the brainstem, although these levels normalized in plasma. In agreement, levels of lipoperoxidation were also maximized in plasma after 15 days of EB treatment. Compared to control, the TBARS levels in plasma of EB-treated animals were 54% and 60% higher in days 7 and 15, respectively (Table 1). No variation in lipoperoxidation levels was observed with propentofylline treatment (PROP) in rats, either in plasma or CNS. Interestingly, by combining EB and PROP treatments, lipoperoxidation also showed similar patterns in plasma and brain tissues with no significant variation within 7 days and a minor increase in day 15 (50.4% and 37.5%, respectively), reaching baseline levels after 31 days (Table 1). Comparing the EB + PROP and EB groups, the lipoperoxidation levels in the EB groups were significantly higher after 15 days (76%).

Table 1. Levels of lipid oxidation and total iron content in plasma or brainstem tissue of rats treated with ethidium bromide (EB) and/or propentofylline (PROP) for 7, 15, and 31 days. (* $p < 0.05$; ** $p < 0.01$).

	Control	EB	PROP	PROP + EB
(i) Plasma				
TBARS (μmol·mL^{-1})				
7 d	13.1 ± 2.4	20.2 ± 2.4 (*)	11.8 ± 0.9	15.4 ± 1.5
15 d	n.d.	21.0 ± 2.9 (*)	15.1 ± 2.6	19.7 ± 6.4 (*)
31 d	n.d.	10.8 ± 1.1	12.9 ± 2.6	12.4 ± 2.1
(ii) Brainstem tissue				
TBARS (μmol·mg prot^{-1})				
7 d	0.64 ± 0.04	1.28 ± 0.27 (**)	0.54 ± 0.06	0.72 ± 0.09
15 d	n.d.	1.55 ± 0.28 (**)	0.63 ± 0.05	0.88 ± 0.05 (*)
31 d	n.d.	1.06 ± 0.13 (**)	0.52 ± 0.05	0.72 ± 0.07
Iron content (μg·mg prot^{-1})				
7 d	88.2 ± 10.5	279.0 ± 60.6 (**)	75.8 ± 24.7	214.5 ± 52.4 (**)
15 d	n.d.	413.4 ± 31.6 (**)	433.3 ± 69.2 (**)	409.7 ± 41.8 (**)
31 d	n.d.	285.3 ± 50.8 (**)	261.0 ± 35.2 (**)	279.6 ± 30.8 (**)

n.d. = not determined.

On the other hand, both EB and PROP (or their combination) caused a major disruption of iron homeostasis in the CNS (Table 1). Maximum levels of "free" iron were measured in the brainstem after 15 days (almost 5-fold higher, independent of the treatment). Between the groups, no differences were observed along the 31 days of evaluation, except for PROP-treated animals after 7 days. The iron content in the brainstem of PROP group was identical to that found in controls after 7 days. Imbalances in iron homeostasis were only observed afterwards, as in all other treated groups (Table 1).

Figure 3 illustrates the antioxidant activities in the brainstem after 7 days of EB, PROP and EB + PROP combined treatments. Although catalase activities were unaltered in all groups (compared to control, Figure 3B), significant changes were observed in FRAP and GR activities (Figure 3A,C, respectively). EB treatment drastically dropped FRAP activity in the nervous tissue after 7 days (-75%, Figure 3A). Interestingly, PROP administration showed a tendency of diminished FRAP activities in the brainstem, but statistically this was not not different ($p = 0.058$; Figure 3A). Undoubtedly, combined EB + PROP treatment reverted the lower FRAP activities found in single EB-treated samples back to control levels (Figure 3A). Regarding GR activities, EB treatment did not affect the enzyme activity in the CNS, although 59% higher GR activity was measured in the EB + PROP group, compared to control (Figure 3C). Single PROP treatment only showed tendencies of higher GR activity compared to control ($p = 0.054$, Figure 3C).

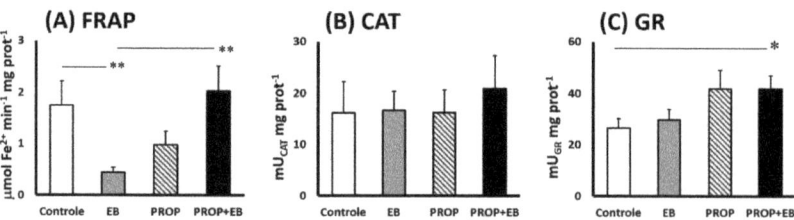

Figure 3. Antioxidant activities in brainstem of Wistar rats after 7 days of treatment (i.p.) with saline solution (control), 0.1% ethydium bromide (EB), 12.5 mg propentofylline·kg^{-1}·day^{-1} (PRO), or both (EB + PROP): (**A**) ferric-reducing activity (FRAP); (**B**) catalase activity (CAT); and (**C**) glutathione reductase activity (GR). (* $p < 0.05$; ** $p < 0.01$).

Concerning thiol-based antioxidant defenses in the CNS, Figure 4 presents levels of reduced (GSH) and oxidized glutathione (GSSG), as well as their ratio expressed as the "reducing power" between experimental groups after 7 days (Figure 4A–C). Minor changes were observed in GSH contents in the brainstem upon the experimental conditions here, except for differences between EB (−65%) and PROP treatments (Figure 4A). Notably, PROP treatment induced significantly higher levels of GSSG, compared to all other experimental groups or control (Figure 4B). GSSG contents in PROP group were 163%, 77%, and 152% higher than control, EB, and EB + PROP groups, respectively (Figure 4B). Finally, the reducing power was significantly diminished with both EB (−60%) and PROP treatments (−65%) but reestablished upon treatment with both EB and PROP combined (Figure 4C).

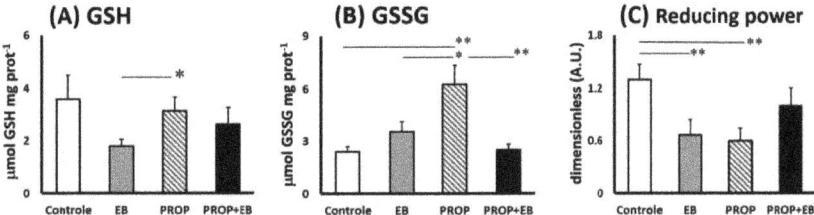

Figure 4. Thiol-based antioxidant defenses in brainstem of Wistar rats after 7 days of treatment (i.p.) with saline solution (control), 0.1% ethydium bromide (EB), 12.5 mg propentofylline·kg^{-1}·day^{-1} (PRO), or both (EB + PROP): (A) reduced glutathione content (GSH); (B) oxidized glutathione content (GSSG); and (C) GSH/GSSG ratio, renowned as "reducing power". (* $p < 0.05$; ** $p < 0.01$).

4. Discussion

Apart from their renowned stimulation effects on the CNS, MTXs have been long suggested as inducers of antioxidant responses in many biological systems [28]. Here, we observed that the synthetic MTX, propentofylline (PROP), also increased antioxidant protection in the brainstem of rats exposed to the gliotoxic agent EB, especially in terms of thiol-based defenses: levels of reduced GSH, redox balance (GSH/GSSG ratio), and GR activities. The data here were in full agreement with other studies from our group that showed that PROP improved oligodendroglial and Schwann cell remyelination and even diminished neuronal dysfunction in chemically induced diabetic Wistar rats [13,14]. These neurodegenerative processes are notably mediated by pathological overproduction of reactive oxygen and nitrogen species (ROS/RNS) [29,30].

Regarding the time course of brainstem injury, previous works showed that EB-treated rats presented demyelinating lesions in the pons and mesencephalon after 7–11 days, which suggested that these regions were extensively exposed to oxidative conditions [31]. Following the progression of the healing process, thinly remyelinated axons could be significantly seen at day 15 [13]. Nonetheless, morphological differences between rats treated or not treated with PROP were clearer from day 21 p.i., as rats treated with PROP presented a greater proportion of oligodendrocyte remyelinated axons compared to the untreated ones. The time course of these previously observed remyelination processes perfectly matched with the progression of lipid oxidation in brainstem and plasma, as shown in Table 1.

Although the mechanism has not been fully unveiled, Table 1 shows that EB-induced injury in rat brainstem was associated with higher release of "free" (labile) iron ions, suggesting a disruption of iron homeostasis [32]. Labile iron ions, when not properly restrained by stocking proteins, such as ferritin and transferrin, catalyze the formation of harmful ROS/RNS, such as hydroxyl (HO•) and alkoxyl radicals (LO•) [33]. This is the main mechanism of the notorious participation of iron ions as biological prooxidant agents [34]. After 7 days of EB administration in the brainstem, the iron concentration was severely increased, a harmful effect that peaked after 15 days, and persisted until 31 days of treatment. The concomitant administration of PROP could not limit iron release in the CNS. In fact, PROP also promoted iron release in a way that was similar to EB-injection within the brainstem. Nevertheless, these results suggest that the chelation of labile iron ions—a preventive antioxidant event—was not the proper mechanism by which PROP protected rat CNS exposed to EB.

Lipid oxidation was inhibited by PROP in EB-treated rats, as shown in Table 1. Interestingly, an identical pattern of lipid oxidation was reproduced in the plasma of animals, suggesting that brain injury generated prooxidant agents (probably the labile iron ions themselves) that disseminated oxidative stress conditions in the plasma and all over the body of the animals. Unfortunately, we did not monitor other biomarkers of oxidative stress in plasma to confirm that.

Data shown in Figures 3 and 4 demonstrate that combined EB + PROP treatments presented similar indices of antioxidant capacity as control groups, especially in terms of FRAP scores and the reducing power (Figures 3A and 4C, respectively). Based on PROP effects over thiol-based antioxidant defenses (Figures 3C and 4A–C), it is very plausible that this positive effect was triggered by the induction of the enzyme glutathione reductase (GR; Figure 3C), which recycles oxidized GSSG molecules back to their reduced form, GSH. Reduced GSH is extensively used for free radical removal (as scavengers of ROS/RNS) and as a conjugation substrate for xenobiotic elimination from animals' bodies (via glutathione-S-transferase; GST) [35]. Interestingly, the treatment with pentoxifylline (an analog of PROP) in mice injected with B16F10 melanoma cells (high energy demanding cells) significantly reduced oxidative stress by also attenuating the altered levels of GSH and lipid peroxides [36]. Accordingly, the natural MXT caffeine also affected GSH levels by increasing glutathione S-transferase activity (GST), causing, in this case, GSH depletion and higher lipid peroxidation indices in high-energy-demanding B16F1 melanoma cells [36]. Moreover, theobromine, another natural MTX (Figure 1), also promoted neuroprotection to the rat brain in a transient global cerebral ischemia-reperfusion model, which was notoriously mediated by ROS/RNS [37]. Despite the bulk of data about the close relationship between MTX activation of the GSH-based antioxidant defenses in brain regions, the proper mechanism is still under debate [38]. Nevertheless, but not surprisingly, the most consistent data about MTX effect on GSH biosynthesis involve the activation of the transcription factors Nrf2, NF-κB, and AP-1, which are the most redox-responsive signaling cascades in animals and humans [39–41]. Figure 5 depicts the oxidative stress conditions observed in rat brainstem (with details of prooxidant and antioxidant markers), treated with EB in the presence or absence of PROP.

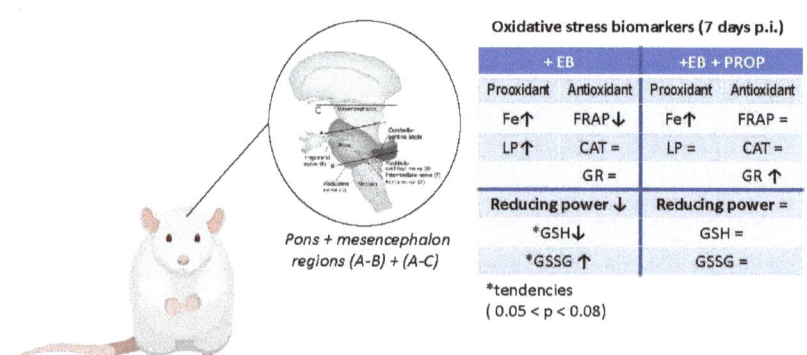

Figure 5. Graphic summary of pro- and antioxidant changes in brainstem (Pons + mesencephalon) of Wistar rats after 7 days of i.p. treatment with 0.1% ethydium bromide (EB) in the presence or absence of 12.5 mg propentofylline·kg^{-1}·day^{-1} (PROP). Where Fe = iron content; LP = lipid oxidation; FRAP = ferric-reducing activity; CAT = catalase activity; GR = glutathione reductase activity; GSH = reduced glutathione; GSSG = oxidized glutathione; reducing power= GSH/GSSG ratio; ↑ = statistical increase; ↓ = statistical decrease; and * (statistical tendency 0.05 < p < 0.08). Adapted from P. Brodal, 2014 [42].

5. Conclusions

In summary, aligning with previous studies from our group and with literature about MTXs, we observed that propentofylline (PROP) improved the thiol-based antioxidant defenses in the rat brainstem by the induction of the enzymatic activity of glutathione reductase (GR), which diminished lipid oxidation progression and rebalanced the redox status in the CNS.

Author Contributions: Conceptualization, S.C.P., M.F.M. and E.F.B.; methodology, S.C.P.; formal analysis, S.C.P., D.E.M.B., C.V.V., M.G. and Á.A.F.P.; resources, E.F.B.; data curation, M.P.B.; writing—original draft preparation, M.P.B.; writing—review and editing, M.P.B., S.C.P., M.F.M. and E.F.B.; supervision, S.C.P. and E.F.B.; project administration & funding acquisition, E.F.B. All authors have read and agreed to the published version of the manuscript.

Funding: This work was supported by (i) the "Coordenação de Aperfeiçoamento de Pessoal de Nível Superior", (CAPES) through the "Programa de Suporte a Pós-Graduação de Instituições de Ensino Particulares" (PROSUP), Brazil, (ii) "Programa Institucional Brasileiro de Iniciação Científica" do Brazilian National Council for Scientific and Technology Development (PIBIC-CNPq), and (iii) the São Paulo Research Foundation (FAPESP) grant BPE #2017/06032-2. The author M.P.B. is a fellow of the Brazilian National Council for Scientific and Technology Development (CNPq: PQ-2 #311839/2021-5, Brazil).

Institutional Review Board Statement: The animal study protocol was approved by the Committee on Care and Use of Laboratory Animal Resources and Brazilian Institutional Ethics Committee, Paulista University (protocol number 182/13, CEUA/ICS/UNIP).

Informed Consent Statement: Not applicable.

Data Availability Statement: The data presented in this study are available on request from the corresponding authors. The data are not publicly available due to potential patent application.

Acknowledgments: The authors are thankful for the technical support from the institutional staff at the Veterinary Complex, Cruzeiro do Sul University, campus São Miguel Paulista, and for I. Braga and C.F.M. Menezes, undergraduate volunteers during assays.

Conflicts of Interest: The authors declare no conflict of interest.

References

1. Franco, R.; Oñatibia-Astibia, A.; Martínez-Pinilla, E. Health benefits of methylxanthines in cacao and chocolate. *Nutrients* **2013**, *5*, 4159–4173. [CrossRef] [PubMed]
2. Goya, L.; Kongor, J.E.; de Pascual-Teresa, S. From Cocoa to Chocolate: Effect of Processing on Flavanols and Methylxanthines and Their Mechanisms of Action. *Int. J. Mol. Sci.* **2022**, *23*, 14365. [CrossRef] [PubMed]
3. Janitschke, D.; Lauer, A.A.; Bachmann, C.M.; Winkler, J.; Griebsch, L.V.; Pilz, S.M.; Theiss, E.L.; Grimm, H.S.; Hartmann, T.; Grimm, M.O.W. Methylxanthines Induce a Change in the AD/Neurodegeneration-Linked Lipid Profile in Neuroblastoma Cells. *Int. J. Mol. Sci.* **2022**, *23*, 2295. [CrossRef] [PubMed]
4. Noschang, C.G.; Krolow, R.; Pettenuzzo, L.F.; Avila, M.C.; Fachin, A.; Arcego, D.; von Pozzer Toigo, E.; Crema, L.M.; Diehl, L.A.; Vendite, D.; et al. Interactions between chronic stress and chronic consumption of caffeine on the enzymatic antioxidant system. *Neurochem. Res.* **2009**, *34*, 1568–1574. [CrossRef]
5. Gołembiowska, K.; Wardas, J.; Noworyta-Sokołowska, K.; Kamińska, K.; Górska, A. Effects of adenosine receptor antagonists on the in vivo LPS-induced inflammation model of Parkinson's disease. *Neurotox. Res.* **2013**, *24*, 29–40. [CrossRef] [PubMed]
6. Sigel, A.; Sigel, H.; Sigel, R.K.O. Coordination Chemistry of Nucleotides and Antivirally Active Acyclic Nucleoside Phosphonates, including Mechanistic Considerations. *Molecules* **2022**, *27*, 2625. [CrossRef]
7. Ichiyama, T.; Hasegawa, S.; Matsubara, T.; Hayashi, T.; Furukawa, S. Theophylline inhibits NF-kappa B activation and I kappa B alpha degradation in human pulmonary epithelial cells. *Naunyn Schmiedebergs Arch. Pharmacol.* **2001**, *364*, 558–561. [CrossRef]
8. Salim, S. Oxidative Stress and the Central Nervous System. *J. Pharmacol. Exp. Ther.* **2017**, *360*, 201–205. [CrossRef]
9. Cobley, J.N.; Fiorello, M.L.; Bailey, D.M. 13 reasons why the brain is susceptible to oxidative stress. *Redox Biol.* **2018**, *15*, 490–503. [CrossRef] [PubMed]
10. Andersen, H.H.; Johnsen, K.B.; Moos, T. Iron deposits in the chronically inflamed central nervous system and contributes to neurodegeneration. *Cell. Mol. Life Sci.* **2014**, *71*, 1607–1622. [CrossRef]
11. Grimm, A.; Eckert, A. Brain aging and neurodegeneration: From a mitochondrial point of view. *J. Neurochem.* **2017**, *143*, 418–431. [CrossRef] [PubMed]

12. Bondan, E.F.; Martins, M.F.; Dossa, P.D.; Viebig, L.B.; Cardoso, C.V.; Martins, J.L., Jr.; Bernardi, M.M. Propentofylline reduces glial scar development following gliotoxic damage in the rat brainstem. *Arq. Neuropsiquiatr.* **2016**, *74*, 730–736. [CrossRef] [PubMed]
13. Bondan, E.F.; Martins, M.F.; Baliellas, M.D.E.; Gimenez, M.C.F.; Poppe, C.S.; Bernardi, M.M. Effects of propentofylline on CNS remyelination in the rat brainstem. *Microsc. Res. Tech.* **2014**, *77*, 23–30. [CrossRef] [PubMed]
14. Bondan, E.F.; Martins, M.F.; Bernardi, M.M. Propentofylline reverses delayed remyelination in streptozotocin-induced diabetic rats. *Arch. Endocrinol. Metab.* **2015**, *59*, 47–53. [CrossRef]
15. Bacchieri, A.; Cioppa, G.D. *Fundamentals of Clinical Research: Bridging Medicine, Statistics and Operations*; Springer: Milano, Italy, 2007.
16. Allen, G.V.; Hopkins, D.A. Topography and synaptology of mamillary body projections to the mesencephalon and pons in the rat. *J. Comp. Neurol.* **1990**, *301*, 214–231. [CrossRef]
17. Christensen, S.D.; Mikkelsen, L.F.; Fels, J.J.; Bodvarsdóttir, T.B.; Hansen, A.K. Quality of plasma sampled by different methods for multiple blood sampling in mice. *Lab. Animals.* **2009**, *43*, 65–71. [CrossRef]
18. Aebi, H. Catalase in vitro. *Method. Enzymol.* **1984**, *105*, 121–126.
19. Carlberg, I.; Mannervik, B. Glutathione reductase. *Methods Enzymol.* **1985**, *113*, 484–490.
20. Bradford, M.M. A rapid and sensitive method for the quantitation of microgram quantities of protein utilizing the principle of protein-dye binding. *Anal. Biochem.* **1976**, *72*, 248–254. [CrossRef]
21. Benzie, I.F.F.; Strain, J.J. The ferric reducing ability of plasma (FRAP) as a measure of "antioxidant power": The FRAP assay. *Anal. Biochem.* **1996**, *239*, 70–76. [CrossRef]
22. Brewer, K.J.; Murphy, W.R., Jr.; Petersen, J.D. Synthesis and characterization of monometallic and bimetallic mixed-ligand complexes of iron(II) containing 2,2′-bipyrimidine or 2,3-bis(2-pyridyl)pyrazine. *Inorg. Chem.* **1987**, *26*, 3376–3379. [CrossRef]
23. Goodwin, J.F.; Murphy, B. The colorimetric determination of iron in biological material with reference to its measurement during chelation therapy. *Clin. Chem.* **1966**, *12*, 58–69. [CrossRef]
24. Rahman, I.; Kode, A.; Biswas, S.K. Assay for quantitative determination of glutathione and glutathione disulfide levels using enzymatic recycling method. *Nat. Protoc.* **2006**, *1*, 3159–3165. [CrossRef]
25. Fraga, C.G.; Leibovitz, B.E.; Tappel, A.L. Lipid peroxidation measured as thiobarbituric acid-reactive substances in tissue slices: Characterization and comparison with homogenates and microsomes. *Free Radic. Biol. Med.* **1988**, *4*, 155–161. [CrossRef]
26. Hoaglin, D.C.; Iglewicz, B. Fine-tuning some resistant rules for outlier labeling. *J. Am. Stat. Assoc.* **1987**, *82*, 1147–1149. [CrossRef]
27. Dixon, W.J. Efficient analysis of experimental observations. *Annu. Rev. Pharmacol. Toxicol.* **1980**, *20*, 441–446. [CrossRef]
28. Janitschke, D.; Lauer, A.A.; Bachmann, C.M.; Grimm, H.S.; Hartmann, T.; Grimm, M.O.W. Methylxanthines and Neurodegenerative Diseases: An Update. *Nutrients* **2021**, *13*, 803. [CrossRef] [PubMed]
29. Polotow, T.G.; Poppe, S.C.; Vardaris, C.V.; Ganini, D.; Guariroba, M.; Mattei, R.; Hatanaka, E.; Martins, M.F.; Bondan, E.F.; Barros, M.P. Redox Status and Neuro Inflammation Indexes in Cerebellum and Motor Cortex of Wistar Rats Supplemented with Natural Sources of Omega-3 Fatty Acids and Astaxanthin: Fish Oil, Krill Oil, and Algal Biomass. *Mar. Drugs.* **2015**, *13*, 6117–6137. [CrossRef]
30. Quincozes-Santos, A.; Santos, C.L.; de Souza Almeida, R.R.; da Silva, A.; Thomaz, N.K.; Costa, N.L.F.; Weber, F.B.; Schmitz, I.; Medeiros, L.S.; Medeiros, L.; et al. Gliotoxicity and Glioprotection: The Dual Role of Glial Cells. *Mol. Neurobiol.* **2021**, *58*, 6577–6592. [CrossRef]
31. Ju, Q.; Li, X.; Zhang, H.; Yan, S.; Li, Y.; Zhao, Y. NFE2L2 Is a Potential Prognostic Biomarker and Is Correlated with Immune Infiltration in Brain Lower Grade Glioma: A Pan-Cancer Analysis. *Oxid. Med. Cell. Longev.* **2020**, *2020*, 3580719. [CrossRef] [PubMed]
32. Singh, N.; Haldar, S.; Tripathi, A.K.; Horback, K.; Wong, J.; Sharma, D.; Beserra, A.; Suda, S.; Anbalagan, C.; Dev, S.; et al. Brain iron homeostasis: From molecular mechanisms to clinical significance and therapeutic opportunities. *Antioxid. Redox Signal.* **2014**, *20*, 1324–1363. [CrossRef]
33. Zhang, N.; Yu, X.; Xie, J.; Xu, H. New Insights into the Role of Ferritin in Iron Homeostasis and Neurodegenerative Diseases. *Mol. Neurobiol.* **2021**, *58*, 2812–2823. [CrossRef] [PubMed]
34. Li, X.; Jankovic, J.; Le, W. Iron chelation and neuroprotection in neurodegenerative diseases. *J. Neural Transm.* **2011**, *118*, 473–477. [CrossRef] [PubMed]
35. Aoyama, K. Glutathione in the Brain. *Int. J. Mol. Sci.* **2021**, *22*, 5010. [CrossRef] [PubMed]
36. Shukla, V.; Gude, R.P. Potentiation of antimetastatic activity of pentoxifylline in B16F10 and B16F1 melanoma cells through inhibition of glutathione content. *Cancer Biother. Radiopharm.* **2003**, *18*, 559–564. [CrossRef] [PubMed]
37. Bhat, J.A.; Gupta, S.; Kumar, M. Neuroprotective effects of theobromine in transient global cerebral ischemia-reperfusion rat model. *Biochem. Biophys. Res. Commun.* **2021**, *571*, 74–80. [CrossRef]
38. Shukla, V.; Gude, R.P. Amelioration of B16F10 melanoma cells induced oxidative stress in DBA/2 mice by pentoxifylline. *J. Exp. Clin. Cancer Res.* **2003**, *22*, 407–410.
39. Kalthoff, S.; Ehmer, U.; Freiberg, N.; Manns, M.P.; Strassburg, C.P. Coffee induces expression of glucuronosyltransferases by the aryl hydrocarbon receptor and Nrf2 in liver and stomach. *Gastroenterology* **2010**, *139*, 1699–1710.e2. [CrossRef]
40. Sugimoto, N.; Miwa, S.; Hitomi, Y.; Nakamura, H.; Tsuchiya, H.; Yachie, A. Theobromine, the primary methylxanthine found in Theobroma cacao, prevents malignant glioblastoma proliferation by negatively regulating phosphodiesterase-4, extracellular signal-regulated kinase, Akt/mammalian target of rapamycin kinase, and nuclear factor-kappa B. *Nutr. Cancer* **2014**, *66*, 419–423. [CrossRef]

41. Lu, S.C. Glutathione synthesis. *Biochim. Biophys. Acta* **2013**, *1830*, 3143–3153. [CrossRef]
42. Brodal, P. *Encyclopedia of the Neurological Sciences*, 2nd ed.; Aminoff, M.J., Daroff, R.B., Eds.; Academic Press: Cambridge, MA, USA, 2014; pp. 936–937, ISBN 9780123851581. [CrossRef]

Disclaimer/Publisher's Note: The statements, opinions and data contained in all publications are solely those of the individual author(s) and contributor(s) and not of MDPI and/or the editor(s). MDPI and/or the editor(s) disclaim responsibility for any injury to people or property resulting from any ideas, methods, instructions or products referred to in the content.

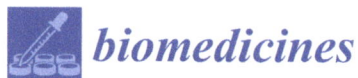

Article

Cognition in Patients with Schizophrenia: Interplay between Working Memory, Disorganized Symptoms, Dissociation, and the Onset and Duration of Psychosis, as Well as Resistance to Treatment

Georgi Panov [1,2,*], Silvana Dyulgerova [1] and Presyana Panova [3]

[1] Psychiatric Clinic, University Hospital for Active Treatment "Prof. Dr. Stoyan Kirkovich", Trakia University, 6000 Stara Zagora, Bulgaria
[2] Medical Faculty, University "Prof. Dr. Asen Zlatarov", 8000 Burgas, Bulgaria
[3] Medical Faculty, Trakia University, 6000 Stara Zagora, Bulgaria; presiana.panova@abv.bg
* Correspondence: gpanov@dir.bg

Citation: Panov, G.; Dyulgerova, S.; Panova, P. Cognition in Patients with Schizophrenia: Interplay between Working Memory, Disorganized Symptoms, Dissociation, and the Onset and Duration of Psychosis, as Well as Resistance to Treatment. *Biomedicines* **2023**, *11*, 3114. https://doi.org/10.3390/biomedicines11123114

Academic Editors: Shaker A. Mousa, Simone Battaglia and Masaru Tanaka

Received: 5 November 2023
Revised: 10 November 2023
Accepted: 17 November 2023
Published: 22 November 2023

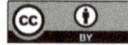

Copyright: © 2023 by the authors. Licensee MDPI, Basel, Switzerland. This article is an open access article distributed under the terms and conditions of the Creative Commons Attribution (CC BY) license (https://creativecommons.org/licenses/by/4.0/).

Abstract: Schizophrenia is traditionally associated with the presence of psychotic symptoms. In addition to these, cognitive symptoms precede them and are present during the entire course of the schizophrenia process. The present study aims to establish the relationship between working memory (short-term memory and attention), the features of the clinical picture, and the course of the schizophrenic process, gender distribution and resistance to treatment. Methods: In total, 105 patients with schizophrenia were observed. Of these, 66 were women and 39 men. Clinical status was assessed using the Positive and Negative Syndrome Scale (PANSS), Brief Psychiatric Rating Scale (BPRS), Dimensional Obsessive–Compulsive Symptom Scale (DOCS), scale for dissociative experiences (DES) and Hamilton Depression Rating Scale (HAM-D)—cognitive functions using the Luria 10-word test with fixation assessment, reproduction and attention analysis. The clinical evaluation of resistance to the treatment showed that 45 patients were resistant to the ongoing medical treatment and the remaining 60 had an effect from the therapy. Results: Our study showed that, in most patients, we found disorders of working memory and attention. In 69.82% of the patients, we found problems with fixation; in 38.1%, problems with reproduction; and in 62.86%, attention disorders. Conducting a regression analysis showed that memory and attention disorders were mainly related to the highly disorganized symptoms scale, the duration of the schizophrenic process and the dissociation scale. It was found that there was a weaker but significant association between the age of onset of schizophrenia and negative symptoms. In the patients with resistant schizophrenia, much greater violations of the studied parameters working memory and attention were found compared to the patients with an effect from the treatment. Conclusion: Impairments in working memory and attention are severely affected in the majority of patients with schizophrenia. Their involvement is most significant in patients with resistance to therapy. Factors associated with the highest degree of memory and attention impairment were disorganized symptoms, duration of schizophrenia, dissociative symptoms and, to a lesser extent, onset of illness. This analysis gives us the right to consider that the early and systematic analysis of cognition is a reliable marker for tracking both clinical dynamics and the effect of treatment.

Keywords: schizophrenia; resistant schizophrenia; working memory; attention; fixation; reproduction; disorganized symptoms; dissociation; short-term memory; working memory

1. Introduction

The classical understanding of schizophrenia considers it a chronic mental illness with a varied clinical presentation and unclear etiology. The clinical presentation is related both to the presence of psychotic (delusions and hallucinations) and negative symptoms, but also to the presence of other clinical phenomena [1–3]. Apart from purely mental symptoms associated with abnormal changes in neuronal networks [4–7], inflammatory disorders associated with metabolic ones are also present in schizophrenia, as a cause and effect of the imbalance between the processes of neuroregeneration and neurodegeneration [8,9]. Traditionally, and in a therapeutic aspect, the dopamine hypothesis has been accepted, which tries to explain both the achieved therapeutic response during treatment with antipsychotic drugs and the development of possible refractoriness to the treatment [10,11]. Resistance as a clinical phenomenon is a challenge in all mental illnesses. Analysis of its prevalence shows a high percentage of 20–60% of patients [12]. No significant difference was observed in patients with schizophrenia. The big problem has always been how we define resistant cases. Over time, different criteria have been used to define resistant patients [13–15]. In search of a unified statement to be used in practice, a consensus statement was created to define resistant cases [16].

The median that runs longitudinally through the picture of schizophrenia drawn in this way is the cognitive disturbances that appear first in the course of the schizophrenic process and persist over time; at the end of the disease, their gradation to the development of demented symptoms is observed [17–19]. Some authors make an association between the development of cognitive symptoms in schizophrenia and frontotemporal dementia [17].

It was established that the cognitive deficit (which is entirely deducible) is the cause of the catastrophic psychosocial outcome of schizophrenia. Throughout the disease, a reduction in IQ from the norm of 100 to 70–85 has been reported [20–22]. Cognitive symptoms are also the primary tool for adaptation to the dynamically changing reality. In this sense, cognition is also the primary mechanism through which adaptation takes place [23,24]. Respectively and vice versa, their violation is the basis of their maladaptation and loss of social connectivity [25].

Cognitive deficits are the earliest and most socially significant symptoms of schizophrenia. They creep before the onset of the disease in the prodromal stage and are present at the debut of the disease [25,26]. They are a significant feature but, in clinical practice, they are not seen as core clinical symptoms, as we traditionally consider positive and negative symptoms [27,28]. Cognitive deficits worsen with the onset of the first psychotic episode, with research showing that they then return to baseline and remain relatively stable throughout the illness (of course, relative to the time of follow-up) [29,30]. When analyzing cognitive functions, we most often analyze the short-term memory and attention of the patient. The relationships between working memory (short-term memory in action) and attention are complex and overlapping [31–33].

Cognitive impairment is usually unresponsive to antipsychotic therapy. Therapeutic interventions have yielded conflicting results [28,34]. In addition to attempts at medication (at this stage without any particular result), various cognitive-rehabilitation techniques are used to improve cognitive functioning in patients with schizophrenia. Some authors have found positive and promising results using these methods [35], while others remain more skeptical about the results of their use [36]. A sizeable contemporary meta-analysis including 8851 patients shows that the use of cognitive remediation in patients with schizophrenia has a beneficial effect in terms of cognitive functioning [37,38]. These data give grounds for the European Psychiatric Association to make a consensus statement regarding the treatment of cognitive disorders in schizophrenia [39]. It is also necessary to take into account the fact that, in order to achieve recovery in patients with schizophrenia, it is necessary to bear in mind two main domains—clinical remission and social functioning [40]. Social functioning is also directly inferred from patients' cognitive resources.

Data on the progression of cognitive impairment in schizophrenia are conflicting. Some studies show no cognitive deterioration over time, at least for the observed period (of one year) after the onset of the disorder. These observations lead some authors to believe that an underlying neurodegenerative process was not observed, as gradient changes in neurocognition were also not observed [41,42]. Other studies have also shown that no gradient deterioration is observed when conducting long-term longitudinal studies.

There is evidence of improvement after the patient goes into clinical remission [43]. A nine-year follow-up finding confirmed the improvement in cognition during the first year found in other studies. The fact that the authors note is that, over the next five years, the curve of neurocognition flattens out and then falls again to be level at year 9 with the level of the first testing (before the improvement) [44]. Other researchers also concluded that relative stability in cognitive function was observed during the first ten years of treatment [45]. In the most extended study of cognition in patients with schizophrenia and hyperactivity disorder—13 years—it was concluded that, over time, there was a reduction in verbal memory and a general stagnation in attention and the speed of cognitive processes [46]. These studies show that, over a certain period, cognitive abilities in patients with schizophrenia recovered by reaching a certain level (that is, for a certain period they are a static phenomenon) and, after about 9–10 years, they again observed deterioration with a tendency to reach the initial values registered at the beginning of the disease [46]. Another meta-analysis showed that gradient morphological and neurocognitive changes were observed over time compared to an observed control group [47]. On the other hand, other researchers consider that it is necessary to take into account the presence of antipsychotic treatment, which can also contribute to the development of neuromorphological and neurocognitive disorders [48].

When we talk about cognition, we usually start using different terms, which do not lead to greater clarity. Given this fact, we stick to the main components that can be registered quickly in clinical practice—short-term memory and attention. The term working memory is also often used. However, it refers to short-term memory and its use in solving everyday problems, which also raises the question of participation in attention [49]. Working memory is a cornerstone in the schizophrenic process and its disorders are considered the most pronounced in these patients [50–53]. These and many other data give grounds for some authors to consider consciousness as a memory function developed from it in the course of evolution [54].

Analysis of attention shows that its disturbance is a fundamental cognitive deficit in patients with schizophrenia [55]. The authors consider that attention is an indicator that should be fundamental to measuring the condition and effectiveness of treatment in patients with schizophrenia. They found that attention was directly related to and inferred from the state of working memory [56]. In search of a practical approach to assessing cognition, the authors used the assessment of short-term memory and attention. Attention was assessed with memory curve analysis when conducting a memory assessment test [57,58].

A relationship between memory impairments and the degree of dissociation was found. Increased dissociation was associated with more significant memory impairments [59]. On the other hand, other authors have found that dissociation decreases with age in cognitively and non-cognitively impaired individuals [60].

These data gave us the basis to look for the relationships between memory and attention disorders in patients with treatment resistance, and, in those with a clinical effect, to establish as well the relationship with the course and clinical peculiarities of the gender distribution of the schizophrenic process in patients with schizophrenia.

2. Methods

2.1. Clinical Contingent

We analyzed 105 patients with schizophrenia. The gender distribution showed that 66 were female and 39 were male. The patients were admitted for treatment in a Psychiatric Clinic of the University Hospital in the city of Stara Zagora after the appearance of consecutive psychotic episodes. Patients were examined in the clinic's outpatient practice and, after providing informed consent, were admitted for treatment and condition assessment. When analyzing their condition and inclusion in the study, inclusion and exclusion criteria were used. The patients were recruited and followed up from 2017 to 2022. The initial analysis and observation were carried out in hospital conditions, and, later, the observation and follow-up of their condition were carried out in outpatient conditions.

Inclusion criteria for patients with resistant schizophrenia [16] are as follows:
1. Assessment of symptoms with the PANSS and BPRS scale [61,62].
2. Prospective monitoring for at least 12 weeks.
3. Administration of at least two antipsychotic medication trials at a dose corresponding to or greater than 600 mg chlorpromazine equivalents.
4. Reduction of symptoms when assessed with the PANSS and BPRS scale by less than 20% for the observed period.
5. The assessment of social dysfunction using the SOFAS scale is below 60.

Criteria for patients with schizophrenia in clinical remission are those who have met the criteria of the published consensus on remission in schizophrenia [63].

The exclusion criteria are as follows:
1. Mental retardation.
2. Psychoactive substance abuse.
3. Presence of organic brain damage.
4. Concomitant progressive neurological or severe somatic diseases.
5. Expressed personality change (according to the diagnostic toolkit of DSM 5 and ICD 10). [64,65].
6. Score of MMSE (Mini-Mental State Examination) below 25 points.
7. Pregnancy and breastfeeding.

2.2. Assessment

Research has been used to assess cognitive impairment using the 10-word test [57,58]. This test is widely used and verified in many countries [66]. The methodology includes stimulus material, which the experimenter has developed himself. It is a set of 10 words, which should be common and short (from 1 to 2 syllables and should not be close in meaning). The two main memory processes are studied: (a) memorization (fixation) and (b) reproduction.

When experimenting, suitable conditions are necessary: A calm environment without interruption of the experiment, silence and a set of 10 words (monosyllabic or bisyllabic) that have no logical connection with each other. The instruction used by the experimenter consists of several stages: First explanation: "I will now read you ten words/words are read at intervals of one second in a clear voice. Listen carefully! When the reading finishes. Immediately repeat the words you have memorized. Their order does not matter. Got it?". After the repetition, the experimenter places crosses under the reproduced words in the protocol. The instruction continues with a second explanation: "Now I will read the exact words to you again, and you must then repeat them. Furthermore, the ones told the first time and those missed altogether in whatever order wanted". The experimenter again puts crosses under each repeated word. "One more time!" is required, and further repetitions of the set of words follow but without any instruction. If the subject says words that do not exist in the set, the experimenter records them by noting in which order these words are reproduced. If the person repeats the same word from the set several times in the protocol, many points are placed next to the cross as the number of times the examinee repeats this word. After five repetitions of the set of ten words, the experiment was terminated. Based on the data from the repetitions, an evaluation of the obtained memory curve is also made—unstable "zigzag", plateau type, asthenic or average—giving information about the state of active attention [58].

Stimulus material (two examples):
1. meat, glass, road, egg, birch, jam, goat, flag, sky, bag
2. house, horse, mushroom, honey, brother, forest, chair, bread, labor, oak

2.3. Statistical Analyses

Statistical package SPSS version 26 was used. The methods used were tailored to the specifics and objectives of the study. Non-parametric methods of analysis were used

Mann–Whitney U test [67], correlation analysis and regression analysis). The regression analysis was conducted with the dependent variables being the studied fixation and reproduction. Independent variables were age, disease onset, duration of schizophrenia process, sex, weight, height, body mass index, PANSS positive, negative and disorganized symptoms, Dissociation Scale, Depression Scale and Obsessive–Compulsive Symptoms Scale. A correlation analysis was also conducted to find a relationship between the analyzed quantities.

The same cohort of patients was also investigated concerning other clinical characteristics such as depressive complaints, obsessive–compulsive and dissociative symptoms, lateralization of brain processes, the effect of the administration of the first antipsychotic medication and the gender-associated role in patients with schizophrenia [68–75].

All patients gave written informed consent before admission to the clinical settings and performing diagnostic tests and therapy. The study was conducted following the Declaration of Helsinki and approved by the Ethical Committee of University Hospital "Prof. Dr. Stoyan Kirkovich" Stara Zagora, protocol code TR3–02-242/30 December 2021.

3. Results

Of 105 patients, 45 have resistant schizophrenia, and the remaining 60 are in clinical remission. The gender distribution showed that 66 were women and 39 were men. The alignments according to the effects of treatment concerning age, onset of illness, duration of schizophrenia, BMI, height, education and handedness are presented in Table 1.

Table 1. Distribution of patients' age, age of onset of schizophrenia, duration of schizophrenia, BMI, height, education and handedness in both groups of patients.

	Resistant SZ	Clinical Remission	Resistant SZ
Age (years)		36.98	37.25
Age of onset of SZ (years)		23.04	27.37
Duration of SZ (years)		14.31	9.87
BMI		26.6022	27.2217
Height		170.11	167.38
Education (years)		11.33	11.60
Handedness (right/left)		42/3	56/4
Sex (M/F)		20/25	19/41

3.1. Assessment of Fixation

Among the 105 patients, we found fixation values within the normal range in 32 (30.18%). In the remaining 73 patients (69.82%), the fixation values were below this norm.

The mean fixation score for all patients we observed was 75.07, SD 15.561, with the minimum and maximum values being 45 and 100%, respectively. When analyzing the gender distribution, we found that, for females, the mean value of fixation was 77.33, with a standard deviation of 15.472. The minimum and maximum values on the scale were 48 and 100 points, respectively. Results for males showed a mean fixation value of 71.23. The standard deviation was 15.141, and the minimum and maximum values were 45 and 100, respectively.

The analysis of statistical significance showed a lack of statistical significance; the obtained value of "p" is in a borderline range, $p = 0.052$ (Table 2, Figure 1).

Table 2. Distribution of male and female fixation values.

	Fixation Score		
Gender	Mean	N	Std. Deviation
f	77,33	66	15,472
m	71,23	39	15,141
Total	75,07	105	15,561

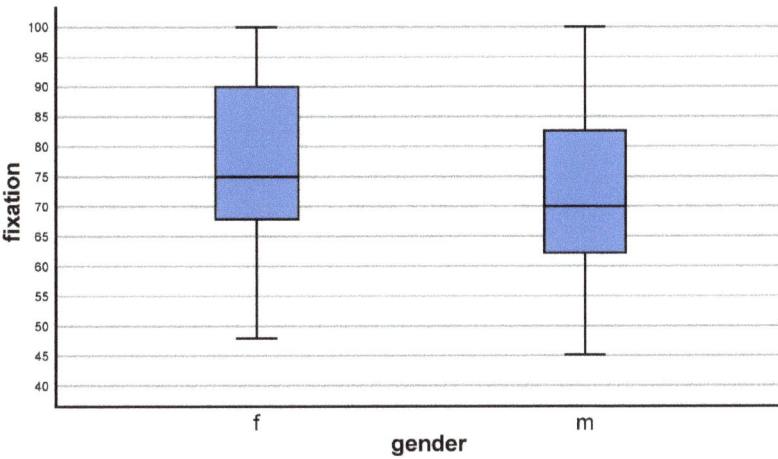

Figure 1. Distribution of male and female fixation values.

When evaluating fixation in patients with resistant symptoms (RS), we found that the average value of fixation in them was 65.18%. The standard deviation was 11.161, and the minimum and maximum values were 45 and 100.

When evaluating the fixation in the patients in CR (clinical remission), we found an average fixation value of 82.48%. The standard deviation was 14.263, and the minimum and maximum values were 45 and 100, respectively.

From these results in the patients with R.S., it is evident that the fixation disorders in them as an average value can be described as moderately pronounced (although in the upper range of the assessment moderate). We see patients with lower fixation in the range of significant impairment and those within the normal range.

The data for patients in clinical remission show that the average value of 82.48 is at the upper end of mild disorders (near the lower end of the norm) (Application 1, Appendix A).

The comparison between the two groups showed the presence of a highly statistically significant difference ($p < 0.001$ ***) (Table 3, Figure 2).

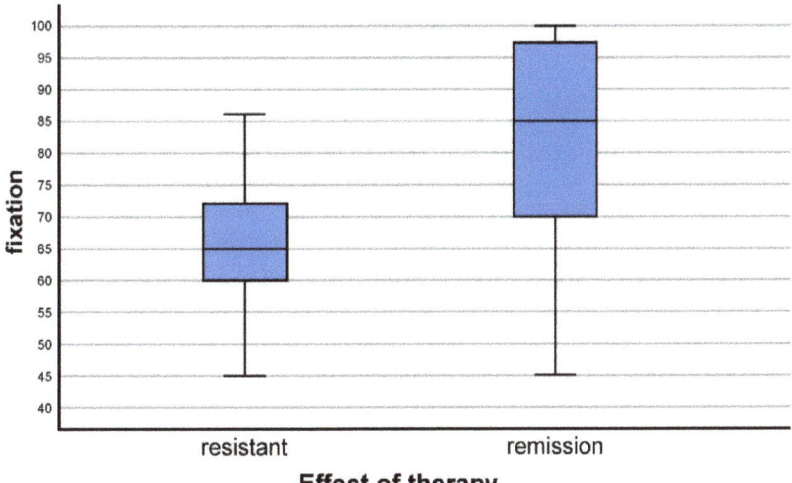

Figure 2. Relationship between fixation values in patients with resistance and those with treatment effect.

Table 3. Presentation of statistical significance of differences between patients with resistance and those with therapy effect according to fixation value.

Mann–Whitney U	467,000
Asymp. Sig. (2-tailed)	0.000 (***)

In order to comprehensively analyze the influence of additional factors, such as the PANSS scales, body mass index, education, the onset of the disease, its duration, the age of the patients, Dissociation Rating Scale, Hamilton depression rating scale, Obsessive-Compulsive Symptoms Rating Scale, on fixation, we conducted a multiple regression analysis.

Three factors influenced fixation status significantly. Factors recorded were the PANSS—disorganized symptoms scale, the duration of the illness and the dissociative symptoms scale (Table 4).

Table 4. Relationship between fixation with the PANSS—disorganized symptoms, duration of schizophrenia and the level of dissociation.

	R2	β	t	p (Sig)
Step 1 PANSS disorganized	0.338	0.889	7.259	0.000 (***)
Step 2 PANSS disorganized Duration of Sch	0.388	0.350	6.865 2.880	0.000 (***)
Step 3 PANSS disorganized Duration of Sch Dissociation score	0.411	0.130	4.869 2.646 1.988	0.000 (***)

Our data show that disorganized symptoms, duration of the schizophrenic process and high dissociation scale are the factors associated with a high degree of fixation involvement. There is also a statistically significant difference between patients with resistance to the treatment and those with an effect from it.

We looked for a relationship between the effect of fixation, the onset of the disease and the duration of the schizophrenic process by conducting a correlation analysis. We found a correlation between the fixation disorder, early onset of the disease, and the duration of the schizophrenic process. The results are presented in Table 5.

Table 5. Assessment of the relationship between fixation disorders and the onset of schizophrenia process and its duration.

		Onset of the Sch	Duration of Sch
Fixation	Pearson Correlation	−0.274 **	−0.325 **
	Sig. (2-tailed)	0.005	0.001

It is clear from the table that the duration of the schizophrenic process is a factor associated with a higher probability of fixation disorders, as both factors have clinically significant statistical significance in terms of their influence.

3.2. Reproduction

We observed 65 (61.90%) of the patients with reproduction values within the normal range. In the remaining 40 patients (38.1%), the reproduction values were below this norm.

The distribution by gender showed that the measured points on the reproduction scale for females was 88.44. The standard deviation was 16.471, with the minimum and maximum values being 50 and 100, respectively.

For males, the reproduction scale analysis showed a mean value of 83.56, with a standard deviation slightly higher than that of females—18.223. The minimum and maximum values were 45 and 100, respectively.

Statistical analysis showed no statistically significant difference ($p > 0.05$). In patients with resistant schizophrenia, the mean value on the reproduction scale was 77.07 and the standard deviation was 16.708, with a minimum value of 45 and a maximum of 100.

In responders to therapy, the mean value of the reproduction scale was 93.9, the standard deviation was 13.872, and the minimum and maximum values were 50 and 100. Statistical analysis using the Mann–Whitney U test for statistical dependence revealed a high correlation (Mann–Whitney U; 607.000; $p < 0.001$ ***).

In order to comprehensively analyze the influence of additional factors such as the PANSS scales, body mass index, education, the onset of the disease, its duration, the age of the patients, Dissociation Rating Scale, Hamilton depression rating scale and Obsessive–Compulsive Symptoms Rating Scale on reproduction, we conducted a multiple regression analysis (Table 6).

Table 6. Relationship between reproduction and the PANSS—disorganized and PANSS—negative symptoms.

	R2	β	T	p (sig)
Step 1 PANSS disorganized	0.321	0.889	6.972	0.000 (***)
Step 2 PANSS disorganized PANSS negative	0.351	0.350	3.251 2.190	0.000 (***)

Analysis of the relationship between reproduction and the duration of schizophrenia showed the presence of a relatively weak correlative dependence. No correlation was found between reproduction and disease onset (Table 7).

Table 7. Relationship of reproduction with the duration and onset of schizophrenia process.

		Reproduction	Onset of the Sch	Duration of Sch
Reproduction	Pearson Correlation Sig. (2-tailed)	1	0.153 0.120	−0.199 * 0.041

3.3. Attention

The analysis of attention in the observed patients was carried out based on an outlined memory curve during the study to reproduce the results.

This analysis showed that, among the observed patients, 41 had an unstable (zigzag) memory curve, 17 had a plateau-type memory curve, 8 had an asthenic memory curve and 39 (37.14%) had a usually presented one.

In total, 66 (62.86%) were found to have an attention disorder. The distribution of the type of memory curve (attention) by gender is presented in Table 8 and Figure 3.

Table 8. Relationship of the type of attention disturbances with the distribution by gender.

		Assessed Memory Curve (Attention)				
		Unstable	Plateau	Asthenic	Normal	Total
Gender	f	23	9	6	28	66
	m	18	8	2	11	39
Total		41	17	8	39	105

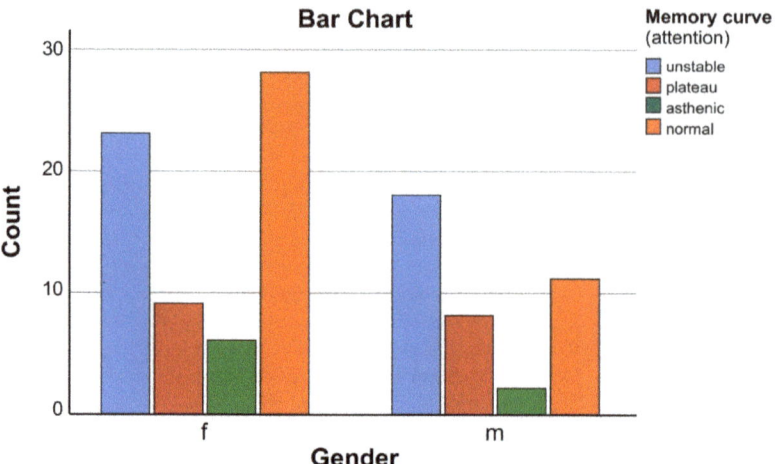

Figure 3. Relationship of the type of attention disturbances with the distribution by gender.

A statistical analysis showed that no statistically significant difference was observed in males and females regarding the type of memory curve and the involvement of attention in this process ($p > 0.05$).

When comparing the patients with schizophrenia according to the effect of the treatment, the following distribution was found (Table 9, Figure 4).

Table 9. Distribution of the type of memory curve in patients with resistance and those with an effect of the therapy.

		Assessed Memory Curve				
		Unstable	Plateau	Asthenic	Normal	Total
Treatment effect	resistant	29	11	2	3	45
	remission	12	6	6	36	60
	Total	41	17	8	39	105

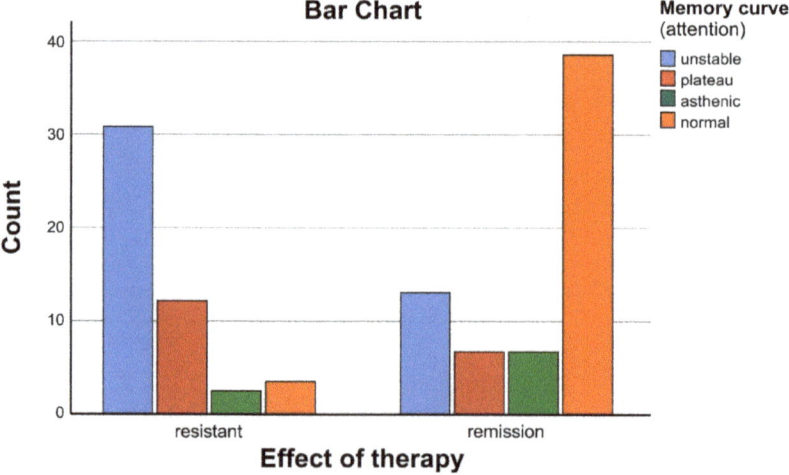

Figure 4. Distribution of the type of memory curve in patients with resistance and those with an effect of the therapy.

From the presented table and graph of the distribution of the type of attention engagement in these patients, it was found that, in the patients with resistance, more than half had an unstable type of memory curve, which is related to instability, i.e., inability to maintain active attention during the task at hand. Regression analysis assessing the influence of other factors such as height, weight, BMI, disease onset, duration, depression scale, dissociation scale, obsessive–compulsive symptoms, and the PANSS positive, negative and disorganized symptoms scales showed that disorganized symptoms and the onset of the disease are the factors influencing the attention disorders to the highest degree (Figures 5 and 6, Table 10).

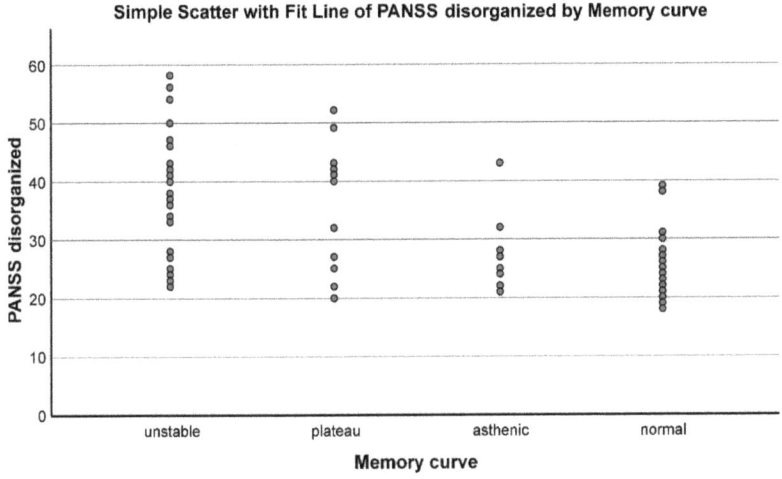

Figure 5. Relationship of attention disorders and PANSS—disorganized symptoms.

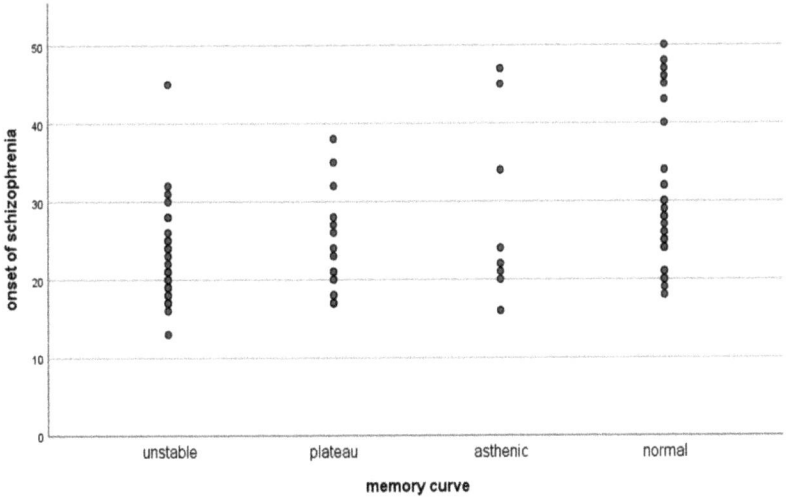

Figure 6. Relationship of attention disorders and the onset of schizophrenia.

Table 10. Relationship between attention disorders and the PANSS—disorganized symptoms and the onset of schizophrenia.

	R2	β	t	p (Sig)
Step 1 PANSS disorganized	0.375	0.613	7.865	0.000 (***)
Step 2 PANSS disorganized Onset of Sch	0.445	0.561 0.268	7.469 3.587	0.000 (***)

4. Discussion

Our research shows that, when assessing working memory and attention, there is no statistically significant difference between males and females. It is noteworthy that, in general, males perform slightly worse than females without reaching a statistically significant difference. These results, on the one hand, confirm the data of other authors on the lack of difference between males and females regarding the cognitive functions studied [76]. Other authors found a difference, with males showing more severe cognitive deficits than females [77]. Our results also show that males have lower scores on the cognitive test assessment without reaching a statistically significant difference to verify these differences. These differences may also be because, in our study, individuals of the female gender predominate, which is most likely also due to the inclusion and exclusion criteria we used. Other evidence also suggests that cognitive impairment is more common in males [78]. We found a significant difference in schizophrenia patients compared to the general population in terms of short-term memory—fixation and reproduction. Our results show that short-term memory impairments are more pronounced for fixation and less so for reproduction in patients with schizophrenia. Data from the literature indicate that cognitive impairment is generally observed in about 80% of patients with schizophrenia [79,80]. Our observation reflects only short-term memory and attention, as the disorders we found were of a lower percentage. In 69% of the patients, there is an impairment of fixation, in 38.1% an impairment of reproduction and, in 62.85%, a violation of attention. The difference in the percentages found (in our low-scoring study) is most likely due to the stricter exclusion criteria and the fact that we are limited to an analysis of short-term memory and attention. When comparing patients with resistance and those with a treatment effect, we found a significant difference in all measures, which was most pronounced in terms of fixation. Our observations confirm the results of other authors on the presence of differences between patients with and without deficits, and that deficits in memory and attention are associated with a poor prognosis [81,82]. The data from the literature show that the cognitive deficit is observed even before the onset of psychosis [83,84] and remains stable for a certain period [41,42,45], and after ten years a deterioration can be observed, usually associated with other factors such as BMI metabolic disorders as well as those involving other organs and systems [46]. The patients we analyzed from the two groups did not show differences in weight and BMI, so these factors cannot be assumed to influence cognitive performance [75].

The analysis of other researchers shows a different trend: cognitive symptoms develop in the first 10–20 years, after which their trajectory does not differ much from that of the main population [85]. These analyses, as well as our observations, pose the question of whether differences in cognition are not observed at the beginning of the disease, which predetermines the later resistance to treatment. Our observation is of patients with an average disease duration of 10.2 years. These observations of ours pose the question whether, on the one hand, the longer duration of the disease in patients with resistance (on average 14.31 years) is not also related to a re-started deterioration of cognition (observed after the 10th year) or, on the other hand, the difference in cognitive performance was present from the beginning of the disease in them?

We find an association of the cognitive impairments we measured with disorganized symptoms, which some authors find criteria for a high probability of resistance [86–89]. With our observations, we cannot support the results of other authors that all PANSS subscales are associated with cognitive impairment [90,91]. We report an association between cognitive symptoms and a high degree of dissociation. On the other hand, there is an established relationship between a high degree of dissociation and resistance in patients with schizophrenia [69]. We find cognitive impairments in terms of working memory and attention. What is necessary to note is the fact that, in more than half of the patients with resistance to the treatment, we find an unstable (zigzag type) memory curve, which indicates an instability or what we can express as a dissociation (fragmentation) of attention while completing the assigned task. We also established a relationship between the unstable type of memory curve and disorganized symptoms in patients with schizophrenia. We found that this relationship further provides an opportunity to elucidate the etiology of disorganized symptoms. The lack of active attention (established instability and fragmentation) is also associated with working memory disorders, which leads to disruption of the continuum in behavior and speech. These results shed light on the relationships between dissociation, resistance, disorganized symptoms and registered cognitive impairment. Regression analysis showed that attention disorders are also dependent on the onset of the disease. This observation of ours confirms the conclusion of other authors that attention is a factor associated with the severity of the schizophrenia process, and is an essential marker for the therapeutic dynamics and prognosis of the disease [55,56,92]. These results pose the question of searching for more complex therapeutic interventions in the treatment of patients [93].

On the other hand, we find impairments in working memory with an underlying fixation impairment. That gives us reason to disagree with the opinion of other authors about the possible similarity of dementia in patients with schizophrenia with frontotemporal dementia [17]. Memory impairment is not one of the cardinal symptoms of frontotemporal dementia or, if present, it occurs later in the nosological process [94,95]. On the other hand, both in schizophrenia and in other diseases, there are data on morphological changes in brain structures but they do not always correspond to the clinical picture, both in patients with schizophrenia and in some neurological diseases [96–98]. We find mainly problems with memory and attention. However, on the other hand, given that cognitive problems appear early before the onset of the acute psychotic state, the question of proximity to frontotemporal dementia can hardly be raised.

5. Limitations

The limitation in our study is also related to the need for more patients to make a complete verification of the obtained results. On the one hand, females predominate, which does not provide complete clarity on the gender differences concerning the identified cognitive disorders. On the other hand, we analyze short-term memory, and the question remains open whether these are also the early characteristics of cognitive disorders at the onset of psychosis and whether these fixation and reproduction disorders associated with a characteristic shape of the memory curve did not appear later in the course of schizophrenia process. Of course, our research shows that the duration of the schizophrenic process is a factor associated with cognitive disorders. However, this association does not answer the question of the extent to which differences in early cognitive impairment play a role in resistance to treatment. Thus, the question remains open as to whether the differences in cognitive impairment in patients with resistance and those in therapeutic remission were not present at the onset of psychosis or developed gradually during the progression of the psychotic state.

On the other hand, the question remains open as to whether we have chosen the most appropriate cognitive tool to analyze the examined patients. We use Luria's 10-word test. This test is not very different from the tests created based on the ideas of George A. Miller with his magic number—7 [99]. Whether it is the best cognitive tool is a question that is difficult for anyone to answer, as is proposing the ideal and universal one. We use a cognitive tool that has been used in clinical practice in Bulgaria for almost 30 years to assess patients with schizophrenia, with which we have practice and experience.

6. Conclusions

We registered the presence of disorders in working memory—fixation and reproduction, as well as disorders in active attention in the studied patients with schizophrenia. These disorders are significantly more pronounced in patients with resistance to treatment. The cognitive symptoms we found were dependent on disease onset, duration of schizophrenia, high degree of dissociation and pronounced disorganized symptoms. Do not the data on a significantly greater disturbance of cognitive symptoms in patients with resistance give us the right to consider resistant schizophrenia as a more "organic" disease, in which the disturbance of cognition is the reason for the lack of effect of antipsychotic medications that do not affect cognitive symptoms (there is also the opposing view – [48]). Our research makes it possible to conclude that the early assessment of cognitive symptoms would enable the prediction of the course of the disease, the search for early therapeutic interventions and the discussion of additional strategies regarding cognitive disorders.

Author Contributions: Conceptualization, data collection and analysis are by G.P.; data collection and analysis are by S.D.; and writing, editing and graphics are by P.P. All authors listed have made a substantial, direct and intellectual contribution to the work. All authors have read and agreed to the published version of the manuscript.

Funding: This research received no external funding.

Institutional Review Board Statement: The study was conducted following the Declaration of Helsinki and approved by the Ethical Committee of University Hospital "Prof. Dr. Stoyan Kirkovich" Stara Zagora, protocol code TR3-02-242/30 December 2021.

Informed Consent Statement: Informed consent was obtained from all subjects involved in the study.

Data Availability Statement: The raw data supporting the conclusions of this article will be made available by the authors upon reasonable request.

Acknowledgments: We would like to express our gratitude to all those who helped us while writing this manuscript. Thanks to all the peer reviewers for their opinions and suggestions.

Conflicts of Interest: The authors declare no conflict of interest.

Appendix A

Application 1: (Memory Impairment Rating Scale)
Scale of Prof. Dr. K. Mechkov
Degree Percent Deviation
I over 84 no/norm/
II 84–68 slightly
III 68–51 moderate
IV 51–34 significantly
V 34–17 severe
VI under 17 very heavy

References

1. Tanaka, M.; Vécsei, L. Editorial of Special Issue "Crosstalk between Depression, Anxiety, and Dementia: Comorbidity in Behavioral Neurology and Neuropsychiatry. *Biomedicines* **2021**, *9*, 517. [CrossRef] [PubMed]
2. Bitter, I.; Mohr, P.; Raspopova, N.; Szulc, A.; Samochowiec, J.; Micluia, I.V.; Skugarevsky, O.; Herold, R.; Mihaljevic-Peles, A.; Okribelashvili, N.; et al. Assessment and Treatment of Negative Symptoms in Schizophrenia-A Regional Perspective. *Front Psychiatry* **2022**, *12*, 820801. [CrossRef] [PubMed]
3. Stoyanov, D. Advances in the Diagnosis and Management of Psychosis. *Diagnostics* **2023**, *13*, 1517. [CrossRef] [PubMed]
4. Stoyanov, D.; Aryutova, K.; Kandilarova, S.; Paunova, R.; Arabadzhiev, Z.; Todeva-Radneva, A.; Kostianev, S.; Borgwardt, S. Diagnostic Task Specific Activations in Functional MRI and Aberrant Connectivity of Insula with Middle Frontal Gyrus Can Inform the Differential Diagnosis of Psychosis. *Diagnostics* **2021**, *11*, 95. [CrossRef] [PubMed]
5. Stoyanov, D.; Kandilarova, S.; Borgwardt, S.; Stieglitz, R.D.; Hugdahl, K.; Kostianev, S. Psychopathology Assessment Methods Revisited: On Translational Cross-Validation of Clinical Self-Evaluation Scale and fMRI. *Front. Psychiatry* **2018**, *9*, 21. [CrossRef]

6. Tanaka, M.; Tóth, F.; Polyák, H.; Szabó, Á.; Mándi, Y.; Vécsei, L. Immune Influencers in Action: Metabolites and Enzymes of the Tryptophan-Kynurenine Metabolic Pathway. *Biomedicines* **2021**, *9*, 734. [CrossRef]
7. Moustafa, S.R.; Al-Rawi, K.F.; Stoyanov, D.; Al-Dujaili, A.H.; Supasitthumrong, T.; Al-Hakeim, H.K.; Maes, M. The Endogenous Opioid System in Schizophrenia and Treatment Resistant Schizophrenia: Increased Plasma Endomorphin 2, and κ and μ Opioid Receptors Are Associated with Interleukin-6. *Diagnostics* **2020**, *10*, 633. [CrossRef]
8. Masumo, Y.; Kanahara, N.; Kogure, M.; Yamasaki, F.; Nakata, Y.; Iyo, M. Dopamine supersensitivity psychosis and delay of clozapine treatment in patients with treatment-resistant schizophrenia. *Int. Clin. Psychopharmacol.* **2022**, *38*, 102–109. [CrossRef]
9. Helaly, A.M.N.; Ghorab, D.S.E.D. Schizophrenia as metabolic disease. What are the causes? *Metab Brain Dis.* **2023**, *38*, 795–804. [CrossRef]
10. Stojanov, D. A Pharmacogenetic and Dynamical Model of the Resistance to Antipsychotic Treatment of Schizophrenia. *Biotechnol. Biotechnol. Equip.* **2006**, *20*, 169–170. [CrossRef]
11. Tanaka, M.; Vécsei, L. Editorial of Special Issue 'Dissecting Neurological and Neuropsychiatric Diseases: Neurodegeneration and Neuroprotection'. *Int. J. Mol. Sci.* **2022**, *23*, 6991. [CrossRef] [PubMed]
12. Howes, O.D.; Thase, M.E.; Pillinger, T. Treatment resistance in psychiatry: State of the art and new directions. *Mol Psychiatry* **2022**, *27*, 58–72. [CrossRef] [PubMed]
13. Demjaha, A.; Murray, R.M.; McGuire, P.K.; Kapur, S.; Howes, O.D. Dopamine synthesis capacity in patients with treatment-resistant schizophrenia. *Am. J. Psychiatry* **2012**, *169*, 1203–1210. [CrossRef] [PubMed]
14. Barnes, T.R. Evidence-based guidelines for the pharmacological treatment of schizophrenia: Recommendations from the British Association for Psychopharmacology. *J. Psychopharmacol.* **2011**, *25*, 567–620. [CrossRef] [PubMed]
15. Verma, S.; Chan, L.L.; Chee, K.S.; Chen, H.; Chin, S.A.; Chong, S.A.; Chua, W.; Fones, C.; Fung, D.; Khoo, C.L.; et al. Ministry of Health clinical practice guidelines: Schizophrenia. *Singap. Med. J.* **2011**, *52*, 521–525, quiz 526.
16. Howes, O.D.; McCutcheon, R.; Agid, O.; de Bartolomeis, A.; van Beveren, N.J.; Birnbaum, M.L.; Bloomfield, M.A.; Bressan, R.A.; Buchanan, R.W.; Carpenter, W.T.; et al. Treatment-Resistant Schizophrenia: Treatment Response and Resistance in Psychosis (TRRIP) Working Group Consensus Guidelines on Diagnosis and Terminology. *Am. J. Psychiatry* **2017**, *174*, 216–229. [CrossRef]
17. de Vries, P.J.; Honer, W.G.; Kemp, P.M.; McKenna, P.J. Dementia as a complication of schizophrenia. *J. Neurol. Neurosurg. Psychiatry* **2001**, *70*, 588–596. [CrossRef]
18. McCutcheon, R.A.; Keefe, R.S.E.; McGuire, P.K. Cognitive impairment in schizophrenia: Etiology, pathophysiology, and treatment. *Mol. Psychiatry* **2023**, *28*, 1902–1918. [CrossRef]
19. Richmond-Rakerd, L.S.; D'Souza, S.; Milne, B.J.; Caspi, A.; Moffitt, T.E. Longitudinal associations of mental disorders with dementia: 30-year analysis of 1.7 million New Zealand citizens. *JAMA Psychiatry* **2022**, *48109*, 333–340. [CrossRef]
20. Green, M.F.; Horan, W.P.; Lee, J. Nonsocial and social cognition in schizophrenia: Current evidence and future directions. *World Psychiatry* **2019**, *18*, 146–161. [CrossRef]
21. Javitt, D.; Sweet, R. Auditory dysfunction in schizophrenia: Integrating clinical and basic features. *Nat. Rev. Neurosci.* **2015**, *16*, 535–550. [CrossRef] [PubMed]
22. Keefe, R.S.E.; Fox, K.H.; Harvey, P.D.; Cucchiaro, J.; Siu, C.; Loebel, A. Characteristics of the MATRICS Consensus Cognitive Battery in a 29-site antipsychotic schizophrenia clinical trial. *Schizophr. Res.* **2011**, *125*, 161–168. [CrossRef]
23. Taylor, S.E. Adjustment to threatening events: A theory of cognitive adaptation. *Am. Psychol.* **1983**, *38*, 1161–1173. [CrossRef]
24. Taylor, S.E.; Brown, J.D. Illusion and well-being: A social psychological perspective on mental health. *Psychol. Bull.* **1988**, *103*, 193–210. [CrossRef]
25. Wójciak, P.; Rybakowski, J. Clinical picture, pathogenesis and psychometric assessment of negative symptoms of schizophrenia. *Psychiatr. Pol.* **2018**, *52*, 185–197. [CrossRef] [PubMed]
26. Bozikas, V.P.; Andreou, C. Longitudinal studies of cognition in first episode psychosis: A systematic review of the literature. *Aust. N. Z. J. Psychiatry* **2011**, *45*, 93–108. [CrossRef]
27. Shah, J.; Eack, S.M.; Montrose, D.M.; Tandon, N.; Miewald, J.M.; Prasad, K.M.; Keshavan, M.S. Multivariate prediction of emerging psychosis in adolescents at high risk for schizophrenia. *Schizophr. Res.* **2012**, *141*, 189–196. [CrossRef]
28. Biedermann, F.; Fleischhacker, W.W. Psychotic disorders in DSM-5 and ICD-11. *CNS Spectr.* **2016**, *21*, 349–354. [CrossRef]
29. Vidailhet, P. Premier épisode psychotique, troubles cognitifs et remédiation [First-episode psychosis, cognitive difficulties and remediation]. *Encephale* **2013**, *39* (Suppl. S2), S83–S92. (In French) [CrossRef]
30. Hashimoto, K. Recent Advances in the Early Intervention in Schizophrenia: Future Direction from Preclinical Findings. *Curr. Psychiatry Rep.* **2019**, *21*, 75. [CrossRef]
31. Oberauer, K. Working Memory and Attention—A Conceptual Analysis and Review. *J. Cogn.* **2019**, *2*, 36. [CrossRef] [PubMed]
32. Oberauer, K. Design for a working memory. *Psychol. Learn. Motiv. Adv. Res. Theory* **2009**, *51*, 45–100. [CrossRef]
33. Oberauer, K. Control of the contents of working memory—A comparison of two paradigms and two age groups. *J. Exp. Psychol. Learn. Mem. Cogn.* **2005**, *31*, 714–728. [CrossRef]
34. Kaar, S.J.; Natesan, S.; McCutcheon, R.; Howes, O.D. Antipsychotics: Mechanisms underlying clinical response and side-effects and novel treatment approaches based on pathophysiology. *Neuropharmacology* **2020**, *172*, 107704. [CrossRef] [PubMed]
35. Hogarty, G.E.; Flesher, S. Developmental theory for a cognitive enhancement therapy of schizophrenia. *Schizophr. Bull.* **1999**, *25*, 677–692. [CrossRef] [PubMed]

36. Bellack, A.S. Cognitive rehabilitation for schizophrenia—Is it possible—Is it necessary. *Schizophr. Bull.* **1992**, *8*, 43–50. [CrossRef] [PubMed]
37. Vita, A.; Barlati, S.; Ceraso, A.; Nibbio, G.; Ariu, C.; Deste, G.; Wykes, T. Effectiveness, Core Elements, and Moderators of Response of Cognitive Remediation for Schizophrenia: A Systematic Review and Meta-analysis of Randomized Clinical Trials. *JAMA Psychiatry* **2021**, *78*, 848–858. [CrossRef] [PubMed]
38. Lejeune, J.A.; Northrop, A.; Kurtz, M.M. A Meta-analysis of Cognitive Remediation for Schizophrenia: Efficacy and the Role of Participant and Treatment Factors. *Schizophr. Bull.* **2021**, *47*, 997–1006. [CrossRef]
39. Vita, A.; Gaebel, W.; Mucci, A.; Sachs, G.; Barlati, S.; Giordano, G.M.; Nibbio, G.; Nordentoft, M.; Wykes, T.; Galderisi, S. European Psychiatric Association guidance on treatment of cognitive impairment in schizophrenia. *Eur. Psychiatry* **2022**, *65*, e57. [CrossRef]
40. Vita, A.; Barlati, S. Recovery from schizophrenia: Is it possible? *Curr. Opin. Psychiatry* **2018**, *31*, 246–255. [CrossRef]
41. Rund, B.R. A review of longitudinal studies of cognitive functions in schizophrenia patients. *Schizophr. Bull.* **1998**, *24*, 425–435. [CrossRef] [PubMed]
42. Rund, B.R. Is there a degenerative process going on in the brain of people with Schizophrenia? *Front. Hum. Neurosci.* **2009**, *3*, 36. [CrossRef] [PubMed]
43. Rund, B.R.; Sundet, K.; Asbjørnsen, A.; Egeland, J.; Landrø, N.I.; Lund, A.; Roness, A.; Stordal, K.I.; Hugdahl, K. Neuropsychological test profiles in schizophrenia and non-psychotic depression. *Acta Psychiatr. Scand.* **2006**, *113*, 350–359. [CrossRef] [PubMed]
44. Stirling, J.; White, C.; Lewis, S.; Hopkins, R.; Tantam, D.; Huddy, A.; Montague, L. Neurocognitive function and outcome in first-episode schizophrenia: A 10-year follow-up of an epidemiological cohort. *Schizophr. Res.* **2003**, *65*, 75–86. [CrossRef] [PubMed]
45. Hoff, A.L.; Svetina, C.; Shields, G.; Stewart, J.; DeLisi, L.E. Ten year longitudinal study of neuropsychological functioning subsequent to a first episode of schizophrenia. *Schizophr. Res.* **2005**, *78*, 27–34. [CrossRef]
46. Øie, M.; Sundet, K.; Ueland, T. Neurocognition and functional outcome in early-onset schizophrenia and attention-deficit/hyperactivity disorder: A 13-year follow-up. *Neuropsychology* **2011**, *25*, 25–35. [CrossRef]
47. Heilbronner, U.; Samara, M.; Leucht, S.; Falkai, P.; Schulze, T.G. The Longitudinal Course of Schizophrenia Across the Lifespan: Clinical, Cognitive, and Neurobiological Aspects. *Harv. Rev. Psychiatry* **2016**, *24*, 118–128. [CrossRef]
48. Fusar-Poli, P.; Smieskova, R.; Kempton, M.J.; Ho, B.C.; Andreasen, N.C.; Borgwardt, S. Progressive brain changes in schizophrenia related to antipsychotic treatment? A meta-analysis of longitudinal MRI studies. *Neurosci. Biobehav. Rev.* **2013**, *37*, 1680–1691. [CrossRef]
49. Cowan, N. What are the differences between long-term, short-term, and working memory? *Prog. Brain Res.* **2008**, *169*, 323–338. [CrossRef]
50. Heinrichs, R.W.; Zakzanis, K.K. Neurocognitive deficit in schizophrenia: A quantitative review of the evidence. *Neuropsychology* **1998**, *12*, 426–445. [CrossRef]
51. Guo, J.Y.; Ragland, J.D.; Carter, C.S. Memory and cognition in schizophrenia. *Mol. Psychiatry* **2019**, *24*, 633–642. [CrossRef]
52. Lee, J.; Park, S. Working memory impairments in schizophrenia: A meta-analysis. *J. Abnorm. Psychol.* **2005**, *114*, 599–611. [CrossRef]
53. Saykin, A.J.; Gur, R.C.; Gur, R.E.; Mozley, P.D.; Mozley, L.H.; Resnick, S.M.; Kester, D.B.; Stafiniak, P. Neuropsychological function in schizophrenia. Selective impairment in memory and learning. *Arch. Gen. Psychiatr.* **1991**, *48*, 618–624. [CrossRef]
54. Budson, A.E.; Richman, K.A.; Kensinger, E.A. Consciousness as a Memory System. *Cogn. Behav. Neurol.* **2022**, *35*, 263–297. [CrossRef] [PubMed]
55. Fioravanti, M.; Carlone, O.; Vitale, B.; Cinti, M.E.; Clare, L. A meta-analysis of cognitive deficits in adults with a diagnosis of schizophrenia. *Neuropsychol. Rev.* **2005**, *15*, 73–95. [CrossRef] [PubMed]
56. Luck, S.J.; Gold, J.M. The construct of attention in schizophrenia. *Biol. Psychiatry* **2008**, *64*, 34–39. [CrossRef] [PubMed]
57. Luria, A.R. *Higher Cortical Functions in Man*; Haigh, B., Ed.; Basic Books; Moscow University Press: New York, NY, USA, 1962.
58. Mechkov, K. *Medical Psychology*; Izdatelstvo "Pik": Veliko Tarnovo, Bulgaria, 1995.
59. 59. Özdemir, O.; Güzel Özdemir, P.; Boysan, M.; Yilmaz, E. The Relationships Between Dissociation, Attention, and Memory Dysfunction. *Noro Psikiyatr Ars.* **2015**, *52*, 36–41. [CrossRef] [PubMed]
60. Walker, R.; Gregory, J.; Oakley, S.; Jr Bloch, R.; Gardner, M. Reduction in dissociation due to aging and cognitive deficit. *Compr. Psychiatry* **1996**, *37*, 31–36. [CrossRef]
61. Overall, J.E.; Gorham, D.R. The Brief Psychiatric Rating Scale. *Psychol. Rep.* **1962**, *10*, 799–812. [CrossRef]
62. Kay, S.R.; Fiszbein, A.; Opler, L.A. The positive and negative syndrome scale (PANSS) for schizophrenia. *Schizophr. Bull.* **1987**, *13*, 261–276. [CrossRef]
63. Andrean, N.C.; Carpenter, W.T., Jr.; Kane, J.M.; Lasser, R.A.; Marder, S.R.; Weinberger, D.R. Remission in schizophrenia: Proposed criteria and rationale for consensus. *Am. J. Psychiatry* **2005**, *162*, 441–449. [CrossRef] [PubMed]
64. Edition, F. *Diagnostic and Statistical Manual of Mental Disorders*; American Psychiatric Association: Washington, DC, USA, 2013.
65. World Health Organization. *Division of Mental Health*; The ICD-10; WHO: Geneva, Switzerland, 1994.
66. Lezak, M.D. *Neuropsychological Assessment*, 3rd ed.; Oxford University Press: Oxford, UK, 1995.
67. Mann, H.B.; Whitney, D.R. On a Test of Whether One of Two Random Variables Is Stochastically Larger than the Other. *Ann. Math. Stat.* **1947**, *18*, 50–60. [CrossRef]

68. Panov, G.; Panova, P. Obsessive-compulsive symptoms in patient with schizophrenia: The influence of disorganized symptoms, duration of schizophrenia, and drug resistance. *Front. Psychiatry* 2023, *14*, 1120974. [CrossRef] [PubMed]
69. Panov, G. Dissociative Model in Patients with Resistant Schizophrenia. *Front. Psychiatry* 2022, *13*, 845493. [CrossRef] [PubMed]
70. Panov, G. Comparative Analysis of Lateral Preferences in Patients with Resistant Schizophrenia. *Front. Psychiatry* 2022, *13*, 868285. [CrossRef]
71. Panov, G. Gender-associated role in patients with schizophrenia. Is there a connection with the resistance? *Front. Psychiatry* 2022, *13*, 845493. [CrossRef]
72. Panov, G. Higher Depression Scores in Patients with Drug-Resistant Schizophrenia. *J. Integr. Neurosci.* 2022, *21*, 126. [CrossRef] [PubMed]
73. Panov, G.P. Early Markers in Resistant Schizophrenia: Effect of the First Antipsychotic Drug. *Diagnostics* 2022, *12*, 803. [CrossRef]
74. Panov, G.; Djulgerova, S.; Panova, P. The effect of education level and sex differences on resistance to treatment in patients with schizophrenia. *Bulg. Med.* 2022, *12*, 22–29.
75. Panov, G.; Djulgerova, S.; Panova, P. Comparative anthropometric criteria in patients with resistant schizophrenia. *Bulg. Med.* 2022, *12*, 30–39.
76. Chen, M.; Zhang, L.; Jiang, Q. Gender Difference in Cognitive Function Among Stable Schizophrenia: A Network Perspective. *Neuropsychiatr. Dis. Treat.* 2022, *18*, 2991–3000. [CrossRef] [PubMed]
77. Han, M.; Huang, X.F.; Chen, D.C.; Xiu, M.H.; Hui, L.; Liu, H.; Kosten, T.R.; Zhang, X.Y. Gender differences in cognitive function of patients with chronic schizophrenia. *Prog. Neuro-Psychopharmacol. Biol. Psychiatry* 2012, *39*, 358–363. [CrossRef] [PubMed]
78. Giordano, G.M.; Bucci, P.; Mucci, A.; Pezzella, P.; Galderisi, S. Gender Differences in Clinical and Psychosocial Features Among Persons with Schizophrenia: A Mini Review. *Front. Psychiatry* 2021, *12*, 789179. [CrossRef] [PubMed]
79. McEvoy, J.P. The costs of schizophrenia. *J. Clin. Psychiatry* 2007, *68*, 4–7.
80. Harvey, P.D.; Bosia, M.; Cavallaro, R.; Howes, O.D.; Kahn, R.S.; Leucht, S.; Müller, D.R.; Penadés, R.; Vita, A. Cognitive dysfunction in schizophrenia: An expert group paper on the current state of the art. *Schizophr. Res. Cogn.* 2022, *29*, 100249. [CrossRef]
81. Kucharska-Mazur, J.; Podwalski, P.; Rek-Owodziń, K.; Waszczuk, K.; Sagan, L.; Mueller, S.T.; Michalczyk, A.; Misiak, B.; Samochowiec, J. Executive Functions and Psychopathology Dimensions in Deficit and Non-Deficit Schizophrenia. *J. Clin. Med.* 2023, *12*, 1998. [CrossRef]
82. Green, M.F.; Kern, R.S.; Heaton, R.K. Longitudinal studies of cognition and functional outcome in schizophrenia: Implications for MATRICS. *Schizophr. Res.* 2004, *72*, 41–51. [CrossRef] [PubMed]
83. Rapoport, J.L.; Giedd, J.N.; Gogtay, N. Neurodevelopmental model of schizophrenia: Update 2012. *Mol. Psychiatry* 2012, *17*, 1228–1238. [CrossRef]
84. Davidson, M.; Reichenberg, A.; Rabinowitz, J.; Weiser, M.; Kaplan, Z.; Mark, M. Behavioral and intellectual markers for schizophrenia in apparently healthy male adolescents. *Am. J. Psychiatry* 1999, *156*, 1328–1335. [CrossRef]
85. van Haren, N.E.M.; Pol, H.E.H.; Schnack, H.G.; Cahn, W.; Brans, R.; Carati, I.; Rais, M.; Kahn, R.S. Progressive brain volume loss in schizophrenia over the course of the illness: Evidence of maturational abnormalities in early adulthood. *Biol. Psychiatry* 2008, *63*, 106–113. [CrossRef]
86. Barone, A.; De Prisco, M.; Altavilla, B.; Avagliano, C.; Balletta, R.; Buonaguro, E.F.; Ciccarelli, M.; D'Ambrosio, L.; Giordano, S.; Latte, G.; et al. Disorganization domain as a putative predictor of Treatment Resistant Schizophrenia (TRS) diagnosis: A machine learning approach. *J. Psychiatr. Res.* 2022, *155*, 572–578. [CrossRef] [PubMed]
87. Metsanen, M.; Wahlberg, K.E.; Hakko, H.; Saarento, O.; Tienari, P. Thought disorder index: A longitudinal study of severity levels and schizophrenia factors. *J. Psychiatr. Res.* 2006, *40*, 258–266. [CrossRef] [PubMed]
88. Reed, R.A.; Harrow, M.; Herbener, E.S.; Martin, E.M. Executive function in schizophrenia: Is it linked to psychosis and poor life functioning? *J. Nerv. Ment. Dis.* 2002, *190*, 725–732. [CrossRef] [PubMed]
89. Shenton, M.E.; Kikinis, R.; Jolesz, F.A.; Pollak, S.D.; LeMay, M.; Wible, C.G.; Hokama, H.; Martin, J.; Metcalf, D.; Coleman, M.; et al. l. Abnormalities of the left temporal lobe and thought disorder in schizophrenia. A quantitative magnetic resonance imaging study. *N. Engl. J. Med.* 1992, *327*, 604–612. [CrossRef]
90. O'Leary, D.S.; Flaum, M.; Kesler, M.L.; Flashman, L.A.; Arndt, S.; Andreasen, N.C. Cognitive correlates of the negative, disorganized, and psychotic symptom dimensions of schizophrenia. *J. Neuropsychiatry Clin. Neurosci.* 2000, *12*, 4–15. [CrossRef] [PubMed]
91. 91. Ruben, C.; Gur, R.C.; Gur, R.E. Memory in health and in schizophrenia. *Dialogues Clin. Neurosci.* 2013, *15*, 399–410. [CrossRef]
92. González-Andrade, A.; López-Luengo, B.; Álvarez, M.M.R.; Santiago-Ramajo, S. Divided Attention in Schizophrenia: A Dual Task Paradigm. *Am. J. Psychol.* 2021, *134*, 187–200. [CrossRef]
93. Ivanova, E.; Panayotova, T.; Grechenliev, I.; Peshev, B.; Kolchakova, P.; Milanova, V. A Complex Combination Therapy for a Complex Disease-Neuroimaging Evidence for the Effect of Music Therapy in Schizophrenia. *Front. Psychiatry* 2022, *13*, 795344. [CrossRef]
94. Younes, K.; Miller, B.L. Frontotemporal Dementia: Neuropathology, Genetics, Neuroimaging, and Treatments. *Psychiatr. Clin. North Am.* 2020, *43*, 331–344. [CrossRef]
95. Bang, J.; Spina, S.; Miller, B.L. Frontotemporal dementia. *Lancet* 2015, *386*, 1672–1682. [CrossRef]

96. Laskaris, L.; Mancuso, S.; Shannon Weickert, C.; Zalesky, A.; Chana, G.; Wannan, C.; Bousman, C.; Baune, B.T.; McGorry, P.; Pantelis, C.; et al. Brain morphology is differentially impacted by peripheral cytokines in schizophrenia-spectrum disorder. *Brain Behav. Immun.* **2021**, *95*, 299–309. [CrossRef] [PubMed]
97. Bortolon, C.; Macgregor, A.; Capdevielle, D.; Raffard, S. Apathy in schizophrenia: A review of neuropsychological and neuroanatomical studies. *Neuropsychologia* **2018**, *118 Pt B*, 22–33. [CrossRef]
98. Nyatega, C.O.; Qiang, L.; Adamu, M.J.; Kawuwa, H.B. Gray matter, white matter and cerebrospinal fluid abnormalities in Parkinson's disease: A voxel-based morphometry study. *Front. Psychiatry* **2022**, *13*, 1027907. [CrossRef] [PubMed]
99. Cowan, N. George Miller's magical number of immediate memory in retrospect: Observations on the faltering progression of science. *Psychol. Rev.* **2015**, *122*, 536–541. [CrossRef] [PubMed]

Disclaimer/Publisher's Note: The statements, opinions and data contained in all publications are solely those of the individual author(s) and contributor(s) and not of MDPI and/or the editor(s). MDPI and/or the editor(s) disclaim responsibility for any injury to people or property resulting from any ideas, methods, instructions or products referred to in the content.

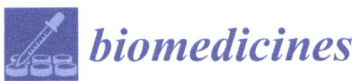

Article

The Blood Concentration of Metallic Nanoparticles Is Related to Cognitive Performance in People with Multiple Sclerosis: An Exploratory Analysis

Marcela de Oliveira [1,*], Felipe Balistieri Santinelli [2], Paulo Noronha Lisboa-Filho [1] and Fabio Augusto Barbieri [3]

1. Medicine and Nanotechnology Applied Physics Group (GFAMN), Department of Physics and Meteorology, School of Sciences, São Paulo University (Unesp), Bauru 17033-360, SP, Brazil; paulo.lisboa@unesp.br
2. REVAL Rehabilitation Research Center, Faculty of Rehabilitation Sciences, Hasselt University, 3500 Hasselt, Belgium; felipe.balistierisantinelli@uhasselt.be
3. Human Movement Research Laboratory (MOVI-LAB), Department of Physical Education, School of Sciences, São Paulo State University (Unesp), Bauru 17033-360, SP, Brazil; fabio.barbieri@unesp.br
* Correspondence: marcela.oliveira@unesp.br

Abstract: The imbalance in the concentration of metallic nanoparticles has been demonstrated to play an important role in multiple sclerosis (MS), which may impact cognition. Biomarkers are needed to provide insights into the pathogenesis and diagnosis of MS. They can be used to gain a better understanding of cognitive decline in people with MS (pwMS). In this study, we investigated the relationship between the blood concentration of metallic nanoparticles (blood nanoparticles) and cognitive performance in pwMS. First, four mL blood samples, clinical characteristics, and cognitive performance were obtained from 21 pwMS. All participants had relapse–remitting MS, with a score of ≤4.5 points in the expanded disability status scale. They were relapse-free in the three previous months from the day of collection and had no orthopedic, muscular, cardiac, and cerebellar diseases. We quantified the following metallic nanoparticles: aluminum, chromium, copper, iron, magnesium, nickel, zinc, and total concentration. Cognitive performance was measured by mini-mental state examination (MMSE) and the symbol digit modalities test (SDMT). Pearson's and Spearman's correlation coefficients and stepwise linear regression were calculated to assess the relationship between cognitive performance and blood nanoparticles. We found that better performance in SDMT and MMSE was related to higher total blood nanoparticles (r = 0.40; $p < 0.05$). Also, better performance in cognitive processing speed and attention (SDMT) and mental state (MMSE) were related to higher blood iron (r = 0.44; $p < 0.03$) and zinc concentrations (r = 0.41; $p < 0.05$), respectively. The other metallic nanoparticles (aluminum, chromium, copper, magnesium, and nickel) did not show a significant relationship with the cognitive parameters ($p > 0.05$). Linear regression estimated a significant association between blood iron concentration and SDMT performance. In conclusion, blood nanoparticles are related to cognitive performance in pwMS. Our findings suggest that the blood concentration of metallic nanoparticles, particularly the iron concentration, is a promising biomarker for monitoring cognitive impairment in pwMS.

Keywords: cognition; multiple sclerosis; processing speed of information; attention; memory; nanoparticles; metal; neuropsychological tests; biomarkers; blood

Citation: de Oliveira, M.; Santinelli, F.B.; Lisboa-Filho, P.N.; Barbieri, F.A. The Blood Concentration of Metallic Nanoparticles Is Related to Cognitive Performance in People with Multiple Sclerosis: An Exploratory Analysis. Biomedicines 2023, 11, 1819. https://doi.org/10.3390/biomedicines11071819

Academic Editors: Simone Battaglia and Masaru Tanaka

Received: 12 April 2023
Revised: 27 May 2023
Accepted: 20 June 2023
Published: 25 June 2023

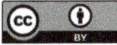

Copyright: © 2023 by the authors. Licensee MDPI, Basel, Switzerland. This article is an open access article distributed under the terms and conditions of the Creative Commons Attribution (CC BY) license (https://creativecommons.org/licenses/by/4.0/).

1. Introduction

Multiple sclerosis (MS) is characterized by a demyelination process that occurs within the central nervous system (CNS), resulting in brain damage and atrophy [1]. Although MS is commonly associated with sensory and motor symptoms [2], cognitive impairment is a frequent manifestation already found in the early stages of the disease [3]. Cognitive impairment is a significant contributor to work-related problems and job loss and indicates a higher risk of future disability worsening [3,4]. The prevalence of cognitive impairment in people with MS (pwMS) ranges from 34% to 65% [5]. Cognitive impairment can be found across all MS phenotypes: 20–25% of individuals with a clinically isolated syndrome, 30–45% of individuals with relapsing–remitting MS, and 50–75% of individuals with secondary progressive MS display cognitive deficits [5,6]. The main cognitive domains affected by MS include cognitive processing speed, visual and verbal memory, executive function, and visuospatial processing [7]. However, changes in cognitive performance in MS are often overlooked, leading to delays in treatment adaptations and hindering the monitoring of disease progression.

Understanding the causes of cognitive deficits and precisely determining cognitive impairment are critical for the effective treatment and management of MS. In a recent study by Rademacher et al. [8], an overview was provided on the use of biological markers to investigate their association with performance on cognitive tests in pwMS. Previous studies have suggested that inflammatory activity and neuro-axonal loss may play a role in cognitive function in MS [2]. Also, cognitive deficits such as defective cognitive processing speeds and impaired learning and memory have been linked to regional grey matter atrophy, the disruption of neural networks, and a lack of compensatory mechanisms in MS, as demonstrated by functional magnetic resonance imaging (MRI) [3]. High levels of iron deposition in the pulvinar, putamen, caudate nucleus, and globus pallidus have also been correlated with reduced cognitive performance in pwMS [9]. While these findings provide valuable insights to explain cognitive impairment in MS, brain imaging analysis protocols (e.g., MRI) can be expensive, inaccessible to all, and require complex techniques. Thus, the development of more affordable and accessible methods for diagnosis and assessment may aid in the early detection and treatment of cognitive impairment in MS.

Diagnosing cognitive impairment in individuals with MS can be challenging. For example, clinicians must consider various factors such as psychiatric comorbidities, medication side effects, and MS symptoms that may negatively impact cognitive performance when making a diagnosis [3]. The mini-mental state examination (MMSE) and the symbol digit modalities test (SDMT) are commonly used tests to screen for cognitive deficits in MS. Considering that information processing speed and attention may be impaired early in MS [10], the SDMT seems to be the most effective single tool to assess cognition even in the initial stages of the disease [3,7]. The SDMT is widely recommended due to its sensitivity, reliability, and predictive validity in pwMS [3,7]. However, it should be noted that while the SDMT assesses information processing speed and attention effectively, it is not specific enough to evaluate other cognitive domains such as working memory, short- and long-term memory, paired-associate learning, and visual scanning, which are also important for overall cognitive performance.

Another commonly used tool, the MMSE, can provide screening of mental state, including memory and executive function. However, it is not sensitive or specific enough to comprehensively evaluate cognition in MS [10]. While simple neuropsychological tests are helpful for routine care for pwMS, they are not sufficient on their own to fully evaluate cognition in MS and do not present unified cut-off scores for cognitive impairment in MS [11] due to the involvement of multiple cognitive domains [10]. Therefore, the identification of biomarkers to complement the diagnosis of cognitive impairment is emergent in MS. Biomarkers can provide a more comprehensive and complete assessment of cognitive performance and aid in monitoring cognitive impairment over time. Integration of biomarkers into the diagnostic process has the potential to enhance the understanding and management of cognitive impairment in MS.

The role of an imbalance in the concentration of metallic nanoparticles in MS degeneration has been established [12]. Metallic elements are known to be neuroactive and can affect various parts of the body, including the CNS [13]. An imbalance in the concentration of metallic nanoparticles may have adverse effects on cellular function, leading to oxidative stress, cell death, and brain damage [9]. Previous studies have reported that around 90% of neurodegenerative diseases are associated with exposure to potentially toxic elements, including metals found in manufacturing, contaminating ecosystems, arable soils, air, and food [14]. Oliveira et al. [12] demonstrated a decrease in the blood concentration of beryllium, copper, chromium, cobalt, nickel, magnesium, and iron, as well as an increase in lead concentrations in pwMS. The low levels of metallic elements in the body play a critical role in various metabolic processes, the development of the nervous system, and the myelination of nerve fibers [15]. In addition, these low blood values may suggest the accumulation of these elements in the CNS, including brain iron accumulation [16]. Therefore, considering that the concentration of metallic nanoparticles has been proposed as a potential cause of neurodegeneration in MS [12], it is plausible to hypothesize that the blood concentration of metallic nanoparticles could also be related to cognitive impairment in pwMS. However, the specific role of the blood concentration of metallic nanoparticles in explaining cognitive dysfunction remains unclear and has not been extensively explored yet. On the other hand, there is promising potential for the use of nanomaterials in the treatment and diagnosis of MS, although their applications are still in their infancy [17]. In this manuscript, we present an exploratory investigation into the relationship between the blood concentration of metallic nanoparticles and cognitive performance, specifically focusing on information processing speed, attention, memory, and executive function in pwMS.

2. Materials and Methods

2.1. Participants

Two power analyses (G*power©) were calculated to determine the sample size of the study. The first analysis indicated a minimum of 19 participants required for correlation (power of 80%, alpha of 0.05, and Cohen's effect size for a large correlation of 0.60). The second analysis indicated a minimum of 13 participants required for linear regression (power of 80%, alpha of 0.05, Cohen's effect size for a large correlation of 0.64, and 2 predictors) [18,19]. Thus, 21 individuals with MS between 18–42 years of age were enrolled in the present study. The inclusion criteria were as follows: (i) a score of $\leq$4.5 points on the expanded disability status scale (EDSS) [20], (ii) relapse-free in the three previous months from the day of evaluation, and (iii) the absence of orthopedic, muscular, cardiac, and cerebellar diseases. All participants exhibited the relapse–remitting type of MS in accordance with the revised McDonald criteria [21]. Additionally, participants with other diseases that could potentially interfere with the method analysis were excluded.

2.2. Study Protocol and Data Analysis

The evaluation assessment procedures were performed in a single visit and standardized in the morning. First, height and weight were measured, and a blood sample was collected. This was followed by clinical evaluation and cognitive tests. The procedures were approved by the School of Sciences ethics committee of the São Paulo State University (3 November 2018—identification code: CAAE #99191318000005398), and all participants signed an informed consent form before data collection.

Four milliliters (mL) of whole blood samples were obtained from all subjects following standard procedures. The samples were collected in dry tubes without an anticoagulant factor for the quantification of blood metallic nanoparticles. Subsequently, all samples were freeze-dried and stored deep-frozen until use. The analyses were conducted in accordance with the recommendations outlined in Oliveira et al.'s study [12]. In brief, approximately 0.2 g (equivalent to ~1.2 mL) of freeze-dried whole blood was added to a mixture containing 3 mL of nitric acid and 2 mL of hydrogen peroxide. The samples were then placed in closed vessels and digested using microwave-assisted digestion techniques, following these steps: (i) 15 min of temperature ramp up to 180 °C and (ii) 15 min duration at 180 °C. This type of procedure has been found to be highly effective for digesting organic samples and biological fluids [22]. After, the digested samples were diluted using a 1.2/25 (v/v) ratio and filled up to 25 mL with deionized water. The diluted samples were then analyzed using inductively coupled plasma—optical emission spectrometry (ICP-OES). The ICP technique, known for its high sensibility, wide dynamic range, and multi-element capability, has been widely utilized for quantifying various elements in bodily fluids [23]. Its application ensures accurate measurement of metals in the blood samples of this study. The reference whole blood sample was digested under the same conditions as the study samples and blank samples. Hydrogen peroxide and nitric acid were considered as blanks in the analytical method. The concentration of metallic elements, including aluminum, chromium, copper, iron, magnesium, nickel, and zinc, was quantified using ICP-OES. Also, the total blood concentration of metallic nanoparticles for each participant was calculated by summing the blood concentration of each metallic nanoparticle.

The EDSS [20], provided by the participants' neurologists, was used for quantifying disability. This scale classifies individuals on a scale of 1 to 10. Scores from 1.0 to 4.5 indicate pwMS who are capable of walking without assistance, while scores from 5.0 to 10 represent individuals with walking impairment. Additionally, information regarding the time since the last relapse (relapse time) and MS onset (disease duration from onset) was also obtained.

The SDMT [24] and MMSE [25] were measured by trained staff to assess the cognitive level of the participants. The SDMT measures cognitive processing speed and attention. It involves a substitution task using a coding key with nine different abstract symbols, each paired with a numeral. A series of these symbols is presented below the key, and the participants are required to respond verbally with the corresponding number for each symbol. Prior to the actual test, the participants completed a practice session consisting of 10 items. During the practice session, any errors made by the participants were corrected by the evaluator, who explained the substitution of the symbol with its corresponding numeral based on the key. The actual test comprises completing as many as 110 items with a time limit of 90 s. The number of correct substitutions/responses made within this timeframe was recorded as the individual's score. The SDMT has been previously validated for use in MS [7]. MMSE measures mental state and evaluates various aspects of cognitive status, including executive function, attention, language, memory, orientation, and visuospatial proficiency. It consists of an 11-question assessment that measures cognitive function across five areas: orientation, registration, attention and calculation, recall, and language. The maximum score achievable for MMSE is 30. MMSE has become widely adopted as a short screening tool for providing cognitive impairment in clinical, research, and community settings [26].

2.3. Statistical Analysis

Statistical analysis was conducted using IBM SPSS software version 26 (IBM Corporation, Armory, NY, USA), with a significance level set at $p < 0.05$. The normality of the cognitive data was assessed using the Shapiro–Wilk test. The SDMT exhibited a normal distribution ($p = 0.201$), while MMSE showed a non-normal distribution ($p = 0.01$). For the SDMT, Pearson's correlation coefficient was applied to examine the relationship between cognitive performance and the blood concentration of metallic nanoparticles. For MMSE, Spearman's correlation coefficient was used. The strength of the correlation was classified as weak ($0 < r < 0.3$), moderate ($0.3 \leq r < 0.5$), or strong ($r \geq 0.5$) [27]. Blood concentrations of metallic nanoparticles that exhibited significant correlation with cognitive variables were included in a stepwise linear regression model.

3. Results

The individual, clinical, and cognition characteristics and blood concentration of metallic nanoparticles are presented in Table 1. Additionally, individual data for the participants' characteristics and blood concentration of metallic nanoparticles are shown in the Supplementary Material (Table S1).

Table 1. Means, standard deviations, maximum and minimum values of individual, clinical, and cognition characteristics, and the study participants' blood concentration of metallic nanoparticles.

Individual Characteristics	
Sex (female/male)	12/9
Age (years)	32 ± 7 (45–18)
Height (m)	1.68 ± 0.02 (1.89–1.55)
Body mass (kg)	74.4 ± 3.1(94.6–51.1)
Clinical characteristics	
EDSS (points)	2.5 ± 1.1 (4.5–1.0)
Relapse time (months)	38 ± 30 (94–3)
Multiple sclerosis onset (months)	92 ± 77 (276–5)
Cognitive characteristics	
SDMT (points)	50.49 ± 10.70 (65–23)
MMSE (points)	29.05 ± 0.80 (30–28)
Blood concentration of metallic nanoparticles	
Aluminum (ug/L)	7.56 ± 2.52 (16.18–4.39)
Copper (ug/L)	0.98 ± 0.39 (1.78–0.44)
Chromium (ug/L)	0.39 ± 0.11 (0.65–0.29)
Iron (ug/L)	297.16 ± 43.84 (363.58–190.74)
Magnesium (ug/L)	28.69 ± 5.59 (41.77–20.03)
Nickel (ug/L)	0.31 ± 0.48 (1.69–0.04)
Zinc (ug/L)	3.20 ± 0.85 (4.58–1.63)
Total (ug/L)	338.30 ± 42.23 (404.92–235.56)

EDSS—expanded disability status scale; SDMT—symbol digit modalities test; MMSE—mini-mental state examination.

The SDMT and MMSE were related to the blood concentration of metallic nanoparticles (Figure 1). Specifically, better cognitive performance on the SDMT was moderately related to higher blood iron concentration and total blood concentration of metallic nanoparticles. In addition, magnesium and copper showed a relationship that approached the threshold of significance, indicating a trend towards a moderately negative relationship with the SDMT ($p = 0.06$ and 0.07, respectively). In the case of MMSE, better cognitive performance was moderately related to higher blood zinc concentration and total blood concentration of metallic nanoparticles. The relationship with iron concentration also approached significance ($p = 0.07$), suggesting a tendency towards a moderate association with MMSE. The other metallic nanoparticles, including aluminum, chromium, copper, magnesium, and nickel, did not show a significant association with the cognitive parameters in our study ($p > 0.05$).

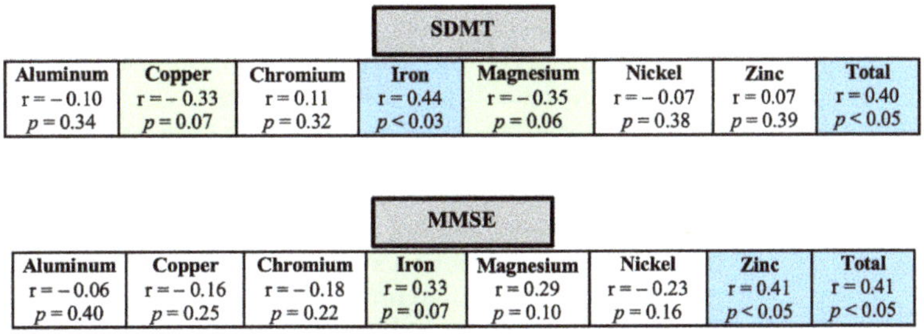

SDMT							
Aluminum	Copper	Chromium	Iron	Magnesium	Nickel	Zinc	Total
r = −0.10	r = −0.33	r = 0.11	r = 0.44	r = −0.35	r = −0.07	r = 0.07	r = 0.40
p = 0.34	p = 0.07	p = 0.32	p < 0.03	p = 0.06	p = 0.38	p = 0.39	p < 0.05

MMSE							
Aluminum	Copper	Chromium	Iron	Magnesium	Nickel	Zinc	Total
r = −0.06	r = −0.16	r = −0.18	r = 0.33	r = 0.29	r = −0.23	r = 0.41	r = 0.41
p = 0.40	p = 0.25	p = 0.22	p = 0.07	p = 0.10	p = 0.16	p < 0.05	p < 0.05

Figure 1. Relationship between cognitive performance (SDMT—symbol digit modalities test and MMSE—mini-mental state examination) and blood concentration of metallic nanoparticles in pwMS. The r and p-values are presented for each metallic nanoparticle. A blue square indicates a significant correlation while a green square indicates a tendency towards a significant correlation. Total—total blood concentration of metallic nanoparticles.

The linear regression analysis revealed a significant association between blood iron concentration and SDMT performance. The blood iron concentration explained 19.1% of the variance in the SDMT performance (Figure 2). No relationship was observed between MMSE performance and blood concentration of any metallic nanoparticles.

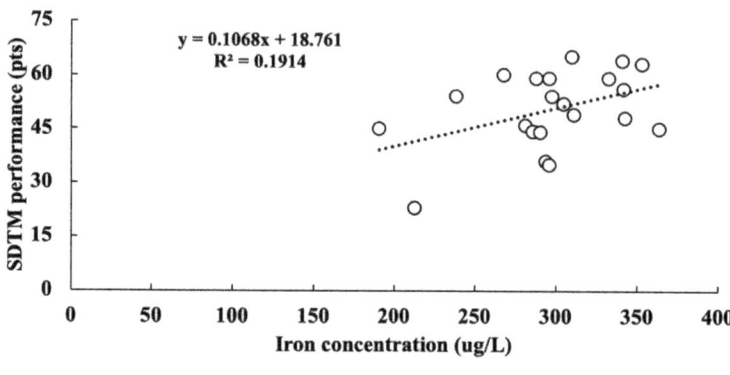

Predictors	Unstandardized β coefficient	Standardized β coefficient	Adjusted R^2	t	p-value
Constant - SDTM					
Iron concentration	0.11	0.43	0.19	2.12	0.04
Total of metallic nanoparticles concentration	-	-	-	-1.18	0.25

Figure 2. The relative contribution of blood iron concentration to the symbol digit modality test (SDMT) performance.

4. Discussion

Our study provided evidence supporting our hypothesis that a lower blood concentration of metallic nanoparticles is associated with reduced cognitive performance in pwMS. Specifically, we found that higher iron and zinc blood concentrations were moderately related to better cognitive performance on the SDMT and MMSE, respectively. Also, the blood iron concentration was a predictor of cognitive processing speed and attention performance (SDMT), explaining 19.1% of the variance in these cognitive abilities. These findings highlight the potential of the blood concentration of metallic nanoparticles as a biomarker for detecting cognitive impairment and complementing the diagnosis and monitoring of cognitive deficits in pwMS.

There is a substantial gap between candidate/validated biomarkers and clinically useful biomarkers in MS, particularly concerning cognitive impairment. Having accurate and neurobiologically plausible biomarkers can greatly enhance diagnostics, predict disease outcomes, and facilitate the monitoring of MS progression [2]. During the cognitive decline preceding progressive MS, pwMS experience early or late subclinical cognitive decline. This decline is associated with a distinct set of biomarkers that can offer valuable insights into both diagnosis and treatment approaches [28]. Our findings may suggest that the blood concentration of metallic nanoparticles holds potential as a biomarker for identifying cognitive impairment in pwMS. Metals play essential roles in various biochemical processes and the normal functioning of the CNS [29]. Transition metals, such as copper, manganese, iron, and zinc, are known to be present in active protein sites serving as metabolic co-factors for structural and catalytic functions. They are also increasingly recognized for their involvement as second messengers in cell signaling [30]. In a previous study conducted by our group [12], we demonstrated decreased blood concentrations of beryllium, copper, chromium, cobalt, nickel, magnesium, and iron, along with an increased lead concentration in pwMS. In addition, the role of metals as risk factors in the etiopathogenesis of neurodegenerative diseases is now recognized, as well as their potential involvement to cause neuronal damage in MS [31]. Thus, it is plausible to propose that the imbalance in blood concentrations of metallic nanoparticles may serve as a biomarker in MS.

Specifically for cognitive impairment, Brummer et al. [2] reported that higher levels of serum neurofilament light chain, which is a marker of neuro-axonal injury, were correlated with worse information processing speed, a key deficit underlying cognitive dysfunction in MS [3]. Serum neurofilament light chain levels have emerged as a fluid biomarker for neuro-axonal damage in MS and have been shown to predict disability progression [32]. Recently, a systematic review and meta-analysis identified several potential molecular biomarkers, such as neurofilament light chain and vitamin D, for cognitive performance in pwMS [8]. Our study adds to the understanding of the potential role of metallic nanoparticles in cognitive performance.

Metals play an indispensable role in reducing neuronal–axonal damage. For example, iron, copper, and zinc metals are crucial co-factors in the metalloproteins involved in myelin synthesis and neurotransmitter synthesis within the CNS [29,33]. In addition, the blood–brain barrier controls the transport of metal elements into the brain [34], which is regulated by the homeostasis of metals, especially zinc [35]. Specifically, metal ions interact with specific receptors in the endothelial lining, such as DMT1 and zinc transporters (ZIP8 and ZIP10), to cross the barrier and directly interact with cellular components in the CNS [31]. This interaction can lead to mitochondrial imbalance and increased production of reactive oxygen species, contributing to oxidative stress [31]. Disruption of metal homeostasis changes the permeability of the blood-brain barrier, allowing increased translocation of metals from the blood into the brain, which can exacerbate oxidative stress and other processes [36]. This imbalance in oxidative stress can trigger a pro-inflammatory response in microglia, characterized by the production of cytokines like IL-1, IL-6, and TNF-alpha, ultimately affecting neuronal viability and myelin production [31]. It is important to consider that the concentration of metals in the blood may indirectly reflect their concentration in the brain and be associated with neurodegeneration processes [37], including cognitive damage. For example, in our study, we observed a reduction in the blood concentration of metallic nanoparticles, which may suggest a higher brain concentration of these nanoparticles. Previous studies have linked higher brain concentrations of metallic nanoparticles to cognitive impairment [38]. Therefore, investigating the relationship between the blood concentration of metallic nanoparticles and the cognitive status of individuals with MS holds promise as a tool for monitoring cognitive progression in MS.

Lesion burden has been identified as a predictor of cognitive disability in MS. Metal deposition is one of the factors contributing to brain lesions, which can have adverse effects on cellular function, including altering protein production and inducing cell death [39]. In addition, Metal ions such as zinc, iron, and copper have also been implicated in the aggregation of Aβ-amyloid and α-synuclein, triggering neurodegeneration [40]. Specifically, we showed that higher blood iron concentration was related to better attention and information processing speed (SDMT), while higher blood zinc concentration was related to better mental state (e.g., memory and executive function) (MMSE). Considering that the metal concentration in the blood and brain are interrelated, with higher levels in the blood corresponding to lower levels in the brain, and vice versa, our findings corroborated with Fujiwara et al.'s study [38], which showed a moderate association between increased iron levels in the globus pallidus and lower cognitive composite scores, including attention and information processing speed, in pwMS. However, it is worth mentioning that Modica et al. [9] did not find a relationship between iron concentration and attention and information processing speed in pwMS when accounting for regional atrophy. Thus, one may argue that the relationship between iron concentration and cognitive performance, particularly in attention and information processing speed, is still a topic of debate. Nonetheless, previous studies have shown that altered iron levels contribute to poor myelination, which is correlated with cognitive decline [41], underscoring the importance of iron concentration in cognitive impairment.

Regarding zinc, the alterations in blood zinc concentration in pwMS are still conflicting: no alteration [42] vs. reduced concentration [15] compared to controls. Despite the inconsistencies in blood zinc concentration, it is important to note that alterations in zinc levels can have detrimental effects on neuronal cells, with both elevated and reduced levels being potentially neurotoxic and contributing to neurodegeneration [35]. Changes in blood zinc concentration may lead to increased extracellular zinc and decreased functioning of zinc in synaptic processes, which has been associated with cognitive decline [43]. Moreover, zinc distribution in the brain is region-specific, with certain areas such as the cerebral cortex and the hippocampus playing a role in cognitive processing [44]. It is worth mentioning that our study is the first to establish a relationship between blood zinc concentration and cognitive status in individuals with MS. However, further research is necessary to validate our findings and gain a better understanding of the potential effects of altered blood zinc concentration on cognition in pwMS.

In short, our findings highlight the potential of blood concentration of metallic nanoparticles, particularly blood iron concentration, as a promising tool for monitoring cognitive impairment in pwMS. The analysis of metallic nanoparticle levels may be one of the ways to confirm cognitive impairment in people with MS, helping in both the diagnosis and monitoring of cognitive performance. In addition, our findings have significant implications for the lifestyle of pwMS. These findings emphasize the importance of reducing metal exposure from the environment, food, and industry to mitigate potential adverse effects. Thus, conducting longitudinal studies would provide valuable insights into the stability and progression of the relationship between metals and cognitive patterns over time in MS. Monitoring cognitive performance and metallic nanoparticle concentrations longitudinally would strengthen the robustness of our findings. Despite promising results, our study should be analyzed cautiously and considered preliminary. Although we had an effective sample size, the inclusion of a small sample of pwMS may impact the statistical power of our analysis. However, we observed moderate correlations and significant relationships (regression) even with a small sample, which is promising. Furthermore, future studies should expand on this analysis by including a broader range of metals, such as manganese, cobalt, and lead. Also, our findings should be validated with a larger sample size and across the full spectrum of MS disability levels, as our study focused on individuals with low-to-moderate disability (EDSS 1 to 4.5). In addition, our sample has no greater cognitive decline. Testing if our findings are consistent in pwMS with more pronounced cognitive decline is critical.

5. Conclusions

In conclusion, our study demonstrated a significant relationship between the blood concentration of metallic nanoparticles and cognitive performance in pwMS. Specifically, we found that a higher blood iron concentration is associated with better cognitive processing speed and attention, as measured by the SDMT. Also, blood zinc concentration is related to higher mental states, including memory and executive function, as measured by MMSE. These findings suggest that the blood concentration of metallic nanoparticles holds promise as a biomarker for cognitive impairment in pwMS.

Supplementary Materials: The following supporting information can be downloaded at: https://www.mdpi.com/article/10.3390/biomedicines11071819/s1, Table S1: Values of individual, clinical, and cognition characteristics, and the study's participants' blood concentration of metallic nanoparticles.

Author Contributions: Conceptualization, M.d.O. and F.B.S.; methodology, M.d.O. and F.B.S.; formal analysis, F.B.S.; investigation, M.d.O., F.B.S., P.N.L.-F. and F.A.B.; data curation, M.d.O. and F.A.B.; writing—original draft preparation, F.A.B. and M.d.O.; writing—review and editing, all authors; supervision, F.A.B.; project administration, F.A.B.; funding acquisition, M.d.O., F.B.S., P.N.L.-F. and F.A.B. All authors have read and agreed to the published version of the manuscript.

Funding: This work was supported by the São Paulo Research Foundation (FAPESP—grant number 2018/18078-0, and 2017/20032-5). Partial funding by Pró-Reitoria de Pesquisa Unesp (number 4440).

Institutional Review Board Statement: The study was approved by the School of Sciences ethics committee of the São Paulo State University (3 November 2018—identification code: CAAE #99191318000005398).

Informed Consent Statement: Informed consent was obtained from all subjects involved in the study.

Data Availability Statement: The data presented in this study are available in this article.

Conflicts of Interest: The authors declare no conflict of interest.

References

1. Dutta, R.; Trapp, B.D. Mechanisms of Neuronal Dysfunction and Degeneration in Multiple Sclerosis. *Prog. Neurobiol.* **2011**, *93*, 1–12. [CrossRef]
2. Brummer, T.; Muthuraman, M.; Steffen, F.; Uphaus, T.; Minch, L.; Person, M.; Zipp, F.; Groppa, S.; Bittner, S.; Fleischer, V. Improved Prediction of Early Cognitive Impairment in Multiple Sclerosis Combining Blood and Imaging Biomarkers. *Brain Commun.* **2022**, *4*, fcac153. [CrossRef] [PubMed]
3. Benedict, R.H.B.; Amato, M.P.; DeLuca, J.; Geurts, J.J.G. Cognitive Impairment in Multiple Sclerosis: Clinical Management, MRI, and Therapeutic Avenues. *Lancet Neurol.* **2020**, *19*, 860–871. [CrossRef] [PubMed]
4. Frndak, S.E.; Kordovski, V.M.; Cookfair, D.; Rodgers, J.D.; Weinstock-Guttman, B.; Benedict, R.H.B. Disclosure of Disease Status among Employed Multiple Sclerosis Patients: Association with Negative Work Events and Accommodations. *Mult. Scler.* **2015**, *21*, 225–234. [CrossRef]
5. Ruano, L.; Portaccio, E.; Goretti, B.; Niccolai, C.; Severo, M.; Patti, F.; Cilia, S.; Gallo, P.; Grossi, P.; Ghezzi, A.; et al. Age and Disability Drive Cognitive Impairment in Multiple Sclerosis across Disease Subtypes. *Mult. Scler. J.* **2017**, *23*, 1258–1267. [CrossRef]
6. Johnen, A.; Landmeyer, N.C.; Bürkner, P.-C.; Wiendl, H.; Meuth, S.G.; Holling, H. Distinct Cognitive Impairments in Different Disease Courses of Multiple Sclerosis—A Systematic Review and Meta-Analysis. *Neurosci. Biobehav. Rev.* **2017**, *83*, 568–578. [CrossRef] [PubMed]
7. Benedict, R.H.; DeLuca, J.; Phillips, G.; LaRocca, N.; Hudson, L.D.; Rudick, R. Validity of the Symbol Digit Modalities Test as a Cognition Performance Outcome Measure for Multiple Sclerosis. *Mult. Scler. J.* **2017**, *23*, 721–733. [CrossRef]
8. Rademacher, T.-D.; Meuth, S.G.; Wiendl, H.; Johnen, A.; Landmeyer, N.C. Molecular Biomarkers and Cognitive Impairment in Multiple Sclerosis: State of the Field, Limitations, and Future Direction—A Systematic Review and Meta-Analysis. *Neurosci. Biobehav. Rev.* **2023**, *146*, 105035. [CrossRef]
9. Modica, C.M.; Zivadinov, R.; Dwyer, M.G.; Bergsland, N.; Weeks, A.R.; Benedict, R.H.B. Iron and Volume in the Deep Gray Matter: Association with Cognitive Impairment in Multiple Sclerosis. *Am. J. Neuroradiol.* **2015**, *36*, 57–62. [CrossRef]
10. Oset, M.; Stasiolek, M.; Matysiak, M. Cognitive Dysfunction in the Early Stages of Multiple Sclerosis—How Much and How Important? *Curr. Neurol. Neurosci. Rep.* **2020**, *20*, 22. [CrossRef]
11. Migliore, S.; Ghazaryan, A.; Simonelli, I.; Pasqualetti, P.; Squitieri, F.; Curcio, G.; Landi, D.; Palmieri, M.G.; Moffa, F.; Filippi, M.M.; et al. Cognitive Impairment in Relapsing-Remitting Multiple Sclerosis Patients with Very Mild Clinical Disability. *Behav. Neurol.* **2017**, *2017*, 7404289. [CrossRef]
12. de Oliveira, M.; Gianeti, T.M.R.; da Rocha, F.C.G.; Lisboa-Filho, P.N.; Piacenti-Silva, M. A Preliminary Study of the Concentration of Metallic Elements in the Blood of Patients with Multiple Sclerosis as Measured by ICP-MS. *Sci. Rep.* **2020**, *10*, 13112. [CrossRef] [PubMed]
13. Crichton, R.R.; Dexter, D.T.; Ward, R.J. Metal Based Neurodegenerative Diseases—From Molecular Mechanisms to Therapeutic Strategies. *Coord. Chem. Rev.* **2008**, *252*, 1189–1199. [CrossRef]
14. Cabral Pinto, M.M.S.; Marinho-Reis, A.P.; Almeida, A.; Ordens, C.M.; Silva, M.M.V.G.; Freitas, S.; Simões, M.R.; Moreira, P.I.; Dinis, P.A.; Diniz, M.L.; et al. Human Predisposition to Cognitive Impairment and Its Relation with Environmental Exposure to Potentially Toxic Elements. *Environ. Geochem. Health* **2018**, *40*, 1767–1784. [CrossRef] [PubMed]
15. Nirooei, E.; Kashani, S.M.A.; Owrangi, S.; Malekpour, F.; Niknam, M.; Moazzen, F.; Nowrouzi-Sohrabi, P.; Farzinmehr, S.; Akbari, H. Blood Trace Element Status in Multiple Sclerosis: A Systematic Review and Meta-Analysis. *Biol. Trace Elem. Res.* **2021**, *200*, 13–26. [CrossRef]

16. Chen, P.; Miah, M.R.; Aschner, M. Metals and Neurodegeneration. *F1000Research* **2016**, *5*, 366. [CrossRef]
17. Singh, A.V.; Khare, M.; Gade, W.N.; Zamboni, P. Theranostic Implications of Nanotechnology in Multiple Sclerosis: A Future Perspective. *Autoimmune Dis.* **2012**, *2012*, 160830. [CrossRef]
18. Faul, F.; Erdfelder, E.; Lang, A.-G.; Buchner, A. G*Power 3: A Flexible Statistical Power Analysis Program for the Social, Behavioral, and Biomedical Sciences. *Behav. Res. Methods* **2007**, *39*, 175–191. [CrossRef]
19. Sullivan, G.M.; Feinn, R. Using Effect Size—Or Why the P Value Is Not Enough. *J. Grad. Med. Educ.* **2012**, *4*, 279–282. [CrossRef]
20. Kurtzke, J.F. Rating Neurologic Impairment in Multiple Sclerosis: An Expanded Disability Status Scale (EDSS). *Neurology* **1983**, *33*, 1444. [CrossRef]
21. Thompson, A.J.; Banwell, B.L.; Barkhof, F.; Carroll, W.M.; Coetzee, T.; Comi, G.; Correale, J.; Fazekas, F.; Filippi, M.; Freedman, M.S.; et al. Diagnosis of Multiple Sclerosis: 2017 Revisions of the McDonald Criteria. *Lancet Neurol.* **2018**, *17*, 162–173. [CrossRef] [PubMed]
22. Gonzalez, M.H.; Souza, G.B.; Oliveira, R.V.; Forato, L.A.; Nóbrega, J.A.; Nogueira, A.R.A. Microwave-Assisted Digestion Procedures for Biological Samples with Diluted Nitric Acid: Identification of Reaction Products. *Talanta* **2009**, *79*, 396–401. [CrossRef] [PubMed]
23. Bocca, B.; Forte, G.; Petrucci, F.; Senofonte, O.; Violante, N.; Alimonti, A. Development of Methods for the Quantification of Essential and Toxic Elements in Human Biomonitoring. *Ann. Ist. Super. Sanita* **2005**, *41*, 165–170. [PubMed]
24. Boringa, J.B.; Lazeron, R.H.; Reuling, I.E.; Adèr, H.J.; Pfennings, L.; Lindeboom, J.; de Sonneville, L.M.; Kalkers, N.F.; Polman, C.H. The Brief Repeatable Battery of Neuropsychological Tests: Normative Values Allow Application in Multiple Sclerosis Clinical Practice. *Mult. Scler.* **2001**, *7*, 263–267. [CrossRef]
25. Folstein, M.F.; Folstein, S.E.; McHugh, P.R. "Mini-Mental State". A Practical Method for Grading the Cognitive State of Patients for the Clinician. *J. Psychiatr. Res.* **1975**, *12*, 189–198. [CrossRef]
26. Arevalo-Rodriguez, I.; Smailagic, N.; Roqué I Figuls, M.; Ciapponi, A.; Sanchez-Perez, E.; Giannakou, A.; Pedraza, O.L.; Bonfill Cosp, X.; Cullum, S. Mini-Mental State Examination (MMSE) for the Detection of Alzheimer's Disease and Other Dementias in People with Mild Cognitive Impairment (MCI). *Cochrane Database Syst. Rev.* **2015**, *2015*, CD010783. [CrossRef]
27. Cohen, J. *Statistical Power Analysis for the Behavioral Sciences*, 2nd ed.; Routledge: New York, NY, USA, 1988.
28. LoPresti, P. Serum-Based Biomarkers in Neurodegeneration and Multiple Sclerosis. *Biomedicines* **2022**, *10*, 1077. [CrossRef]
29. Dales, J.-P.; Desplat-Jégo, S. Metal Imbalance in Neurodegenerative Diseases with a Specific Concern to the Brain of Multiple Sclerosis Patients. *Int. J. Mol. Sci.* **2020**, *21*, 9105. [CrossRef]
30. Barnham, K.J.; Bush, A.I. Biological Metals and Metal-Targeting Compounds in Major Neurodegenerative Diseases. *Chem. Soc. Rev.* **2014**, *43*, 6727–6749. [CrossRef]
31. Ferrero, M.E. Neuron Protection by EDTA May Explain the Successful Outcomes of Toxic Metal Chelation Therapy in Neurodegenerative Diseases. *Biomedicines* **2022**, *10*, 2476. [CrossRef]
32. Bittner, S.; Oh, J.; Havrdová, E.K.; Tintoré, M.; Zipp, F. The Potential of Serum Neurofilament as Biomarker for Multiple Sclerosis. *Brain* **2021**, *144*, 2954–2963. [CrossRef]
33. Hametner, S.; Dal Bianco, A.; Trattnig, S.; Lassmann, H. Iron Related Changes in MS Lesions and Their Validity to Characterize MS Lesion Types and Dynamics with Ultra-High Field Magnetic Resonance Imaging. *Brain Pathol.* **2018**, *28*, 743–749. [CrossRef]
34. Skjørringe, T.; Møller, L.B.; Moos, T. Impairment of Interrelated Iron- and Copper Homeostatic Mechanisms in Brain Contributes to the Pathogenesis of Neurodegenerative Disorders. *Front. Pharmacol.* **2012**, *3*, 169. [CrossRef]
35. Qi, Z.; Liu, K.J. The Interaction of Zinc and the Blood-Brain Barrier under Physiological and Ischemic Conditions. *Toxicol. Appl. Pharmacol.* **2019**, *364*, 114–119. [CrossRef]
36. Johnson, S. The Possible Role of Gradual Accumulation of Copper, Cadmium, Lead and Iron and Gradual Depletion of Zinc, Magnesium, Selenium, Vitamins B2, B6, D, and E Essential Fatty Acids in Multiple Sclerosis. *Med. Hypotheses* **2000**, *55*, 239–241. [CrossRef]
37. Ontaneda, D.; Thompson, A.J.; Fox, R.J.; Cohen, J.A. Progressive Multiple Sclerosis: Prospects for Disease Therapy, Repair, and Restoration of Function. *Lancet* **2017**, *389*, 1357–1366. [CrossRef]
38. Fujiwara, E.; Kmech, J.A.; Cobzas, D.; Sun, H.; Seres, P.; Blevins, G.; Wilman, A.H. Cognitive Implications of Deep Gray Matter Iron in Multiple Sclerosis. *AJNR. Am. J. Neuroradiol.* **2017**, *38*, 942–948. [CrossRef] [PubMed]
39. Williams, R.; Buchheit, C.L.; Berman, N.E.J.; LeVine, S.M. Pathogenic Implications of Iron Accumulation in Multiple Sclerosis. *J. Neurochem.* **2012**, *120*, 7–25. [CrossRef] [PubMed]
40. Molina-Holgado, F.; Hider, R.C.; Gaeta, A.; Williams, R.; Francis, P. Metals Ions and Neurodegeneration. *BioMetals* **2007**, *20*, 639–654. [CrossRef] [PubMed]
41. Bartzokis, G. Age-Related Myelin Breakdown: A Developmental Model of Cognitive Decline and Alzheimer's Disease. *Neurobiol. Aging* **2004**, *25*, 5–62. [CrossRef]
42. da Silva Castro, Á.; da Silva Albuquerque, L.; de Melo, M.L.P.; D'Almeida, J.A.C.; Braga, R.A.M.; de Assis, R.C.; do Nascimento Marreiro, D.; Matos, W.O.; Maia, C.S.C. Relationship between Zinc-Related Nutritional Status and the Progression of Multiple Sclerosis. *Mult. Scler. Relat. Disord.* **2022**, *66*, 104063. [CrossRef] [PubMed]

43. McAllum, E.J.; Finkelstein, D.I. Metals in Alzheimer's and Parkinson's Disease: Relevance to Dementia with Lewy Bodies. *J. Mol. Neurosci.* **2016**, *60*, 279–288. [CrossRef] [PubMed]
44. Choi, B.; Jung, J.; Suh, S. The Emerging Role of Zinc in the Pathogenesis of Multiple Sclerosis. *Int. J. Mol. Sci.* **2017**, *18*, 2070. [CrossRef] [PubMed]

Disclaimer/Publisher's Note: The statements, opinions and data contained in all publications are solely those of the individual author(s) and contributor(s) and not of MDPI and/or the editor(s). MDPI and/or the editor(s) disclaim responsibility for any injury to people or property resulting from any ideas, methods, instructions or products referred to in the content.

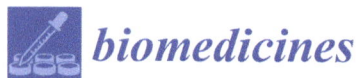

Review

Unraveling Down Syndrome: From Genetic Anomaly to Artificial Intelligence-Enhanced Diagnosis

Aabid Mustafa Koul [1], Faisel Ahmad [2], Abida Bhat [3], Qurat-ul Aein [4], Ajaz Ahmad [5,*], Aijaz Ahmad Reshi [6] and Rauf-ur-Rashid Kaul [7,*]

1. Department of Immunology and Molecular Medicine, Sher-i-Kashmir Institute of Medical Sciences, Srinagar 190006, India
2. Department of Zoology, Central University of Kashmir, Ganderbal, Srinagar 190004, India
3. Advanced Centre for Human Genetics, Sher-i-Kashmir Institute of Medical Sciences, Srinagar 190011, India
4. Department of Human Genetics, Guru Nanak Dev University, Amritsar 143005, Punjab, India; quratain417@gmail.com
5. Departments of Clinical Pharmacy, College of Pharmacy, King Saud University, Riyadh 11451, Saudi Arabia
6. Department of Computer Science, College of Computer Science and Engineering, Taibah University, Madinah 42353, Saudi Arabia; aijazonnet@gmail.com
7. Department of Community Medicine, Sher-i-Kashmir Institute of Medical Sciences, Srinagar 190006, India
* Correspondence: ajukash@gmail.com (A.A.); raufkaul@gmail.com (R.-u.-R.K.)

Abstract: Down syndrome arises from chromosomal non-disjunction during gametogenesis, resulting in an additional chromosome. This anomaly presents with intellectual impairment, growth limitations, and distinct facial features. Positive correlation exists between maternal age, particularly in advanced cases, and the global annual incidence is over 200,000 cases. Early interventions, including first and second-trimester screenings, have improved DS diagnosis and care. The manifestations of Down syndrome result from complex interactions between genetic factors linked to various health concerns. To explore recent advancements in Down syndrome research, we focus on the integration of artificial intelligence (AI) and machine learning (ML) technologies for improved diagnosis and management. Recent developments leverage AI and ML algorithms to detect subtle Down syndrome indicators across various data sources, including biological markers, facial traits, and medical images. These technologies offer potential enhancements in accuracy, particularly in cases complicated by cognitive impairments. Integration of AI and ML in Down syndrome diagnosis signifies a significant advancement in medical science. These tools hold promise for early detection, personalized treatment, and a deeper comprehension of the complex interplay between genetics and environmental factors. This review provides a comprehensive overview of neurodevelopmental and cognitive profiles, comorbidities, diagnosis, and management within the Down syndrome context. The utilization of AI and ML represents a transformative step toward enhancing early identification and tailored interventions for individuals with Down syndrome, ultimately improving their quality of life.

Keywords: Down syndrome; neurodevelopment; cognitive impairment; comorbidity; diagnosis; management; artificial intelligence; machine learning; neurological disorders; intellectual disability

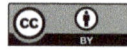

1. Introduction

Down syndrome, first described by John Langdon Down in 1866, is a genetic disorder characterized by the presence of an additional chromosome 21 due to non-disjuntioning during gametogenesis and is reportedly the most common chromosomal abnormality in humans [1–4]. Down syndrome is a genetic disorder characterized by the presence of an extra copy of chromosome 21. It manifests in three main types: trisomy 21, translocation Down syndrome, and mosaicism [5]. Trisomy 21, accounting for the majority of cases, involves an extra copy of chromosome 21 in every cell [6]. Translocation Down syndrome occurs when the extra copy is attached to another chromosome [7]. Mosaicism, the least common type, involves a mixture of cells with two and three copies of chromosome 21 [7–9]. Patients suffering with this disorder show mild to moderate intellectual disability, retarded growth besides other peculiar facial features [10].

The incidence of Down syndrome, ranging from 1 in 319 to 1 in 1000 live births, escalates with advanced maternal age, surpassing 200,000 cases annually globally [11,12]. It is established in the scientific literature that the occurrence of other autosomal trisomy is much more common than trisomy 21 but owing to their poor postnatal survival, Down syndrome takes a lead in being the most frequently occurring live born aneuploidy (trisomy 21) [13]. Differences in the incidence and presentation of Down syndrome based upon the ethnic and geographic background are also reported [14]. Besides the occurrence of non-disjunction in chromosome 21 during gametogenesis, there are other factors that can lead to trisomy 21, including Robertsonian translocation, isochromosome formation, and the presence of a ring chromosome [6]. Isochromosome formation entails the simultaneous separation of two long arms, as opposed to one long and one short arm, and this phenomenon is observed in approximately 2% to 4% of patients [15,16]. In cases of Robertsonian translocation, the long arm of chromosome 21 becomes fused with another chromosome, typically chromosome 14 [17].

Children with Down syndrome exhibit a range of malformations in addition to cognitive impairments resulting from the presence of extra genetic material from chromosome 21 [18,19]. Although the phenotype varies, common characteristics that can lead experts to suspect Down syndrome includes reduced muscular tone (hypotonia), a brachycephalic head shape, a flat nasal bridge, epicanthal folds, the presence of Brushfield spots in the iris, a small mouth, small ears, excess skin at the back of the neck, upward-slanting palpebral fissures, a short fifth finger, a single transverse palmar crease, clinodactyly (abnormal curvature of the fifth finger), and wide spacing between the first and second toes, often accompanied by a deep groove between them [20,21]. The neurodevelopmental and cognitive profiles observed in individuals with Down syndrome are characterized by significant diversity, presenting unique challenges and opportunities for diagnosis, management, and support [22]. Comorbidities associated with Down syndrome further contribute to the complexity of providing comprehensive care to this population [23–25]. Cognitive impairment in individuals with Down syndrome can range from mild (with an IQ between 50 and 70) to moderate (with an IQ between 35 and 50), and occasionally, it can be severe (with an IQ between 20 and 35) [26,27]. Additionally, individuals with Down syndrome face a significant risk of experiencing hearing loss (75%), obstructive sleep apnea (50% to 79%), otitis media (50% to 70%), eye-related issues (60%) including cataracts (15%) and severe refractive errors (50%), congenital heart defects (50%), neurological dysfunction (ranging from 1% to 13%), gastrointestinal atresias (12%), hip dislocation (6%), and thyroid disorders (ranging from 4% to 18%) (Table 1) [28].

Artificial intelligence (AI) and machine learning (ML) have emerged as powerful tools with the potential to revolutionize various fields, including healthcare [29–31]. ML, as a subset of AI, focuses on enabling computers to learn from data and improve their performance on specific tasks without explicit programming [32]. While AI is a broader concept, ML plays a crucial role in the implementation of intelligent systems [33–35]. In recent years, AI and ML have gained significant attention in healthcare due to their potential to enhance diagnosis, prediction, and treatment planning for various conditions, including DS [36]. These technologies can analyze complex medical data, identify patterns and trends, and provide valuable insights for healthcare professionals and families affected by DS [36]. ML holds promise in the field of Down syndrome by facilitating early diagnosis, predicting associated medical conditions, and enhancing educational interventions [37]. By leveraging ML algorithms to analyze large datasets of genetic and clinical information, researchers and healthcare professionals can gain valuable insights that contribute to personalized care and improved outcomes for individuals with Down syndrome [36]. Given the diverse neurodevelopmental and cognitive profiles in individuals with Down syndrome and the complexities posed by associated comorbidities, this review aims to comprehensively analyze the existing literature. It specifically focuses on neurodevelopmental and cognitive features, comorbidities, and current approaches to diagnosis and management in Down syndrome. Additionally, it explores the potential role of ML and AI in enhancing Down syndrome care, emphasizing the need for careful evaluation and further research. By synthesizing the available information, this review aims to inform and guide healthcare practitioners in their efforts to provide effective and individualized care to individuals with Down syndrome.

Table 1. Down syndrome associated complications.

S. No.	Down Syndrome Associated Complications	Occurrence
1.	Cataracts	15%
2.	Congenital heart ailments	40–50%
3.	Dental eruption (Delayed)	23%
4.	Gastrointestinal atresias	12%
5.	Hearing issues	75%
6.	Hip dislocation	6%
7.	Neurological Impairment	1–13%
8.	Otitis media	50–70%
9.	Refractive errors	50%
10.	Sleep apnea (Obstructive)	50–75%
11.	Thyroid disorders	4–18%
12.	Vision impairments	60%

2. Diagnostics

The prospective for the growth and socialization of Down syndrome affected individual has now been realized and improved with early intervention techniques, thereby timely support for DS affected children is extensively implemented [38–40]. With the introduction of first trimester screening, the options of diagnostics for Down syndrome have improved significantly. In addition to maternal age, the assessment includes nuchal translucency ultrasonography, along with the measurement of maternal serum human chorionic gonadotropin and plasma protein A in relation to the pregnancy [41–43]. The second-trimester screening incorporates the maternal age-related risk and involves measuring maternal serum hCG, unconjugated estriol, α-fetoprotein (AFP), and inhibin levels [44–46]. The first-trimester screening achieves a detection rate for Down syndrome ranging from 82% to 87%, while the second-trimester screening achieves an 80% detection rate. When both the first and second-trimester screenings are combined, often referred to as integrated screening, the detection rate increases to approximately 95% [47–49]. Early diagnosis, intervention, and ongoing support are crucial for individuals with Down syndrome to reach their full potential and lead fulfilling lives [50]. Early childhood intervention programs, involving a multidisciplinary approach, provide comprehensive support in areas such as speech, motor skills, cognition, and social-emotional development [50,51]. Individualized education plans (IEPs) tailor educational goals and accommodations to each child's unique needs, promoting inclusive learning and skill development [9,50]. Medical management, including regular check-ups and proactive care for associated health conditions, ensures optimal health outcomes [52–54]. By emphasizing the importance of early interventions and support strategies, we highlight the need to empower individuals with Down syndrome and promote their development across multiple domains [9,50].

2.1. Prenatal Diagnostics

Parental awareness plays a crucial role in the context of Down syndrome, as it is essential for parents to possess a comprehensive understanding of the potential conditions associated with Down syndrome [55,56]. Such awareness can significantly contribute to the accurate diagnosis and appropriate treatment of this disorder [57,58]. The introduction of cell-free prenatal screening and the parallel sequencing of maternal plasma cell-free DNA (cfDNA) has brought about a profound transformation in the standard approach to prenatal Down syndrome diagnosis [47]. The utilization of non-invasive prenatal screening has the potential to reduce the need for invasive tests such as amniocentesis or chorionic villus sampling [59]. Furthermore, soft markers, including the absence or small size of the nasal bone, increased nuchal fold thickness, and enlarged ventricles, can be detected through ultrasound examinations performed between the 14th and 24th weeks of gestation [60,61]. An elevated fetal nuchal translucency measurement is indeed associated with an increased risk of Down syndrome. Increased fetal detection of Down syndrome offers important benefits despite the limited need for fetal or neonatal intervention in most cases [62]. Early detection enables comprehensive prenatal counseling, facilitating informed decision-making for expectant parents and access to specialized care and support. It respects individual autonomy, allowing families to make choices aligned with their values [63].

Moreover, increased detection contributes to research and advancements in prenatal care and treatments, driving improved outcomes for individuals with Down syndrome [50,62,63]. By accumulating data and insights, it enables the development of innovative interventions, early interventions, and support strategies. Therefore, advocating for increased fetal detection is crucial, as it empowers parents, facilitates specialized care, respects personal choices, and fuels research advancements [63]. In addition to these advancements, various methods are employed for prenatal diagnosis, with traditional cytogenic analysis remaining widely used in many countries. Nevertheless, some rapid molecular assays, such as fluorescent in situ hybridization (FISH), quantitative fluorescence PCR (QF-PCR), and multiplex probe ligation assay (MLPA), are also utilized for prenatal diagnosis [7]. Prenatal diagnosis provides valuable information about the chromosomal abnormality, but it does not directly inform us about the specific cognitive and neurodevelopmental traits that individuals with Down syndrome will exhibit [1]. Understanding this variability requires comprehensive research that explores cognitive profiles, strengths, and challenges in individuals with Down syndrome, considering environmental influences and personalized experiences [22,64]. It is crucial to acknowledge that while prenatal diagnosis provides valuable information about the chromosomal abnormality, it does not directly inform us about the wide variability in neurodevelopmental and cognitive characteristics that will be unique to each person with Down syndrome [65]. Indeed, the neurodevelopmental and cognitive profiles in individuals with Down syndrome exhibit significant diversity [66,67]. While the presence of an extra copy of chromosome 21 contributes to shared characteristics, such as intellectual disability and certain physical features, the specific cognitive abilities, strengths, and challenges can vary widely among individuals [68]. Factors such as genetic variations and individual differences contribute to this variability. In order to provide a comprehensive understanding of Down syndrome, it is crucial to consider beyond prenatal diagnosis [69]. Additional assessments, evaluations, and ongoing monitoring are necessary to capture the individual's specific cognitive and neurodevelopmental traits. This includes evaluating cognitive abilities, language skills, motor development, adaptive functioning, and social-emotional aspects [69]. It emphasizes the need for personalized and individualized interventions that address the unique strengths, challenges, and needs of each person [65]. By considering the wide range of cognitive and neurodevelopmental profiles, practitioners can provide more effective and tailored support for individuals with Down syndrome [65,66]. Many countries have chosen to incorporate prenatal diagnosis into their healthcare systems, offering prospective parents an opportunity to make informed choices aligned with their personal values [70]. This encompasses decisions regarding whether to proceed with a pregnancy or consider termination of pregnancy (TOP). The integration of prenatal diagnosis respects individual autonomy by empowering families to navigate complex decisions in accordance with their unique values and beliefs. In recognizing the diversity of international practices, it is important to emphasize that the availability of prenatal diagnosis is not universally linked to the sole option of termination. Rather, it serves as a means to provide comprehensive information, fostering an environment where families can make decisions that align with their individual circumstances and ethical considerations [71,72].

2.2. Artificial Intelligence (AI)-Based Diagnosis

Medical lab tests, investigation of medical history, and genetic testing are all commonly used methods to diagnose Down syndrome. To help with the diagnosing process, artificial intelligence (AI) and machine learning (ML) approaches can be quite useful [30,35]. A variety of clinical data can be analyzed using AI and ML algorithms, which can be trained to identify patterns that might be symptomatic of Down syndrome. Incorporating ML techniques into Down syndrome detection holds significant potential for enhancing accuracy, efficiency, and accessibility [64,68,73]. The integration of machine learning (ML) into cell-free prenatal screening and maternal plasma cell-free DNA sequencing for Down syndrome diagnosis will present a transformative paradigm with significant motivations and potential enhancements. Early detection may be improved, and the potential for reduced false positives addresses concerns related to unnecessary interventions. ML's adaptive nature ensures continuous improvement, contributing to the evolution of more precise and reliable prenatal Down syndrome predictions. ML algorithms enable the analysis of large datasets encompassing clinical and genetic information, potentially identifying subtle markers and patterns that improve detection accuracy beyond traditional methods [74]. Integrating multiple data sources, including maternal age, biochemical markers, and ultrasound measurements, ML-based predictive models can yield more sophisticated risk assessments and enable precise counseling for expectant parents [35]. ML methods offer broader accessibility and cost-effectiveness compared to invasive procedures like amniocentesis or chorionic villus sampling, as they primarily rely on non-invasive data sources such as maternal blood samples and medical records. Furthermore, ML techniques can be automated and scaled, facilitating widespread implementation and reducing the economic burden associated with DS screening [35,74]. While current diagnostic methods for Down syndrome exhibit high accuracy rates, incorporating ML methods can provide additional advantages in terms of improved accuracy, risk assessment, counseling, and broader accessibility. By leveraging ML algorithms to analyze comprehensive datasets, healthcare providers can enhance DS detection and deliver more personalized care [35]. These motivations and benefits of ML methods in Down syndrome detection will be further emphasized in the revised manuscript, supporting the advocacy for their integration. ML and AI can help with the diagnosis in the following ways:

2.2.1. Facial Recognition

AI programs can be trained to identify facial characteristics that are commonly linked to Down syndrome [75]. ML models can recognize distinct features like an upward slope in the eyes, a flattened face profile, and a tiny nose by looking at facial images. These algorithms may precisely identify these features, assisting in diagnosis of Down syndrome [76].

2.2.2. Genetic Screening

AI and ML can help with the analysis of genetic algorithm data to identify the early risk of Down syndrome [77]. Medical experts may input a person's genetic sequence into an ML model, which can then compare it with a very large dataset of genetic profiles known to be associated with Down syndrome [36]. The system can assess the likelihood of Down syndrome and accurately identify biological markers.

2.2.3. Analysis of Medical Data

AI algorithms can process patient medical records [78] to find patterns and links with Down syndrome. This analysis includes historical test results, developmental milestones, and symptoms. A huge collection of patient information can be used to train machine learning models to spot patterns or warning signs that are typical of the ailment [79]. It can thus aid medical professionals in developing more precise and effective diagnosis [80].

2.2.4. Support for Prenatal Diagnosis

AI and ML can also help with Down syndrome prenatal diagnosis [49]. Artificial intelligence (AI) systems can spot possible indicators of Down syndrome in a growing fetus by examining ultrasound images [81] or blood test data. Because of the early detection, parents and medical professionals can better anticipate and support the child's requirements.

2.2.5. Decision Support Systems for Healthcare

By making timely and accurate recommendations based on patient data, AI and ML can serve as decision support tools for healthcare professionals [82]. ML models can predict the risk of Down syndrome through incorporating clinical and genomic data analysis, enabling healthcare practitioners to make well-informed decisions about additional diagnostic procedures or specialist referrals [83]. It is significant to remember that a medical practitioner should always validate the final diagnosis [84]. The purpose of AI and ML in the diagnosis of Down syndrome is to support medical practitioners by offering insightful information and improving the precision and effectiveness of the diagnostic procedure.

3. Cognitive Challenges in Down Syndrome

Cognitive functioning is the collective term for a variety of mental processes, such as retention, acquisition, reasoning, problem-solving, adaptability, and attention. Cognitive functioning, which ranges from profound to borderline intellectual capacity, is a hallmark of Down syndrome (DS) [8,85–87]. Most Down syndrome sufferers have moderate to severe intellectual disabilities. Cognitive growth goes on all the way through childhood, adolescence, and the first few years of adulthood. The loss of skills that are commonly associated with dementia gradually follows this. When compared to visual information, people with Down syndrome consistently have trouble understanding verbal information. Learning, memory, and language problems that cause mild to severe intellectual disability are characteristics of Down's syndrome [85,86,88,89].

3.1. Speech, Mental Abilities, and Memory Retention

The cognitive profiles of those with the disease differ, with maintained visuospatial short-term memory, associative learning, implicit long-term memory, poor morphosyntax, verbal short-term memory, and explicit memory. Individuals with Down syndrome are better at pictorial tasks equated to verbal short-term memory tasks [8,90]. Although infants show less vocal response and environmental alertness than older children and adults, early language milestones are often met within an age-expected range. It has been shown that youngsters acquire their first words later than anticipated [85,86]. At the outset, it is usually recognized as a characteristic to have a small vocabulary, thoughtful communication, and pragmatism in language. The usage of multi-word sentences is delayed as linguistic demands rise, and strange communication patterns emerge. Persistent language problems are noticed after a child is five. The language profiles of school-aged children reveal a noteworthy lag in the progression of expressive language when compared to receptive language. This discrepancy is most pronounced in the domains of expressive syntax and phonological processing, where the most substantial delays are observed [87,91,92]. Syntactic insufficiency is mainly evident in late infancy and the start of puberty. Adults have less phonological processing, morphosyntax, and articulation issues with language, but their semantic, pragmatic, and communicative goals remain largely unaltered. Learning, memory, and other cognitive processes can all suffer from impaired language comprehension processing [86,88,93,94].

3.2. Processing Speed, Inhibition, and Attention

The executive functions (EFs), which control behavior and cognition, include things like attention, inhibition, and processing speed. Higher level executive function includes skills like strategic planning, impulse control, systematic search, flexibility of thought and action, and the ability to blend what one wants with what they can do [94]. Teenagers with Down syndrome perform worse on tests of attention, perceptual quickness, response time, and motor control when compared to peers with similar mental ability. These limitations persist as individuals age, making it more challenging to allocate tasks, retain attention, and respond reliably to situations [95,96]. Poor response inhibition is evident across the whole developmental lifespan, with vocally mediated inhibition tasks being more difficult and having poor inhibition of irrelevant information. Response time assessments yield contradictory results, with faster reaction times compatible with intellectual functioning but slower than those with mental age matching individuals who possess intellectual disability [87,93].

3.3. Short-Term Auditory Memory

The visuospatial working memory system is more developed than the auditory working memory system, and verbal working memory deficits go beyond those seen in those who have difficulty hearing and speaking well [93,97]. Lack of engaged learning may contribute to diminished verbal memory retention in scholastic age adolescents and kids. The ability to recall information correlates with syntax interpretation in both modalities, illustrating the relationship between working memory and linguistic acquisition. When compared to verbal working memory, tasks requiring less information or when the visual and spatial components are assessed separately still have little impact on visual and spatial short-term memory [98,99]. Children with Down syndrome have trouble with problem-solving techniques, and as they become older, they take longer to complete planning activities, even when the results are similar to those of children whose mental ages are matched. Multitasking and time shifting are exceedingly challenging for children and persons with Down syndrome, especially when it comes to vocally mediated tasks [100]. People with Down syndrome commonly experience verbal comprehension, self-monitoring, and executive function deficits, in contrast to other genetic ID-related disorders. Additionally, they erroneously and more slowly assimilate information [93,101–103].

3.4. Organization, Spatial Cognition, and Self-Monitoring

Children with Down syndrome frequently experience difficulties with integrating new knowledge and problem-solving techniques, which delays down their developmental progress. As individuals age, scheduling tasks take longer to accomplish, but their efficiency is comparable to that of mental age matched controls [104]. For kids and people with Down syndrome, multitasking and setting changing are extremely difficult, especially when it comes to vocally mediated activities. Additionally, people with Down syndrome struggle with verbal comprehension and self-awareness, frequently failing to indicate when they have understood something [105,106]. Due to poor monitoring for intrusion mistakes and problems avoiding irrelevant information from interfering with cognitive processes, adults with Down syndrome still have trouble self-monitoring. The profile of visual-spatial ability in people with Down syndrome is uneven, with some parts matching average cognitive capacity and others falling short of projected developmental levels. Though cognitive function is deteriorating, visuospatial abilities are still mostly intact [86,107,108].

3.5. Learning and Long-Term Memory

Children with Down syndrome have distinct degrees of learning ability, with diminished short-term and long-term memory learning abilities [109,110]. They do better at combining rewards with objects and with observational learning, but exhibit trouble with instrumental learning [111,112]. They are more socially inclined and receptive to positive reinforcement, enhancing the success in socially oriented learning. Visual learning is more efficient than verbal learning, which shows that interpersonal abilities are robust. Problems in attention and a high demand for processing contribute to long-term memory problems in Down syndrome at the encoding and retrieval levels [113]. These deficits might be intrinsic in origin rather than just a symptom of a language processing disorder. These inadequacies persist throughout life, but they worsen with advancing years [103].

3.6. Associated Conditions and Disorders

People with Down syndrome are more likely to have a number of different health issues, such as Dementia, autism spectrum disorders, hormonal, glandular issues, sensory impairments, sleep disruption, seizures, and cardiac abnormalities [114,115]. Celiac disease, hypothyroidism, leukemia, congenital heart abnormalities, and diabetes are additional illnesses with increased occurrence in this group [85,86,116,117]. Many people with Down syndrome are born with congenital heart defects, such as atrioventricular septal defect or ventricular septal defect. These heart conditions may necessitate surgical intervention [114]. Hearing issues, including conductive or sensorineural hearing loss, are frequently observed in individuals with Down syndrome. Regular hearing assessments are crucial for early intervention [115]. Ocular problems like cataracts, strabismus (crossed eyes), and refractive errors are more common among those with Down syndrome [118]. Hypothyroidism, which is an underactive thyroid gland, is more prevalent in people with Down syndrome. Routine monitoring of thyroid function is of utmost importance [117].

4. Discussion

Down syndrome, caused by a genetic anomaly (trisomy 21), manifests in characteristic physical features and cognitive delays [9]. Individuals often contend with a range of comorbidities, including heart defects, gastrointestinal issues, and increased susceptibility to infections. These additional health concerns necessitate comprehensive medical care and early interventions to address associated challenges and optimize overall wellbeing [8,9]. Numerous co-morbidities (Figure 1) identified such as congenital heart defects, celiac disease, gastrointestinal defects, seizures, thyroid disease, hematological disorders, autism, and emotional and behavioral disorder (EBD) are known to affect the quality of life in children with Down syndrome [8,119]. Table 2 presents the various specific disorders/diseases as subcategories of these co-morbidities. Individuals with Down syndrome are also predisposed to sleep disorder breathing (SDB) which includes central sleep apnea (CSA), hypoxemia disorder, hypoventilation disorder, and obstructive sleep apnea (OSA) [120,121]. Central airway anatomical features such as small oropharynx, mid-facial hypoplasia, narrow nasopharynx, and macroglossia contribute DS towards increased susceptibility for SDB [122,123]. Many previous studies have reported SDB high prevalence associated with Down syndrome condition compared to the general population [124–126]. Douglas Bush et al., in a retrospective large cohort study (n = 1242), identified high incidence (28%) of pulmonary hypertension with associated co-morbidities such as OSA, chronic hypoxia, recurrent pneumonia, and aspiration in patients with DS [127]. Early management of respiratory disorders contributes towards improved condition and reduced susceptibility of pulmonary hypertension in individuals with Down syndrome. Reports based on co-morbidity epilepsy (seizure disorder) showed increased prevalence in individuals (8.1–26%) with Down syndrome compared to general population (1.5–5%) [128]. Major biological and metabolic factors present in Down syndrome patients contributing to increased seizures include dyskinesia of dendrites, frontal/temporal lobe hypoplasia, abnormal neuronal lamination, glutamatergic receptor GluR5 alteration, and congenital heart disease [129,130]. Following seizures, there is a profound connection with other associated co-morbidity i.e., dementia in Down syndrome patients. Hithersay et al., in a prospective longitudinal study, found individuals in older age and late-onset of epilepsy were associated with increased risk of developing dementia in Down syndrome cases [131]. Another cross-sectional study by Bayen et al. determined high prevalence of dementia in DS adults above 65 years with marked risk of developing Alzheimer disease (AD) [132]. Further, a neuroimaging study by Pujol et al. based on adults with DS showed significant volume reduction in hippocampus and substantia innominata of brain anatomy specifically linked to cognitive impairment and dementia progression [133]. Early diagnosis of dementia and AD in DS individuals is not possible due to pre-existing behavioral and intellectual disorders. Recently, a study by Dekker et al. based on behavioral and psychological symptoms of dementia in Down syndrome (BPSD-DS) scale identified behavioral changes such as anxiety, agitation, depression, sleep disturbance, and apathy had significantly high scores in DS+AD (Down syndrome with AD) compared to DS+Q (Down syndrome with questionable dementia) and without dementia individual study groups [62,134]. Based on other behavioral studies, individuals with DS presented symptoms such as sleep disturbance, anxiety, depression, and apathy as alarming signs for developing AD [135–137]. Other neurodevelopment disorders associated with DS include autism spectrum disorder (ASD) and attention deficit hyperactivity disorder (ADHD), as investigated in recent population based cohort study showing 42% ASD and 34% ADHD prevalence in DS individuals [138]. Pre-existing intellectual disability associated with Down syndrome might be the facilitating factor for the characteristic heterogeneity in ASD symptoms. Congenital heart defects (CHDs) are one of the profound co-morbidities associated with DS as the prevalent cause of infant mortality [139–143]. Baban et al. investigated the frequency of Down syndrome infants (N = 859) for CHD subtypes based on a single center study, reporting a high proportion with CHDs (72.2%) and 4.7% with atypical CHDs [144]. Following research for DS-CHD (DS associated with CHD) trend in infants present less frequency mainly due to selective abortion of fetus or diagnostic improvement for managing antenatal CHD [113,145]. Patients with DS are reported to present two common types of cardiac defects such as atrioventricular septal defect (45%) and ventricular septal defects (20–30%), respectively [71,146]. The prevalence of different co-morbidities associated with Down syndrome varies across the geographical population [147,148]. Further, the majority of co-morbidities generally requires clinical and psychiatric management with not much effect on mortality, except CHD and epilepsy. Future management of patients with DS thus requires proper understanding of the co-morbidities associated for providing appropriate help they need [147,148].

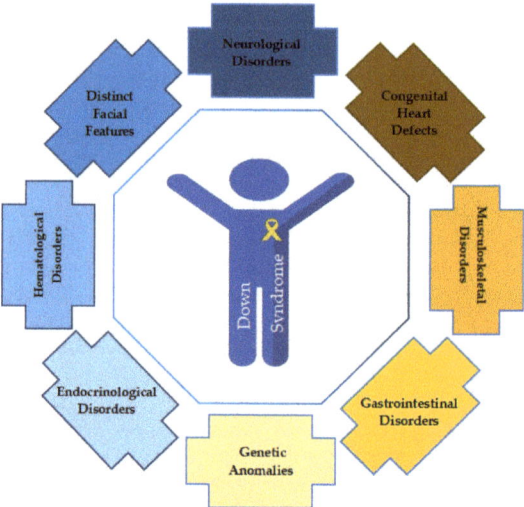

Figure 1. Down syndrome and neurocognitive profiles associated disorders.

Table 2. Co-morbidities and corresponding disorders/diseases.

Co-Morbidity	Disorder/Disease
Neurological Disorders	• Alzheimer disease • Dementia • Excessive flexibility • Intellectual disability • Learning disability • Lennox–Gastaut syndrome • Less concentration • Seizures
Congenital Heart Defects	• AVS defect • Isolate PDA • SA defect • Tetralogy of Fallot • VS defect
Musculoskeletal Disorders	• Broad small hands • Decreased bone mass • Growth retardation • Hypotonia • Short fingers • Short height • Vitamin D deficiency • Small feet
Gastrointestinal Disorders	• Celiac disease • Chronic constipation • Duodenal atresia • Gastroesophagal reflux • Hirschsprung disease • Imperforate anus • Intermittent diarrhea • Intestinal obstruction
Possible Genetic Anomalies	• Mosaicism • Translocation • Trisomy 21
Endocrinological Disorders	• Ambiguous genitalia • Cryptorchidism • Delayed puberty • Micropenis • Hyperthyroidism • Hypothyroidism
Hematological Disorders	• Leukemia • Myelopoiesis • Neutrophilia • Polycythemia • Thrombocytopenia
Distinct Facial Features	• Flattened face and nose • Palmer/Siamese crease • Palpebral fissures • Protruding tongue • Short neck • Slanting eyes • Small head, mouth, and ears

ML algorithms have been employed to analyze large datasets of genetic and clinical information to gain insights into Down syndrome and improve patient care. Down syndrome is a genetic disorder caused by the presence of an extra copy of chromosome 21, leading to cognitive and developmental delays [8]. ML techniques have been used to identify biological markers and patterns associated with Down syndrome. By analyzing genomic data from individuals with Down syndrome and comparing it with data from typically developing individuals, ML algorithms can identify specific genetic variations or expression patterns that are characteristic of the condition [74,149]. These studies present pioneering applications of artificial intelligence (AI) and machine learning (ML) in Down syndrome (DS) research. Another study employs ML to scrutinize clinical records of 106 DS subjects, successfully identifying key features associated with intellectual disability (ID). The models, including random forest and gradient boosting, showcase high accuracy, spotlighting variables linked to cognitive impairment, encompassing hearing, gastrointestinal health, thyroid function, immune system, and vitamin B12 levels [74]. In a second study, addressing executive function decline in adults with DS, data-driven techniques pinpoint constructive praxis, verbal and immediate memory, planning, and written verbal comprehension as crucial predictors for inhibition capacity in 188 adults, providing insights for tailored interventions [149]. This can aid in early diagnosis, genetic counseling, and personalized treatment strategies. Furthermore, ML algorithms can assist in the development of predictive models for assessing the risk of certain medical conditions commonly associated with Down syndrome [73,150]. Another study addresses the frequent occurrence of obstructive sleep apnea (OSA) in individuals with Down syndrome. Using a Logic Learning Machine, the study develops a predictive tool with a cross-validated negative predictive value of 73% for mild OSA and 90% for moderate or severe OSA. This cost-effective model includes survey responses, medication history, anthropometric measurements, vital signs, age, and physical examination findings, offering potential improvements to sleep-related healthcare [73]. ML also plays a role in improving educational interventions and therapies for individuals with Down syndrome [74]. By analyzing data from educational programs, ML algorithms can identify effective teaching strategies, personalize learning approaches, and provide recommendations for individualized educational plans [74]. Additionally, ML-based technologies, such as speech and language processing algorithms, can assist in speech therapy and communication interventions for individuals with Down syndrome [68]. This study provides an in-depth analysis of AI-driven solutions that enhance communication and education for disabled children, concluding with considerations for future developments and ethical concerns associated with these technologies [68]. Together, these studies showcase the multifaceted applications of AI and ML in advancing understanding, diagnosis, and care for individuals with DS. It is important to note that the application of ML in Down syndrome research and healthcare requires careful consideration of ethical and privacy considerations. Ensuring the responsible use of data, protecting privacy, and addressing potential biases in algorithms are crucial aspects that need to be addressed to fully harness the potential of ML in improving the lives of individuals with Down syndrome [151]. These studies collectively illuminate the transformative potential of artificial intelligence (AI) and machine learning (ML) in diverse fields. From enhancing Down syndrome diagnosis by pinpointing key cognitive indicators and predicting inhibitory capacity to predicting sleep apnea risk and advancing assistive technologies for children with special needs, the application of AI and ML showcases promising avenues for precision, efficiency, and innovative solutions. Additionally, these studies also underscore the indispensable role of AI in addressing data challenges across industries, offering valuable insights and strategies for effective implementation. Furthermore, these findings collectively underscore the significant impact of AI and ML in reshaping research, diagnosis, and intervention strategies across various domains.

The present review extends prior research by providing a comprehensive exploration of Down syndrome's multifaceted dimensions. By synthesizing insights into neurodevelopmental aspects, associated comorbidities, and the integration of artificial intelligence (AI), this study offers a significant extension of existing knowledge. The implication of our review lies in its potential to steer future research, emphasizing the need for sophisticated knowledge and technological advancements in AI for a more precise understanding of Down syndrome. The ultimate goal is to leverage AI's potential to enhance diagnostic accuracy, intervention strategies, and therapeutic advancements. However, challenges persist, notably in data quality, interpretability, and ethical considerations. While highlighting AI's transformative merits and potential clinical applications, we acknowledge the limitations and call for future research focusing on refining methodologies and ethical frameworks to maximize AI's benefits in Down syndrome research and care pathways. These technologies can improve screening, diagnosis, and personalized interventions, ultimately benefiting individuals with Down syndrome. However, the responsible and ethical use of ML and AI in Down syndrome care requires ongoing research, validation, and careful consideration of privacy and fairness concerns. This line of research holds immense significance in reshaping our approach to Down syndrome, paving the way for impactful innovations and improving the lives of individuals affected by this condition. By harnessing the power of ML and AI responsibly, practitioners can improve outcomes and provide better care for individuals with Down syndrome. The continued collaboration between researchers, healthcare practitioners, policymakers, and the Down syndrome community will drive further progress towards enhancing the lives and prospects of individuals with Down syndrome. Future studies should delve into these complexities to inform tailored interventions and support systems that promote positive outcomes for individuals with DS and their families.

5. Conclusions

In conclusion, this comprehensive review has highlighted the neurodevelopmental and cognitive characteristics observed in individuals with Down syndrome. The findings underscore the diverse nature of this population, emphasizing the importance of tailored interventions and support techniques. Moreover, emerging research has demonstrated the potential of ML and AI algorithms in accurately identifying individuals at risk of Down syndrome, aiding healthcare practitioners in early detection and intervention. While individuals with Down syndrome may face cognitive challenges, it is crucial to recognize and nurture their unique skills and qualities. By promoting inclusive environments and providing customized support, we can empower individuals with Down syndrome to reach their full potential and enhance their overall quality of life. Looking towards the future, ongoing advancements in research and therapeutic interventions offer promising prospects for individuals with Down syndrome. By further understanding the underlying mechanisms and exploring innovative approaches, we can develop targeted interventions that address specific cognitive and behavioral aspects. This, in turn, will enable individuals with Down syndrome to attain greater levels of autonomy and well-being. Societal progress and awareness play pivotal roles in fostering an inclusive and supportive environment for individuals with Down syndrome. By prioritizing the cultivation of an inclusive society, we can create opportunities for meaningful participation, education, and employment for individuals with Down syndrome. This will contribute to their social integration and overall quality of life.

Author Contributions: Conceptualization, A.M.K., R.-u.-R.K., F.A., A.A. and A.A.R.; methodology, F.A., A.B. and Q.-u.A.; software, A.A.R.; resources, A.M.K., F.A., A.B. and Q.-u.A.; data curation, F.A., A.B. and Q.-u.A.; writing-original draft preparation, A.M.K., F.A. and A.A.R.; writing-review and editing, A.A., A.A.R and R.-u.-R.K. All authors have read and agreed to the published version of the manuscript.

Funding: King Salman Center for Disability Research (KSRG-2023-562).

Informed Consent Statement: Not applicable.

Data Availability Statement: Data are contained within the article.

Acknowledgments: The authors extend their appreciation to the King Salman Center for Disability Research for funding this work through Research Group no KSRG-2023-562.

Conflicts of Interest: The authors declare no conflict of interest.

References

1. Kazemi, M.; Salehi, M.; Kheirollahi, M. Down Syndrome: Current Status, Challenges and Future Perspectives. *Int. J. Mol. Cell. Med.* **2016**, *5*, 125–133.
2. Akhtar, F.; Bokhari, S.R.A. Down Syndrome. In *StatPearls*; Disclosure: Syed Rizwan Bokhari Declares No Relevant Financial Relationships with Ineligible Companies; Treasure Island (FL) Ineligible Companies: St. Petersburg, FL, USA, 2023.
3. Ataman, A.D.; Vatanoglu-Lutz, E.E.; Yildirim, G. Medicine in stamps: History of Down syndrome through philately. *J. Turk. Ger. Gynecol. Assoc.* **2012**, *13*, 267–269. [CrossRef]
4. Down, J. Observations on an ethnic classification of idiots. *Clin. Lect. Rep. Lond. Hosp.* **1866**, *3*, 259–262.
5. Gardiner, K.; Herault, Y.; Lott, I.T.; Antonarakis, S.E.; Reeves, R.H.; Dierssen, M. Down syndrome: From understanding the neurobiology to therapy. *J. Neurosci.* **2010**, *30*, 14943–14945. [CrossRef] [PubMed]
6. Sullivan, K.D.; Lewis, H.C.; Hill, A.A.; Pandey, A.; Jackson, L.P.; Cabral, J.M.; Smith, K.P.; Liggett, L.A.; Gomez, E.B.; Galbraith, M.D.; et al. Trisomy 21 consistently activates the interferon response. *Elife* **2016**, *5*, e16220. [CrossRef] [PubMed]
7. Asim, A.; Kumar, A.; Muthuswamy, S.; Jain, S.; Agarwal, S. "Down syndrome: An insight of the disease". *J. Biomed. Sci.* **2015**, *22*, 41. [CrossRef] [PubMed]
8. Bull, M.J. Down Syndrome. *N. Engl. J. Med.* **2020**, *382*, 2344–2352. [CrossRef] [PubMed]
9. Antonarakis, S.E.; Skotko, B.G.; Rafii, M.S.; Strydom, A.; Pape, S.E.; Bianchi, D.W.; Sherman, S.L.; Reeves, R.H. Down syndrome. *Nat. Rev. Dis. Primers* **2020**, *6*, 9. [CrossRef] [PubMed]
10. Barca, D.; Tarta-Arsene, O.; Dica, A.; Iliescu, C.; Budisteanu, M.; Motoescu, C.; Butoianu, N.; Craiu, D. Intellectual disability and epilepsy in down syndrome. *Maedica* **2014**, *9*, 344–350.
11. Kvarnung, M.; Nordgren, A. Intellectual Disability & Rare Disorders: A Diagnostic Challenge. In *Advances in Experimental Medicine and Biology*; Springer: Berlin/Heidelberg, Germany, 2017; pp. 39–54. [CrossRef]
12. Murthy, S.K.; Malhotra, A.K.; Mani, S.; Shara, M.E.; Al-Rowaished, E.E.; Naveed, S.; Alkhayat, A.I.; Alali, M.T. Incidence of Down syndrome in Dubai, UAE. *Med. Princ. Pract.* **2007**, *16*, 25–28. [CrossRef]
13. Cereda, A.; Carey, J.C. The trisomy 18 syndrome. *Orphanet J. Rare Dis.* **2012**, *7*, 81. [CrossRef] [PubMed]
14. Centers for Disease Control and Prevention (CDC). *Down Syndrome*. 2023. Available online: https://www.cdc.gov/ncbddd/birthdefects/downsyndrome.html (accessed on 22 November 2023).
15. Pota, P.; Grammatopoulou, V.; Torti, E.; Braddock, S.; Batanian, J.R. Instability of isochromosome 4p in a child with pure trisomy 4p syndrome features and entire 4q-arm translocation. *Cytogenet. Genome Res.* **2014**, *144*, 280–284. [CrossRef] [PubMed]
16. Vijay, S.; Sarojam, S.; Raveendran, S.; Syamala, V.; Leelakumari, S.; Narayanan, G.; Hariharan, S. Recurrent isochromosome 21 and multiple abnormalities in a patient suspected of having acute myeloid leukemia with eosinophilic differentiation—A rare case from South India. *Chin. J. Cancer* **2012**, *31*, 45–50. [CrossRef] [PubMed]
17. Hamanoue, H. Genetic Counseling: Chromosomal Structural Rearrangements. In *Fetal Morph Functional Diagnosis*; Springer: Singapore, 2020; pp. 271–296. [CrossRef]
18. Lana-Elola, E.; Watson-Scales, S.D.; Fisher, E.M.; Tybulewicz, V.L. Down syndrome: Searching for the genetic culprits. *Dis. Model. Mech.* **2011**, *4*, 586–595. [CrossRef]
19. Abukhaled, Y.; Hatab, K.; Awadhalla, M.; Hamdan, H. Understanding the genetic mechanisms and cognitive impairments in Down syndrome: Towards a holistic approach. *J. Neurol.* **2023**. [CrossRef]
20. Sharmin, F.; Begum, S.; Jahan, I.; Parvin, R.; Biswas, D.C. Down syndrome with Disorder of Sex development (DSD): A Rare Presentation. *Bangladesh J. Child Health* **2020**, *44*, 48–51. [CrossRef]
21. Ministry of Health. *The Clinical Assessment and Management of Children, Young People and Adults with Down Syndrome Recommended Clinical Practice*; Ministry of Health: Wellington, New Zealand, 2001.
22. Hendrix, J.A.; Amon, A.; Abbeduto, L.; Agiovlasitis, S.; Alsaied, T.; Anderson, H.A.; Bain, L.J.; Baumer, N.; Bhattacharyya, A.; Bogunovic, D.; et al. Opportunities, barriers, and recommendations in down syndrome research. *Transl. Sci. Rare Dis.* **2021**, *5*, 99–129. [CrossRef]
23. Baksh, R.A.; Pape, S.E.; Chan, L.F.; Aslam, A.A.; Gulliford, M.C.; Strydom, A.; Consortium, G.-D. Multiple morbidity across the lifespan in people with Down syndrome or intellectual disabilities: A population-based cohort study using electronic health records. *Lancet Public Health* **2023**, *8*, e453–e462. [CrossRef]
24. Varshney, K.; Iriowen, R.; Morrell, K.; Pillay, P.; Fossi, A.; Stephens, M.M. Disparities and outcomes of patients living with Down Syndrome undergoing healthcare transitions from pediatric to adult care: A scoping review. *Am. J. Med. Genet. A* **2022**, *188*, 2293–2302. [CrossRef]
25. Chicoine, B.; Rivelli, A.; Fitzpatrick, V.; Chicoine, L.; Jia, G.; Rzhetsky, A. Prevalence of Common Disease Conditions in a Large Cohort of Individuals with Down Syndrome in the United States. *J. Patient Cent. Res. Rev.* **2021**, *8*, 86–97. [CrossRef]
26. Klosowska, A.; Kuchta, A.; Cwiklinska, A.; Salaga-Zaleska, K.; Jankowski, M.; Klosowski, P.; Manski, A.; Zwiefka, M.; Anikiej-Wiczenbach, P.; Wierzba, J. Relationship between growth and intelligence quotient in children with Down syndrome. *Transl. Pediatr.* **2022**, *11*, 505–513. [CrossRef] [PubMed]
27. O'Toole, C.; Lee, A.S.; Gibbon, F.E.; van Bysterveldt, A.K.; Hart, N.J. Parent-mediated interventions for promoting communication and language development in young children with Down syndrome. *Cochrane Database Syst. Rev.* **2018**, *10*, CD012089. [CrossRef] [PubMed]

28. Bu, Q.; Qiang, R.; Cheng, H.; Wang, A.; Chen, H.; Pan, Z. Analysis of the Global Disease Burden of Down Syndrome Using YLDs, YLLs, and DALYs Based on the Global Burden of Disease 2019 Data. *Front. Pediatr.* **2022**, *10*, 882722. [CrossRef] [PubMed]
29. Davenport, T.; Kalakota, R. The potential for artificial intelligence in healthcare. *Future Healthc. J.* **2019**, *6*, 94–98. [CrossRef] [PubMed]
30. Bajwa, J.; Munir, U.; Nori, A.; Williams, B. Artificial intelligence in healthcare: Transforming the practice of medicine. *Future Healthc. J.* **2021**, *8*, e188–e194. [CrossRef] [PubMed]
31. Alowais, S.A.; Alghamdi, S.S.; Alsuhebany, N.; Alqahtani, T.; Alshaya, A.I.; Almohareb, S.N.; Aldairem, A.; Alrashed, M.; Bin Saleh, K.; Badreldin, H.A.; et al. Revolutionizing healthcare: The role of artificial intelligence in clinical practice. *BMC Med. Educ.* **2023**, *23*, 689. [CrossRef] [PubMed]
32. Alzubi, J.; Nayyar, A.; Kumar, A. Machine Learning from Theory to Algorithms: An Overview. *J. Phys. Conf. Ser.* **2018**, *1142*, 012012. [CrossRef]
33. Briganti, G. Artificial intelligence: An introduction for clinicians. *Rev. Mal. Respir.* **2023**, *40*, 308–313. [CrossRef]
34. Choi, R.Y.; Coyner, A.S.; Kalpathy-Cramer, J.; Chiang, M.F.; Campbell, J.P. Introduction to Machine Learning, Neural Networks, and Deep Learning. *Transl. Vis. Sci. Technol.* **2020**, *9*, 14.
35. Deo, R.C. Machine Learning in Medicine. *Circulation* **2015**, *132*, 1920–1930. [CrossRef]
36. Zhang, H.-G.; Jiang, Y.-T.; Dai, S.-D.; Li, L.; Hu, X.-N.; Liu, R.-Z. Application of intelligent algorithms in Down syndrome screening during second trimester pregnancy. *World J. Clin. Cases* **2021**, *9*, 4573–4584. [CrossRef] [PubMed]
37. He, F.L.; Lin, B.; Mou, K.; Jin, L.Z.; Liu, J.T. A machine learning model for the prediction of down syndrome in second trimester antenatal screening. *Clin. Chim. Acta* **2021**, *521*, 206–211. [CrossRef] [PubMed]
38. Mohammed Nawi, A.; Ismail, A.; Abdullah, S. The Impact on Family among Down syndrome Children with Early Intervention. *Iran. J. Public Health* **2013**, *42*, 996–1006. [PubMed]
39. NDSS. Early Interventions. Available online: https://ndss.org/resources/early-intervention (accessed on 8 August 2023).
40. Guralnick, M.J. Effectiveness of early intervention for vulnerable children: A developmental perspective. *Am. J. Ment. Retard.* **1998**, *102*, 319–345. [CrossRef] [PubMed]
41. Ong, C.Y.T.; Lee, C.P.; Leung, K.Y.; Lau, E.; Tang, M.H.Y. Human Chorionic Gonadotropin and Plasma Protein-A in Alpha0-Thalassemia Pregnancies. *Obstet. Gynecol.* **2006**, *108*, 651–655. [CrossRef] [PubMed]
42. Russo, M.L.; Blakemore, K.J. A historical and practical review of first trimester aneuploidy screening. *Semin. Fetal Neonatal Med.* **2014**, *19*, 183–187. [CrossRef] [PubMed]
43. Shiefa, S.; Amargandhi, M.; Bhupendra, J.; Moulali, S.; Kristine, T. First Trimester Maternal Serum Screening Using Biochemical Markers PAPP-A and Free beta-hCG for Down Syndrome, Patau Syndrome and Edward Syndrome. *Indian J. Clin. Biochem.* **2013**, *28*, 3–12. [CrossRef]
44. Zhang, X.; Wang, W.; He, F.; Zhong, K.; Yuan, S.; Wang, Z. Proficiency testing of maternal serum prenatal screening in second trimester in China, 2015. *Biochem. Med.* **2017**, *27*, 114–121. [CrossRef]
45. Canick, J.A.; MacRae, A.R. Second trimester serum markers. *Semin. Perinatol.* **2005**, *29*, 203–208. [CrossRef]
46. Ren, F.; Hu, Y.U.; Zhou, H.; Zhu, W.Y.; Jia, L.I.; Xu, J.J.; Xue, J. Second trimester maternal serum triple screening marker levels in normal twin and singleton pregnancies. *Biomed. Rep.* **2016**, *4*, 475–478. [CrossRef]
47. Wald, N.J.; Bestwick, J.P.; Huttly, W.J. Improvements in antenatal screening for Down's syndrome. *J. Med. Screen.* **2013**, *20*, 7–14. [CrossRef]
48. Malone, F.D.; Canick, J.A.; Ball, R.H.; Nyberg, D.A.; Comstock, C.H.; Bukowski, R.; Berkowitz, R.L.; Gross, S.J.; Dugoff, L.; Craigo, S.D.; et al. First-trimester or second-trimester screening, or both, for Down's syndrome. *N. Engl. J. Med.* **2005**, *353*, 2001–2011. [CrossRef]
49. Zournatzi, V.; Daniilidis, A.; Karidas, C.; Tantanasis, T.; Loufopoulos, A.; Tzafettas, J. A prospective two years study of first trimester screening for Down syndrome. *Hippokratia* **2008**, *12*, 28–32. [PubMed]
50. Gori, C.; Cocchi, G.; Corvaglia, L.T.; Ramacieri, G.; Pulina, F.; Sperti, G.; Cagnazzo, V.; Catapano, F.; Strippoli, P.; Cordelli, D.M.; et al. Down Syndrome: How to communicate the diagnosis. *Ital. J. Pediatr.* **2023**, *49*, 18. [CrossRef]
51. Ho, L. Current status of the early childhood developmental intervention ecosystem in Singapore. *Singap. Med. J.* **2021**, *62*, S43–S52. [CrossRef]
52. Paterick, T.E.; Patel, N.; Tajik, A.J.; Chandrasekaran, K. Improving health outcomes through patient education and partnerships with patients. *Bayl. Univ. Med. Cent. Proc.* **2017**, *30*, 112–113. [CrossRef]
53. Wills, J. Health literacy: New packaging for health education or radical movement? *Int. J. Public Health* **2009**, *54*, 3–4. [CrossRef]
54. Nutbeam, D. The evolving concept of health literacy. *Soc. Sci. Med.* **2008**, *67*, 2072–2078. [CrossRef]
55. Bohnstedt, C.; Stenmarker, M.; Olersbacken, L.; Schmidt, L.; Larsen, H.B.; Schmiegelow, K.; Hansson, H. Participation, challenges and needs in children with down syndrome during cancer treatment at hospital: A qualitative study of parents' experiences. *Front. Rehabil. Sci.* **2023**, *4*, 1099516. [CrossRef] [PubMed]
56. Fuca, E.; Galassi, P.; Costanzo, F.; Vicari, S. Parental perspectives on the quality of life of children with Down syndrome. *Front. Psychiatry* **2022**, *13*, 957876. [CrossRef] [PubMed]
57. Rabbani, S.A.; Mossa, M.S.; Al Nuaimi, G.A.; Al Khateri, F.A. Down syndrome: Knowledge and attitudes among future healthcare providers. *J. Taibah Univ. Med. Sci.* **2023**, *18*, 1179–1187. [CrossRef] [PubMed]

58. Telman, G.; Sosnowska-Sienkiewicz, P.; Strauss, E.; Mazela, J.; Mankowski, P.; Januszkiewicz-Lewandowska, D. Why Is Health Care for Children with Down Syndrome So Crucial from the First Days of Life? A Retrospective Cohort Study Emphasized Transient Abnormal Myelopoiesis (TAM) Syndrome at Three Centers. *Int. J. Environ. Res. Public Health* **2022**, *19*, 9774. [CrossRef] [PubMed]
59. Gadsboll, K.; Petersen, O.B.; Gatinois, V.; Strange, H.; Jacobsson, B.; Wapner, R.; Vermeesch, J.R.; Group, N.I.-m.S.; Vogel, I. Current use of noninvasive prenatal testing in Europe, Australia and the USA: A graphical presentation. *Acta Obstet. Gynecol. Scand.* **2020**, *99*, 722–730. [CrossRef] [PubMed]
60. Zalel, Y.; Zemet, R.; Kivilevitch, Z. The added value of detailed early anomaly scan in fetuses with increased nuchal translucency. *Prenat. Diagn.* **2017**, *37*, 235–243. [CrossRef]
61. Zhou, Y.; Wu, S.; Han, J.; Zhen, L.; Yang, X.; Li, R.; Zhang, Y.; Jing, X.; Li, F.; Liu, H. Prenatal diagnosis of ultrasound soft markers in a single medical center of mainland China. *Mol. Cytogenet.* **2023**, *16*, 3. [CrossRef] [PubMed]
62. Hasina, Z.; Wang, C.C. Prenatal and Postnatal Therapies for Down's Syndrome and Associated Developmental Anomalies and Degenerative Deficits: A Systematic Review of Guidelines and Trials. *Front. Med.* **2022**, *9*, 910424. [CrossRef]
63. Inglis, A.; Hippman, C.; Austin, J.C. Prenatal testing for Down syndrome: The perspectives of parents of individuals with Down syndrome. *Am. J. Med. Genet. A* **2012**, *158A*, 743–750. [CrossRef]
64. Channell, M.M.; Mattie, L.J.; Hamilton, D.R.; Capone, G.T.; Mahone, E.M.; Sherman, S.L.; Rosser, T.C.; Reeves, R.H.; Kalb, L.G.; Down Syndrome Cognition, P. Capturing cognitive and behavioral variability among individuals with Down syndrome: A latent profile analysis. *J. Neurodev. Disord.* **2021**, *13*, 16. [CrossRef]
65. Klein, J.A.; Haydar, T.F. Neurodevelopment in Down syndrome: Concordance in humans and models. *Front. Cell Neurosci.* **2022**, *16*, 941855. [CrossRef]
66. Windsperger, K.; Hoehl, S. Development of Down Syndrome Research Over the Last Decades-What Healthcare and Education Professionals Need to Know. *Front. Psychiatry* **2021**, *12*, 749046. [CrossRef]
67. Onnivello, S.; Pulina, F.; Locatelli, C.; Marcolin, C.; Ramacieri, G.; Antonaros, F.; Vione, B.; Caracausi, M.; Lanfranchi, S. Cognitive profiles in children and adolescents with Down syndrome. *Sci. Rep.* **2022**, *12*, 1936. [CrossRef] [PubMed]
68. Zdravkova, K.; Krasniqi, V.; Dalipi, F.; Ferati, M. Cutting-edge communication and learning assistive technologies for disabled children: An artificial intelligence perspective. *Front. Artif. Intell.* **2022**, *5*, 970430. [CrossRef]
69. Thomas, M.S.C.; Alfageme, O.O.; D'Souza, H.; Patkee, P.A.; Rutherford, M.A.; Mok, K.Y.; Hardy, J.; Karmiloff-Smith, A.; Consortium, L. A multi-level developmental approach to exploring individual differences in Down syndrome: Genes, brain, behaviour, and environment. *Res. Dev. Disabil.* **2020**, *104*, 103638. [CrossRef]
70. Stoll, K.; Jackson, J. Supporting Patient Autonomy and Informed Decision-Making in Prenatal Genetic Testing. *Cold Spring Harb. Perspect. Med.* **2020**, *10*, a036509. [CrossRef]
71. Stoll, C.; Dott, B.; Alembik, Y.; Roth, M.-P. Associated congenital anomalies among cases with Down syndrome. *Eur. J. Med. Genet.* **2015**, *58*, 674–680. [CrossRef] [PubMed]
72. Lawson, K.L.; Pierson, R.A. Maternal decisions regarding prenatal diagnosis: Rational choices or sensible decisions? *J. Obstet. Gynaecol. Can.* **2007**, *29*, 240–246. [CrossRef] [PubMed]
73. Skotko, B.G.; Macklin, E.A.; Muselli, M.; Voelz, L.; McDonough, M.E.; Davidson, E.; Allareddy, V.; Jayaratne, Y.S.; Bruun, R.; Ching, N.; et al. A predictive model for obstructive sleep apnea and Down syndrome. *Am. J. Med. Genet. A* **2017**, *173*, 889–896. [CrossRef]
74. Baldo, F.; Piovesan, A.; Rakvin, M.; Ramacieri, G.; Locatelli, C.; Lanfranchi, S.; Onnivello, S.; Pulina, F.; Caracausi, M.; Antonaros, F.; et al. Machine learning based analysis for intellectual disability in Down syndrome. *Heliyon* **2023**, *9*, e19444. [CrossRef]
75. Qin, B.; Liang, L.; Wu, J.; Quan, Q.; Wang, Z.; Li, D. Automatic Identification of Down Syndrome Using Facial Images with Deep Convolutional Neural Network. *Diagnostics* **2020**, *10*, 487. [CrossRef]
76. Srisraluang, W.; Rojnueangnit, K. Facial recognition accuracy in photographs of Thai neonates with Down syndrome among physicians and the Face2Gene application. *Am. J. Med. Genet. Part A* **2021**, *185*, 3701–3705. [CrossRef]
77. Jamshidnezhad, A.; Hosseini, S.M.; Mohammadi-Asl, J.; Mahmudi, M. An intelligent prenatal screening system for the prediction of Trisomy-21. *Inform. Med. Unlocked* **2021**, *24*, 100625. [CrossRef]
78. Reshi, A.A.; Rustam, F.; Mehmood, A.; Alhossan, A.; Alrabiah, Z.; Ahmad, A.; Alsuwailem, H.; Choi, G.S. An Efficient CNN Model for COVID-19 Disease Detection Based on X-Ray Image Classification. *Complexity* **2021**, *2021*, 6621607. [CrossRef]
79. Koivu, K.; Korpimäki, T.; Kivelä, P.; Pahikkala, T.; Sairanen, M. Evaluation of machine learning algorithms for improved risk assessment for Down's syndrome. *Comput. Biol. Med.* **2018**, *98*, 1–7. [CrossRef]
80. Reshi, A.A.; Ashraf, I.; Rustam, F.; Shahzad, H.F.; Mehmood, A.; Choi, G.S. Diagnosis of vertebral column pathologies using concatenated resampling with machine learning algorithms. *PeerJ Comput. Sci.* **2021**, *7*, e547. [CrossRef] [PubMed]
81. Lin, Q.; Zhou, Y.; Shi, S.; Zhang, Y.; Yin, S.; Liu, X.; Peng, Q.; Huang, S.; Jiang, Y.; Cui, C.; et al. How much can AI see in early pregnancy: A multi-center study of fetus head characterization in week 10–14 in ultrasound using deep learning. *Comput. Methods Programs Biomed.* **2022**, *226*, 107170. [CrossRef] [PubMed]
82. Rustam, F.; Reshi, A.A.; Aljedaani, W.; Alhossan, A.; Ishaq, A.; Shafi, S.; Lee, E.; Alrabiah, Z.; Alsuwailem, H.; Ahmad, A.; et al. Vector mosquito image classification using novel RIFS feature selection and machine learning models for disease epidemiology. *Saudi J. Biol. Sci.* **2022**, *29*, 583–594. [CrossRef] [PubMed]

83. Celik, E.; Ilhan, H.O.; Elbir, A. Detection and estimation of down syndrome genes by machine learning techniques. In Proceedings of the 2017 25th Signal Processing and Communications Applications Conference (SIU), Antalya, Turkey, 15–18 May 2017.
84. Hallowell, N.; Badger, S.; McKay, F.; Kerasidou, A.; Nellåker, C. Democratising or disrupting diagnosis? Ethical issues raised by the use of AI tools for rare disease diagnosis. *SSM Qual. Res. Health* **2023**, *3*, 100240. [CrossRef] [PubMed]
85. Bull, M.J. Health Supervision for Children with Down Syndrome. *Pediatrics* **2011**, *128*, 393–406. [CrossRef]
86. Eadie, P.A.; Fey, M.E.; Douglas, J.M.; Parsons, C.L. Profiles of Grammatical Morphology and Sentence Imitation in Children with Specific Language Impairment and Down Syndrome. *J. Speech Lang. Hear. Res.* **2002**, *45*, 720–732. [CrossRef]
87. Brunamonti, E.; Pani, P.; Papazachariadis, O.; Onorati, P.; Albertini, G.; Ferraina, S. Cognitive control of movement in down syndrome. *Res. Dev. Disabil.* **2011**, *32*, 1792–1797. [CrossRef]
88. Ellis, N.R.; Woodley-Zanthos, P.; Dulaney, C.L. Memory for spatial location in children, adults, and mentally retarded persons. *Am. J. Ment. Retard.* **1989**, *93*, 521–526. [PubMed]
89. Ulrich, D.A.; Burghardt, A.R.; Lloyd, M.; Tiernan, C.; Hornyak, J.E. Physical Activity Benefits of Learning to Ride a Two-Wheel Bicycle for Children with Down Syndrome: A Randomized Trial. *Phys. Ther.* **2011**, *91*, 1463–1477. [CrossRef] [PubMed]
90. Lott, I.T.; Dierssen, M. Cognitive deficits and associated neurological complications in individuals with Down's syndrome. *Lancet Neurol.* **2010**, *9*, 623–633. [CrossRef]
91. Vicari, S. Motor Development and Neuropsychological Patterns in Persons with Down Syndrome. *Behav. Genet.* **2006**, *36*, 355–364. [CrossRef]
92. Vicari, S.; Pontillo, M.; Armando, M. Neurodevelopmental and psychiatric issues in Down's syndrome. *Psychiatr. Genet.* **2013**, *23*, 95–107. [CrossRef] [PubMed]
93. Chapman, R.; Hesketh, L. Language, cognition, and short-term memory in individuals with Down syndrome. *Down Syndr. Res. Pract.* **2001**, *7*, 1–7. [CrossRef]
94. Shanahan, M.A.; Pennington, B.F.; Yerys, B.E.; Scott, A.; Boada, R.; Willcutt, E.G.; Olson, R.K.; DeFries, J.C. Processing Speed Deficits in Attention Deficit/Hyperactivity Disorder and Reading Disability. *J. Abnorm. Child Psychol.* **2006**, *34*, 584–601. [CrossRef]
95. Borella, E.; Carretti, B.; Lanfranchi, S. Inhibitory mechanisms in Down syndrome: Is there a specific or general deficit? *Res. Dev. Disabil.* **2013**, *34*, 65–71. [CrossRef]
96. Chen, C.C.; Spanò, G.; Edgin, J.O. The impact of sleep disruption on executive function in Down syndrome. *Res. Dev. Disabil.* **2013**, *34*, 2033–2039. [CrossRef]
97. Marcell, M.M.; Weeks, S.L. Short-term memory difficulties and Down's syndrome. *J. Intellect. Disabil. Res.* **2008**, *32*, 153–162. [CrossRef]
98. Jarrold, C.; Baddeley, A.D.; Phillips, C.E. Verbal Short-Term Memory in Down Syndrome. *J. Speech Lang. Hear. Res.* **2002**, *45*, 531–544. [CrossRef]
99. Karagianni, E.; Drigas, A. Language Development and Mobile Apps for Down Syndrome Children. *Tech. Soc. Sci. J.* **2022**, *34*, 193–213. [CrossRef]
100. Kent, R.D.; Eichhorn, J.; Wilson, E.M.; Suk, Y.; Bolt, D.M.; Vorperian, H.K. Auditory-Perceptual Features of Speech in Children and Adults with Down Syndrome: A Speech Profile Analysis. *J. Speech Lang. Hear. Res.* **2021**, *64*, 1157–1175. [CrossRef] [PubMed]
101. Robles-Bello, M.A.; Sánchez-Teruel, D.; Camacho-Conde, J.A. Variables that Predict the Potential Efficacy of Early Intervention in Reading in Down Syndrome. *Psicol. Educ.* **2020**, *26*, 95–100. [CrossRef]
102. Schworer, E.K.; Voth, K.; Hoffman, E.K.; Esbensen, A.J. Short-term memory outcome measures: Psychometric evaluation and performance in youth with Down syndrome. *Res. Dev. Disabil.* **2022**, *120*, 104147. [CrossRef] [PubMed]
103. Miles, S.; Chapman, R.; Sindberg, H. Sampling Context Affects MLU in the Language of Adolescents with Down Syndrome. *J. Speech Lang. Hear. Res.* **2006**, *49*, 325–337. [CrossRef]
104. Mandal, A.S.; Fama, M.E.; Skipper-Kallal, L.M.; DeMarco, A.T.; Lacey, E.H.; Turkeltaub, P.E. Brain structures and cognitive abilities important for the self-monitoring of speech errors. *Neurobiol. Lang.* **2020**, *1*, 319–338. [CrossRef]
105. Maessen, B.; Zink, I.; Maes, B.; Rombouts, E. The effect of manual movements on stuttering in individuals with down syndrome. *J. Fluen. Disord.* **2023**, *75*, 105958. [CrossRef]
106. Parthimos, T.P.; Karavasilis, E.; Rankin, K.P.; Seimenis, I.; Leftherioti, K.; Papanicolaou, A.C.; Miller, B.; Papageorgiou, S.G.; Papatriantafyllou, J.D. The Neural Correlates of Impaired Self-Monitoring Among Individuals with Neurodegenerative Dementias. *J. Neuropsychiatry Clin. Neurosci.* **2019**, *31*, 201–209. [CrossRef]
107. Traverso, L.; Fontana, M.; Usai, M.C.; Passolunghi, M.C. Response Inhibition and Interference Suppression in Individuals with Down Syndrome Compared to Typically Developing Children. *Front. Psychol.* **2018**, *9*, 660. [CrossRef]
108. Martin, G.E.; Klusek, J.; Estigarribia, B.; Roberts, J.E. Language Characteristics of Individuals with Down Syndrome. *Top. Lang. Disord.* **2009**, *29*, 112–132. [CrossRef]
109. Zhu, P.J.; Khatiwada, S.; Cui, Y.; Reineke, L.C.; Dooling, S.W.; Kim, J.J.; Li, W.; Walter, P.; Costa-Mattioli, M. Activation of the ISR mediates the behavioral and neurophysiological abnormalities in Down syndrome. *Science* **2019**, *366*, 843–849. [CrossRef]
110. Vacca, R.A.; Bawari, S.; Valenti, D.; Tewari, D.; Nabavi, S.F.; Shirooie, S.; Sah, A.N.; Volpicella, M.; Braidy, N.; Nabavi, S.M. Down syndrome: Neurobiological alterations and therapeutic targets. *Neurosci. Biobehav. Rev.* **2019**, *98*, 234–255. [CrossRef]

111. Lukowski, A.F.; Milojevich, H.M.; Eales, L. Cognitive Functioning in Children with Down Syndrome: Current Knowledge and Future Directions. In *Advances in Child Development and Behavior*; Elsevier: Amsterdam, The Netherlands, 2019; pp. 257–289. [CrossRef]
112. Caloway, C.L.; Diercks, G.R.; Keamy, D.; de Guzman, V.; Soose, R.; Raol, N.; Shott, S.R.; Ishman, S.L.; Hartnick, C.J. Update on hypoglossal nerve stimulation in children with down syndrome and obstructive sleep apnea. *Laryngoscope* **2019**, *130*, E263–E267. [CrossRef]
113. Santoro, S.L.; Steffensen, E.H. Congenital heart disease in Down syndrome—A review of temporal changes. *J. Congenit. Cardiol.* **2021**, *5*, 1. [CrossRef]
114. Reller, M.D.; Strickland, M.J.; Riehle-Colarusso, T.; Mahle, W.T.; Correa, A. Prevalence of congenital heart defects in metropolitan Atlanta, 1998–2005. *J. Pediatr.* **2008**, *153*, 807–813. [CrossRef] [PubMed]
115. Roizen, N.J.; Patterson, D. Down's syndrome. *Lancet* **2003**, *361*, 1281–1289. [CrossRef] [PubMed]
116. Morris-Rosendahl, D.J.; Crocq, M.-A. Neurodevelopmental disorders-the history and future of a diagnostic concept. *Dialogues Clin. Neurosci.* **2020**, *22*, 65–72. [CrossRef]
117. Metwalley, K.A.; Farghaly, H.S. Endocrinal dysfunction in children with down syndrome. *Ann. Pediatr. Endocrinol. Metab.* **2022**, *27*, 15–21. [CrossRef] [PubMed]
118. Martin-Perez, Y.; Gonzalez-Montero, G.; Gutierrez-Hernandez, A.L.; Blázquez-Sánchez, V.; Sánchez-Ramos, C. Vision Impairments in Young Adults with Down Syndrome. *Vision* **2023**, *7*, 60. [CrossRef] [PubMed]
119. Patel, L.; Wolter-Warmerdam, K.; Hickey, F. Patterns of Behavior and Medical Comorbidities in Down syndrome. *J. Ment. Health Res. Intellect. Disabil.* **2020**, *13*, 267–280. [CrossRef]
120. Horne, R.S.C.; Wijayaratne, P.; Nixon, G.M.; Walter, L.M. Sleep and sleep disordered breathing in children with down syndrome: Effects on behaviour, neurocognition and the cardiovascular system. *Sleep Med. Rev.* **2019**, *44*, 1–11. [CrossRef]
121. Lal, C.; White, D.R.; Joseph, J.E.; van Bakergem, K.; LaRosa, A. Sleep-Disordered Breathing in Down Syndrome. *Chest* **2015**, *147*, 570–579. [CrossRef]
122. Sibarani, C.R.; Walter, L.M.; Davey, M.J.; Nixon, G.M.; Horne, R.S.C. Sleep-disordered breathing and sleep macro- and micro-architecture in children with Down syndrome. *Pediatr. Res.* **2021**, *91*, 1248–1256. [CrossRef]
123. Subramaniam, D.R.; Mylavarapu, G.; McConnell, K.; Fleck, R.J.; Shott, S.R.; Amin, R.S.; Gutmark, E.J. Compliance Measurements of the Upper Airway in Pediatric Down Syndrome Sleep Apnea Patients. *Ann. Biomed. Eng.* **2016**, *44*, 873–885. [CrossRef] [PubMed]
124. de Miguel-Díez, J.; Villa-Asensi, J.R.; Álvarez-Sala, J.L. Prevalence of Sleep-Disordered Breathing in Children with Down Syndrome: Polygraphic Findings in 108 Children. *Sleep* **2003**, *26*, 1006–1009. [CrossRef] [PubMed]
125. Maris, M.; Verhulst, S.; Wojciechowski, M.; Van de Heyning, P.; Boudewyns, A. Prevalence of Obstructive Sleep Apnea in Children with Down Syndrome. *Sleep* **2016**, *39*, 699–704. [CrossRef] [PubMed]
126. Chawla, J.K.; Cooke, E.; Miguel, M.C.; Burgess, S.; Staton, S. Parents' Experiences of Having a Child with Down Syndrome and Sleep Difficulties. *Behav. Sleep Med.* **2022**, *21*, 570–584. [CrossRef] [PubMed]
127. Bush, D.; Galambos, C.; Ivy, D.D.; Abman, S.H.; Wolter-Warmerdam, K.; Hickey, F. Clinical Characteristics and Risk Factors for Developing Pulmonary Hypertension in Children with Down Syndrome. *J. Pediatr.* **2018**, *202*, 212–219.e2. [CrossRef] [PubMed]
128. Altuna, M.; Giménez, S.; Fortea, J. Epilepsy in Down Syndrome: A Highly Prevalent Comorbidity. *J. Clin. Med.* **2021**, *10*, 2776. [CrossRef] [PubMed]
129. Rho, J.M.; Boison, D. The metabolic basis of epilepsy. *Nat. Rev. Neurol.* **2022**, *18*, 333–347. [CrossRef] [PubMed]
130. Frye, R.E.; Casanova, M.F.; Fatemi, S.H.; Folsom, T.D.; Reutiman, T.J.; Brown, G.L.; Edelson, S.M.; Slattery, J.C.; Adams, J.B. Neuropathological Mechanisms of Seizures in Autism Spectrum Disorder. *Front. Neurosci.* **2016**, *10*, 192. [CrossRef] [PubMed]
131. Hithersay, R.; Startin, C.M.; Hamburg, S.; Mok, K.Y.; Hardy, J.; Fisher, E.M.C.; Tybulewicz, V.L.J.; Nizetic, D.; Strydom, A. Association of Dementia with Mortality Among Adults with Down Syndrome Older Than 35 Years. *JAMA Neurol.* **2019**, *76*, 152–160. [CrossRef]
132. Bayen, E.; Possin, K.L.; Chen, Y.; Cleret de Langavant, L.; Yaffe, K. Prevalence of Aging, Dementia, and Multimorbidity in Older Adults with Down Syndrome. *JAMA Neurol.* **2018**, *75*, 1399–1406. [CrossRef]
133. Pujol, J.; Fenoll, R.; Ribas-Vidal, N.; Martínez-Vilavella, G.; Blanco-Hinojo, L.; García-Alba, J.; Deus, J.; Novell, R.; Esteba-Castillo, S. A longitudinal study of brain anatomy changes preceding dementia in Down syndrome. *Neuroimage Clin.* **2018**, *18*, 160–166. [CrossRef]
134. Dekker, A.D.; Sacco, S.; Carfi, A.; Benejam, B.; Vermeiren, Y.; Beugelsdijk, G.; Schippers, M.; Hassefras, L.; Eleveld, J.; Grefelman, S.; et al. The Behavioral and Psychological Symptoms of Dementia in Down Syndrome (BPSD-DS) Scale: Comprehensive Assessment of Psychopathology in Down Syndrome. *J. Alzheimer's Dis.* **2018**, *63*, 797–819. [CrossRef] [PubMed]
135. Ball, S.L.; Holland, A.J.; Hon, J.; Huppert, F.A.; Treppner, P.; Watson, P.C. Personality and behaviour changes mark the early stages of Alzheimer's disease in adults with Down's syndrome: Findings from a prospective population-based study. *Int. J. Geriatr. Psychiatry* **2006**, *21*, 661–673. [CrossRef]
136. Ball, S.L.; Holland, A.J.; Treppner, P.; Watson, P.C.; Huppert, F.A. Executive dysfunction and its association with personality and behaviour changes in the development of Alzheimer's disease in adults with Down syndrome and mild to moderate learning disabilities. *Br. J. Clin. Psychol.* **2008**, *47*, 1–29. [CrossRef] [PubMed]

137. Pentkowski, N.S.; Rogge-Obando, K.K.; Donaldson, T.N.; Bouquin, S.J.; Clark, B.J. Anxiety and Alzheimer's disease: Behavioral analysis and neural basis in rodent models of Alzheimer's-related neuropathology. *Neurosci. Biobehav. Rev.* **2021**, *127*, 647–658. [CrossRef] [PubMed]
138. Oxelgren, U.W.; Myrelid, Å.; Annerén, G.; Ekstam, B.; Göransson, C.; Holmbom, A.; Isaksson, A.; Åberg, M.; Gustafsson, J.; Fernell, E. Prevalence of autism and attention-deficit–hyperactivity disorder in Down syndrome: A population-based study. *Dev. Med. Child Neurol.* **2016**, *59*, 276–283. [CrossRef] [PubMed]
139. Weijerman, M.E.; van Furth, A.M.; van der Mooren, M.D.; van Weissenbruch, M.M.; Rammeloo, L.; Broers, C.J.M.; Gemke, R.J.B.J. Prevalence of congenital heart defects and persistent pulmonary hypertension of the neonate with Down syndrome. *Eur. J. Pediatr.* **2010**, *169*, 1195–1199. [CrossRef] [PubMed]
140. Paladini, D.; Tartaglione, A.; Agangi, A.; Teodoro, A.; Forleo, F.; Borghese, A.; Martinelli, P. The association between congenital heart disease and Down syndrome in prenatal life. *Ultrasound Obstet. Gynecol.* **2000**, *15*, 104–108. [CrossRef] [PubMed]
141. Bermudez, B.E.B.V.; Medeiros, S.L.; Bermudez, M.B.; Novadzki, I.M.; Magdalena, N.I.R. Down syndrome: Prevalence and distribution of congenital heart disease in Brazil. *Sao Paulo Med. J.* **2015**, *133*, 521–524. [CrossRef]
142. Kim, M.-A.; Lee, Y.S.; Yee, N.H.; Choi, J.S.; Choi, J.Y.; Seo, K. Prevalence of congenital heart defects associated with Down syndrome in Korea. *J. Korean Med. Sci.* **2014**, *29*, 1544–1549. [CrossRef] [PubMed]
143. Al-Aama, J.Y.; Bondagji, N.S.; El-Harouni, A.A. Congenital heart defects in Down syndrome patients from western Saudi Arabia. *Saudi Med. J.* **2012**, *33*, 1211–1215.
144. Baban, A.; Olivini, N.; Cantarutti, N.; Calì, F.; Vitello, C.; Valentini, D.; Adorisio, R.; Calcagni, G.; Alesi, V.; Di Mambro, C.; et al. Differences in morbidity and mortality in Down syndrome are related to the type of congenital heart defect. *Am. J. Med. Genet. Part A* **2020**, *182*, 1342–1350. [CrossRef]
145. Bergström, S.; Carr, H.; Petersson, G.; Stephansson, O.; Bonamy, A.-K.E.; Dahlström, A.; Halvorsen, C.P.; Johansson, S. Trends in Congenital Heart Defects in Infants with Down Syndrome. *Pediatrics* **2016**, *138*, e20160123. [CrossRef]
146. Santos, F.C.G.B.; Croti, U.A.; Marchi, C.H.D.; Murakami, A.N.; Brachine, J.D.P.; Borim, B.C.; Finoti, R.G.; Godoy, M.F.d. Surgical Treatment for Congenital Heart Defects in Down Syndrome Patients. *Braz. J. Cardiovasc. Surg.* **2019**, *34*, 1–7. [CrossRef]
147. Lu, E.; Pyatka, N.; Burant, C.J.; Sajatovic, M. Systematic Literature Review of Psychiatric Comorbidities in Adults with Epilepsy. *J. Clin. Neurol.* **2021**, *17*, 176–186. [CrossRef]
148. Startin, C.M.; D'Souza, H.; Ball, G.; Hamburg, S.; Hithersay, R.; Hughes, K.M.O.; Massand, E.; Karmiloff-Smith, A.; Thomas, M.S.C.; LonDown, S.C.; et al. Health comorbidities and cognitive abilities across the lifespan in Down syndrome. *J. Neurodev. Disord.* **2020**, *12*, 4. [CrossRef]
149. Jojoa-Acosta, M.F.; Signo-Miguel, S.; Garcia-Zapirain, M.B.; Gimeno-Santos, M.; Mendez-Zorrilla, A.; Vaidya, C.J.; Molins-Sauri, M.; Guerra-Balic, M.; Bruna-Rabassa, O. Executive Functioning in Adults with Down Syndrome: Machine-Learning-Based Prediction of Inhibitory Capacity. *Int. J. Environ. Res. Public Health* **2021**, *18*, 785. [CrossRef] [PubMed]
150. Cole, J.H.; Annus, T.; Wilson, L.R.; Remtulla, R.; Hong, Y.T.; Fryer, T.D.; Acosta-Cabronero, J.; Cardenas-Blanco, A.; Smith, R.; Menon, D.K.; et al. Brain-predicted age in Down syndrome is associated with beta amyloid deposition and cognitive decline. *Neurobiol. Aging* **2017**, *56*, 41–49. [CrossRef] [PubMed]
151. Aldoseri, A.; Al-Khalifa, K.N.; Hamouda, A.M. Re-Thinking Data Strategy and Integration for Artificial Intelligence: Concepts, Opportunities, and Challenges. *Appl. Sci.* **2023**, *13*, 7082. [CrossRef]

Disclaimer/Publisher's Note: The statements, opinions and data contained in all publications are solely those of the individual author(s) and contributor(s) and not of MDPI and/or the editor(s). MDPI and/or the editor(s) disclaim responsibility for any injury to people or property resulting from any ideas, methods, instructions or products referred to in the content.

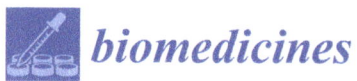

Article

Screening for Neuroprotective and Rapid Antidepressant-like Effects of 20 Essential Oils

Khoa Nguyen Tran [†], Nhi Phuc Khanh Nguyen [†], Ly Thi Huong Nguyen, Heung-Mook Shin * and In-Jun Yang *

Department of Physiology, College of Korean Medicine, Dongguk University, Gyeongju 38066, Republic of Korea; trannguyen053@dgu.ac.kr (K.N.T.); npkhanhnhi@dgu.ac.kr (N.P.K.N.); nguyenthihuongly_t58@hus.edu.vn (L.T.H.N.)
* Correspondence: heungmuk@dongguk.ac.kr (H.-M.S.); injuny@dongguk.ac.kr (I.-J.Y.); Tel.: +82-54-770-2372 (H.-M.S.); +82-54-770-2366 (I.-J.Y.)
[†] These authors contributed equally to this work.

Abstract: Depression is a serious psychiatric disorder with high prevalence, and the delayed onset of antidepressant effects remains a limitation in the treatment of depression. This study aimed to screen essential oils that have the potential for rapid-acting antidepressant development. PC12 and BV2 cells were used to identify essential oils with neuroprotective effects at doses of 0.1 and 1 µg/mL. The resulting candidates were treated intranasally (25 mg/kg) to ICR mice, followed by a tail suspension test (TST) and an elevated plus maze (EPM) after 30 min. In each effective essential oil, five main compounds were computationally analyzed, targeting glutamate receptor subunits. As a result, 19 essential oils significantly abolished corticosterone (CORT)-induced cell death and lactate dehydrogenase (LDH) leakage, and 13 reduced lipopolysaccharide (LPS)-induced tumor necrosis factor alpha (TNF-α) and interleukin 6 (IL-6). From in vivo experiments, six essential oils decreased the immobility time of mice in the TST, in which *Chrysanthemum morifolium* Ramat. and *Myristica fragrans* Houtt. also increased time and entries into the open arms of the EPM. Four compounds including atractylon, α-curcumene, α-farnesene, and selina-4(14),7(11)-dien-8-one had an affinity toward GluN1, GluN2B, and Glu2A receptor subunits surpassed that of the reference compound ketamine. Overall, *Atractylodes lancea* (Thunb.) DC and *Chrysanthemum morifolium* Ramat. essential oils are worthy of further research for fast-acting antidepressants through interactions with glutamate receptors, and their main compounds (atractylon, α-curcumene, α-farnesene, and selina-4(14),7(11)-dien-8-one) are predicted to underlie the fast-acting effect.

Keywords: depression; anxiety; rapid-acting effect; essential oil; glutamate; neurotoxicity; neuroinflammation

Citation: Tran, K.N.; Nguyen, N.P.K.; Nguyen, L.T.H.; Shin, H.-M.; Yang, I.-J. Screening for Neuroprotective and Rapid Antidepressant-like Effects of 20 Essential Oils. *Biomedicines* 2023, 11, 1248. https://doi.org/10.3390/biomedicines11051248

Academic Editors: Simone Battaglia and Masaru Tanaka

Received: 13 March 2023
Revised: 13 April 2023
Accepted: 21 April 2023
Published: 23 April 2023

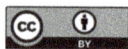

Copyright: © 2023 by the authors. Licensee MDPI, Basel, Switzerland. This article is an open access article distributed under the terms and conditions of the Creative Commons Attribution (CC BY) license (https://creativecommons.org/licenses/by/4.0/).

1. Introduction

Depression is a complex psychiatric disorder, characterized by fatigue, constant feelings of sadness, and loss of pleasure [1]. Statistics show that depression remains a major burden in society, affecting approximately 280 million people worldwide [2]. Several pathological mechanisms of depression have been documented, including alterations in neurotransmitter systems, hypothalamus–pituitary–adrenal (HPA) axis activity, neuroinflammation, and changes in brain structures [3]. Norepinephrine and dopamine are neurotransmitters that play a role in reward processing and motivation, and their abnormal serum levels have been reported in depressed rodents [4]. Although serotonin has been the most extensively studied neurotransmitter in depression, researchers recently offer compelling data rejecting the relationship between serotonin activity to depression [5]. Stress-induced biological alterations, therefore, are receiving more attention as significant contributors to depression [6]. The HPA axis is a complex system that regulates the body's stress response. Dysregulation of the HPA axis and the resulting elevations in corticotrophin-releasing hormone, adrenocorticotropic hormone, and cortisol or corticosterone (CORT) levels have been proposed as key mechanisms underlying the development of depression [7,8]. A dysregulated HPA axis activity is proposed to be accompanied by the overproduction of pro-inflammatory cytokines such as tumor necrosis factor alpha (TNF-α), interleukin (IL)-6, or IL-1β, which leads to the loss of hippocampal neurogenesis and promotion of depression-like behaviors [9,10]. In addition, chronic exposure to glucocorticoids such as cortisol or CORT can lead to dysfunction prefrontal cortex or atrophy of the hippocampus and structural deficits in the dentate gyrus area, which are all brain regions responsible for mood regulation [11,12]. In clinical practice, classical antidepressants exert their effects by inhibiting neurotransmitter-degrading enzymes (monoamine oxidase inhibitors) or inhibiting neurotransmitter reabsorption (selective serotonin reuptake inhibitors (SSRIs), selective serotonin and noradrenaline reuptake inhibitors, and tricyclic antidepressants) [13]. However, safety concerns have been raised, with side effects including weight gain, constipation, drowsiness, or even lethal hypertension [14,15]. Furthermore, the delayed onset of antidepressant action is another major limitation. For instance, acute treatment with SSRIs was found to initially elevate serotonin levels only in the cell body and dendrites, not in axons, which then immediately inhibit serotonin neuronal firing via an action at 5HT1A somatodendritic autoreceptors. In long-term treatment, SSRIs can cause a desensitization of 5HT1A autoreceptors, increasing the firing rate of neurons and serotonin release at axon terminals to postsynaptic receptors [16]. This partly explains the slow onset response of existing antidepressants, which usually take two to three weeks to manifest their effects [17]. Therefore, these limitations lead to an urgent need for safer agents with rapid antidepressant action.

In recent years, there has been a growing interest in research using essential oils due to their purported ability to alleviate a wide range of health issues, including inflammation, cancer, insomnia, anxiety, and depression with fewer side effects [18]. Essential oil is a mixture of secondary metabolites derived from plants [19]. Over 60 components have been identified in essential oils, with major compounds being benzenoids, phenylpropanoids, and terpenoids [20]. Their small, lipophilic components can rapidly and easily penetrate the blood–brain barrier (BBB) to access brain tissues, interacting with the thalamus, cerebral cortex, and limbic system, suggesting their potential use in rapidly reducing the symptoms of anxiety and depression [21,22]. For instance, lavender and citrus essential oil exerted anxiolytic-like and antidepressant-like effects in rodent models by restoring the decrease of monoamine neurotransmitter levels with downregulation of BDNF in serum or in the hippocampus [23–25].

Intranasal administration has been emphasized as a noninvasive method for the rapid management of neuropsychiatric disorders [26]. Intranasal agents directly stimulate the olfactory and trigeminal chemoreceptors, further enhancing the production of neurotransmitters and regulating the neuroendocrine system. In addition, mucosal epithelial pathways with blood vessel-dense nasal mucosa also contribute to rapid substance absorption and subsequent systemic effects, avoiding the hepatic first-pass effect and thus improving drug bioavailability [26,27]. Intranasal delivery of berberine, curcumin, and genipin using a thermosensitive hydrogel system has been reported to improve depressant-like activities in rodent models by enhancing monoamine neurotransmitter concentrations in the hippocampus and striatum. Additionally, at a lower dosage, these treatments exerted superior effects compared with intragastric or intraperitoneal administration [28–30].

Ketamine is a widely known medication that can rapidly alleviate the symptoms of depression through interacting with N-methyl-D-aspartate receptors (NMDARs), including GluN1 and GluN2B receptor subunits [31]. Notably, the GluN2B subunit is involved in many neurological disorders, and therefore significantly responsible for the biophysical and pharmacological properties of the NMDARs [32]. Ifenprodil, a GluN2B-selective NMDAR antagonist, was also found to exert a rapid-acting antidepression-like effect, compared with traditional medications that regulate the monoaminergic system [33]. In addition to NMDARs, the role of alpha-amino-3-hydroxy-5-methyl-4-isoxazole propionic acid receptors (AMPARs) including GluA1 and GluA2 subunits was also revealed in the rapid and long-lasting effects of antidepressants, for instance, ketamine and TAK-653 that potentiate AMPAR activity in maintaining synaptic plasticity [34–36]. Therefore, studies on the rapid action of new antidepressants should consider mechanisms via NMDARs and AMPARs.

Against this background, the present study was performed to identify and recommend essential oils that might have a rapid antidepression-like effect. We examined the in vitro neuroprotective and anti-neuroinflammatory effects of 20 essential oils to investigate their potential antidepression-like effects. Potentially antidepressant essential oils were then evaluated via intranasal administration in ICR mice using the tail suspension test (TST) and elevated plus maze test (EPM). Molecular docking was subsequently performed to predict the interactions between the major compounds in the effective essential oils and NMDAR and AMPAR subunits.

2. Materials and Methods

2.1. Preparation of Essential Oils

Twenty herbs were purchased from Omni Herb (Daegu, Republic of Korea), and each herbal material was immersed in distilled water (1:10 w/w) and hydrodistilled for 4 h using a steam distillation solvent extraction (SDE) apparatus, and the distilled oil was captured in n-hexane (Chemicals Duksan Corp., Ansan, Gyeonggi, Republic of Korea). The oil was dehydrated using a separating funnel, and n-hexane was evaporated. The essential oil was weighed (*Thuja orientalis* L. (0.28% w/w), *Acorus gramineus* Sol. (1.79%), *Foeniculum vulgare* Mill. (1.09%), *Magnolia biondii* Pamp. (0.55%), *Ligusticum striatum* DC. (0.46%), *Prunella vulgaris* L. (0.03%), *Chrysanthemum morifolium* Ramat. (0.28%), *Cinnamomum cassia* (Nees & T.Nees) J.Presl (0.75%), *Zingiber officinale* Roscoe (0.11%), *Santalum album* L. (0.39%), *Nardostachys jatamansi* (D. Don) DC. (1.38%), *Angelica acutiloba* (Siebold & Zucc.) Kitag. (0.20%), *Aucklandia lappa* DC. (0.21%), *Mentha arvensis* L. (yield 0.73%), *Perilla frutescens* (L.) Britton (0.39%), *Syzygium aromaticum* (L.) Merr. & L.M.Perry (6.75%), *Citrus reticulata* Blanco (0.41%), *Atractylodes lancea* (Thunb.) DC. (0.11%), *Agastache rugosa* (Fisch. & C.A.Mey.) Kuntze (0.20%), *Myristica fragrans* Houtt. (0.87%)) and stored at $-20\,^\circ\mathrm{C}$ until further use.

2.2. Animal Experiments and Treatments

Five-week-old male ICR outbred mice weighing 25–29 g were obtained from Koatech Lab Animal Inc. (Pyeongtaek, Gyeonggi, Republic of Korea) and acclimated for one week before the behavioral test. All mice had free access to water and a commercial pellet diet (5L79; PMI Nutrition, St. Louis, MO, USA). All experimental animal procedures were approved by the Institutional Animal Care and Use Committee of Dongguk University (IACUC-2021-15). The mice were randomly divided into the following groups: control group (CON), essential oil treatment groups (EO), and memantine group (MEM), which were offered vehicle (saline and Tween 80, 3% v/v), essential oil (25 mg/kg), and memantine (3 mg/kg), respectively. On the day of the experiment, all animals were habituated to the test room for two hours prior to receiving a 10 µL intranasal administration (CON and EO groups) or 200 µL intraperitoneal injection (MEM group). Thirty minutes after the treatment, a behavioral test was performed.

2.3. Tail Suspension Test (TST)

The effect of essential oils on depression-like behaviors in mice using the TST test was based on the fact that rodents subjected to the short-term, inescapable stress of being suspended by their tail will develop an immobile posture [37]. The tail of the mouse was attached to a bar using 15 cm adhesive tape, and the distance from the bar to the ground was fixed at 50 cm. All 6 min trials were recorded, and the total mobility time of each mouse was measured by manual scoring. The strong shaking of the body and movement of the four limbs akin to running were counted as mobility, whereas small movements that were confined to the front legs but without the involvement of the hind legs were not. The total mobility time was then subtracted from the 360 s of test time and was then stated as the immobility time. After each trial, the suspension box was wiped with 70% ethanol to remove unwanted odors.

2.4. Elevated Plus Maze Test (EPM)

The EPM test, which is based on the innate tendency of rodents to avoid elevated and open spaces and explore novel environments, was performed to assess the anxiety-like behaviors of mice after essential oil treatment [38]. The equipment consisted of four 29 cm × 5 cm arms elevated 40 cm above the ground, with two "closed arms" enclosed by 14 cm black walls. Each mouse was placed in the central area of the maze for a 5-min free exploration period. The arms were cleaned with 70% ethanol after every trial to remove unwanted odors, urine, and feces. The distance traveled, number of entries into, and time spent in the open arms were recorded and analyzed using Smart V3.0 software (Panlab Harvard Apparatus, Holliston, MA, USA).

2.5. Cell Culture and Treatments

PC12 cells (a rat adrenal medullary pheochromocytoma cell line) were cultured in Roswell Park Memorial Institute (RPMI) medium (Welgene Inc., Gyeongsan, Gyeongsangbuk-do, Republic of Korea) supplemented with 10% fetal bovine serum (FBS) (Merck KGaA, Darmstadt, Germany) and 1% penicillin-streptomycin (Thermo Fisher Scientific, Waltham, MA, USA) at 37 °C in a 5% CO_2 humidified environment. PC12 cells were incubated with the SDE extract of each essential oil (0.1 or 1 μg/mL) for 1 h and then stimulated with corticosterone (CORT) (200 μM) for 24 h.

BV2 cells (an immortalized mouse microglial cell line) were cultured in Dulbecco's Modified Eagle Medium (DMEM) supplemented with 10% FBS (Merck KGaA, Darmstadt, Germany) and 1% penicillin-streptomycin (Thermo Fisher Scientific, Waltham, MA, USA) at 37 °C in a 5% CO_2 humidified environment. For the cell viability assay, BV2 cells were treated with the SDE extract of each essential oil (0.1 or 1 μg/mL). To test the anti-neuroinflammatory effects of the essential oils, BV2 cells were pretreated with non-toxic doses of each herb extract for 6 h and then stimulated with lipopolysaccharide (LPS) (1 μg/mL) for 18 h.

2.6. Water-Soluble Tetrazolium Salt Assay (WST)

The effects of the essential oils on the viability of PC12 and BV2 cells were examined using the EZ-Cytox assay kit (DoGenBio, Seoul, Republic of Korea). Cells were seeded at a density of 5×10^4 cells/100 μL/well in 96-well plates and incubated at 37 °C and 5% CO_2 for 24 h. After treating the cells and incubating for 24 h, 10 μL of the WST solution was added to each well, and the plates were incubated for 3–4 h. Absorbances were measured at a detection wavelength of 450 nm and a reference wavelength of 650 nm using a Tecan microplate reader (Männedorf, Switzerland).

2.7. Lactate Dehydrogenase Assay (LDH)

LDH released into the culture supernatant was measured using an EZ-LDH assay kit (DoGenBio, Seoul, Republic of Korea). PC12 cells were seeded and incubated under the same conditions as those used for the WST assay. After 24 h of treatment, the cell culture plates were centrifuged at $600 \times g$ for 5 min. Subsequently, 10 μL of supernatant from each well was transferred to a new 96-well plate and mixed with 100 μL of LDH reaction mixture for 30 min in darkness. LDH levels in the culture medium were determined by measuring the absorbance at 450 nm (reference wavelength, 650 nm) using a Tecan microplate reader (Männedorf, Switzerland).

2.8. Enzyme-Linked Immunosorbent Assay (ELISA)

The levels of inflammatory cytokines TNF-α and IL-6 secreted by BV2 cells in the culture media were measured to evaluate the anti-inflammatory activity of the essential oils. The cells were seeded at a density of 2×10^5 cells/1 mL/well in 12-well plates and incubated at 37 °C and 5% CO_2 for one day. 24 h after treatments, cell culture media were collected and centrifuged at 1500× g rpm for 10 min at 4 °C to remove particulates. The next steps were performed using ELISA kits (LABISKOMA, Seoul, Republic of Korea) following the manufacturer's protocols. The absorbance at 450 nm was measured to detect cytokine levels, using a Tecan microplate reader (Männedorf, Switzerland).

2.9. Molecular Docking

The crystal structures of the GluN1 and GluN2B-NMDAR subunits and GluA2-AMPAR subunit (PDB ID:5H8Q, 5EWM, and 5ZG3, respectively) were downloaded from the Protein Data Bank (RCSB PDB) as previously described [39–41]. Then, all the heteroatoms and water molecules of the proteins were removed. Finally, Kollman charges were added to the proteins, and the macromolecules were exported into a PDBQT format for molecular docking. Information about the main compounds of essential oils was collected from the PubMed database and Traditional Chinese Medicine Systems Pharmacology Database and Analysis Platform (TCMSP). Only compounds with a molecular weight $\leq$ 500 Da and blood–brain barrier index $\geq$ 0.3 were selected. The 3D structures of the compounds were retrieved from the PubChem database. All ligands were then converted into PDBQT format using AutoDockTools version 1.5.6 (The Scripps Research Institute, San Diego, CA, USA).

Molecular docking of GluN1, GluN2B, and GluA2 was performed using AutoDock Vina, version 1.2.0 (The Scripps Research Institute, San Diego, CA, USA). According to the native ligand, the grid boxes that covered the active sites of GluN1, GluN2B, and GluA2 were defined using the following parameters: center_x = 14.66, center_y = −14.25, center_z = −25.74, size_x = 30, size_y = 30, and size_z = 30; center_x = 81.00, center_y = 5.90, center_z = −32.42, size_x = 30, size_y = 30, and size_z = 30; and center_x = 33.47, center_y = −55.89, center_z = 19.58, size_x = 30, size_y = 30, and size_z = 30, respectively. Before the docking study was performed, the docking parameters and algorithm were validated by re-docking the native ligand to the target receptor. The re-docked conformation was then superimposed onto the co-crystallized one using Discovery Studio Visualizer 2021 (Dassault Systèmes BIOVIA, San Diego, CA, USA) and the root mean square deviation (RMSD) was calculated. An RMSD lower than 2 Å suggested that the method could consistently predict the natural conformation of the ligand receptor [42,43].

In this study, ketamine, ifenprodil, and TAK-653, allosteric NMDAR antagonists and an allosteric AMPAR potentiator, respectively, were selected as reference compounds to check whether they strongly interacted with proteins inside selected binding pockets. Within the same grid boxes, herbal compounds with good protein affinity were suggested to exert similar effects as the reference compounds. Favorable conformations were selected based on the lowest binding energy. Finally, Discovery Studio Visualizer 2021 was used to visualize the molecular interactions between proteins and ligands.

2.10. Statistical Analysis

All experiments were performed with at least three independent experiments. GraphPad Prism 8.0 (GraphPad Software, San Diego, CA, USA) was used for statistical analysis. The results are presented as means ± standard deviations (SDs) followed by statistical significance (two-tailed unpaired Student's *t*-test) defined as a p-value < 0.05.

3. Results

3.1. Effects of Essential Oils on CORT-Induced Neurotoxicity in PC12 Cells

To determine the appropriate concentration of CORT for inducing cell damage, PC12 cells were incubated for 24 h with 100, 200, 300, and 400 μM CORT. Exposure to CORT reduced survival in a dose-dependent manner by 25, 38, 70, and 85%, respectively (Figure 1A). The cell viability of the 200 μM CORT-treated group decreased to about half that of the control group; this concentration was therefore used in subsequent experiments to induce neurotoxicity.

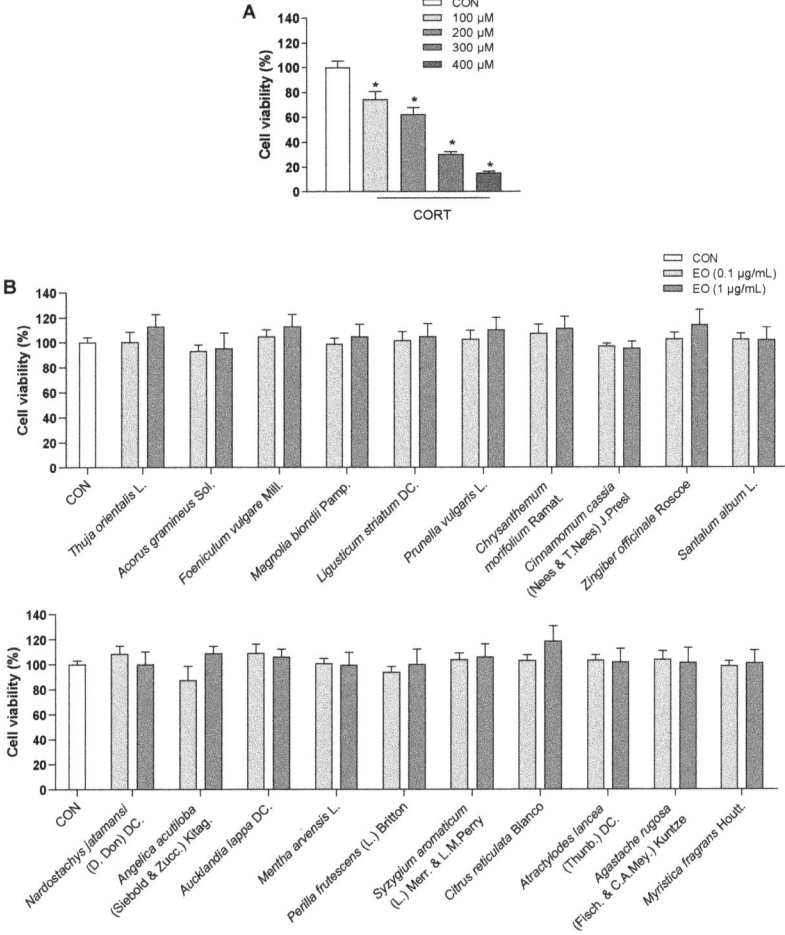

Figure 1. Effects of (**A**) CORT and (**B**) essential oils on the viability of PC12 cells. Results are presented as means ± SDs ($n = 3$ per experiment). * $p < 0.05$ vs. CON.

The effects of 0.1 and 1.0 μg/mL of each essential oil on the viability of PC12 cells were also assessed. As shown in Figure 1B, all essential oils did not cause toxicity to PC12 cells at doses of 0.1 and 1.0 μg/mL; these doses were then used to treat the cells for 1 h prior to incubation with CORT for 24 h. As shown in Figure 2A, compared with the control group, the cell survival rate significantly decreased in the model group treated with 200 μM CORT ($p < 0.05$). *Foeniculum vulgare* Mill., *Chrysanthemum morifolium* Ramat., *Angelica acutiloba* (Siebold & Zucc.) Kitag., *Aucklandia lappa* DC., *Syzygium aromaticum* (L.) Merr. & L.M. Perry, *Citrus reticulata* Blanco, *Atractylodes lancea* (Thunb.) DC., and *Myristica fragrans* Houtt. essential oils showed a dose-response relationship, while *Acorus gramineus* Sol. did not exhibit a protective effect at either of the two doses, and the remaining 11 essential oils exerted an effect only at the higher dose.

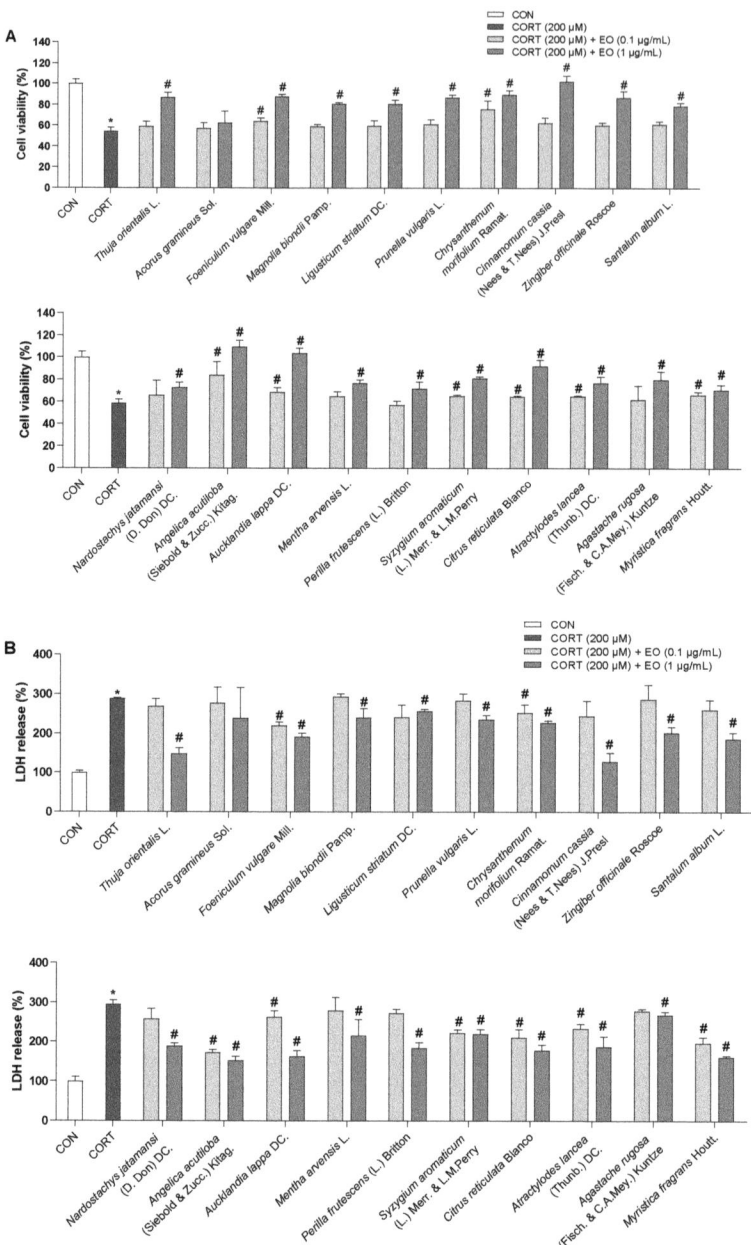

Figure 2. Effects of essential oils on CORT-induced neurotoxicity in PC12 cells. (**A**) Effects of essential oils on the cell viability in CORT-stimulated PC12 cells. (**B**) Effects of essential oils on the LDH release in CORT-stimulated PC12 cells. Results are presented as means ± SDs (n = 3 per experiment). * $p < 0.05$ vs. CON, # $p < 0.05$ vs. CORT-treated cells.

As LDH leakage from cells is widely used as a cellular damage marker, LDH release was measured in the culture medium to assess PC12 cell injury. LDH secreted from cells was significantly increased in the model group compared to that in the control group;

the percentage of LDH leakage increased from 100% (control) to 288 ± 6.9%. However, pretreatment with essential oils reduced LDH leakage (Figure 2B), which was consistent with the data from the WST assay. These results indicated that essential oil pretreatment could prevent CORT-induced injury in PC12 cells.

3.2. Effects of Essential Oils on LPS-Induced Neuroinflammation in BV2 Cells

To test whether essential oil treatments were toxic to the viability of BV2 cells, a WST assay was performed using concentrations of 0.1 and 1.0 µg/mL of each essential oil. From the results, all essential oils did not cause toxicity to BV2 cells at doses of 0.1 and 1.0 µg/mL. Although *Thuja orientalis* L. at 1.0 µg/mL decreased cell viability to approximately 75%, this reduction was not statistically significant (Figure 3). Hence, doses of 0.1 and 1.0 µg/mL of all essential oils were used for the subsequent experiments.

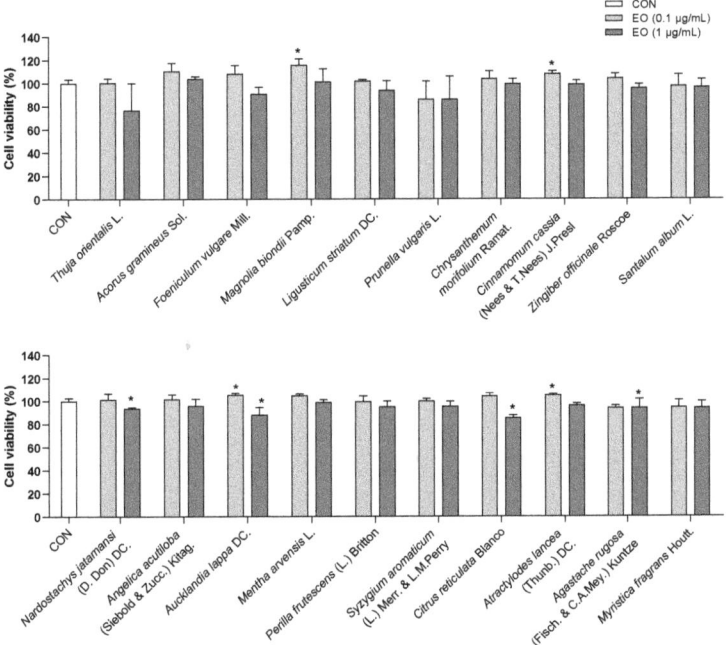

Figure 3. Effects of essential oils on the viability of BV2 cells. Results are presented as means ± SDs (n = 3 per experiment). * p < 0.05 vs. CON.

As shown in Figure 4, LPS (1 µg/mL) remarkably increased the production of the inflammatory cytokines TNF-α and IL-6 compared to that in the control BV2 cells, but this effect was blunted by pretreatment with essential oils at different levels. In particular, 10 essential oils (*Ligusticum striatum* DC., *Cinnamomum cassia* (Nees & T.Nees) J.Presl, *Santalum album* L., *Aucklandia lappa* DC., *Mentha arvensis* L., *Perilla frutescens* (L.) Britton, *Syzygium aromaticum* (L.) Merr. & L.M. Perry, *Citrus reticulata* Blanco, *Atractylodes lancea* (Thunb.) DC., and *Myristica fragrans* Houtt.) reduced IL-6 release, yet only six essential oils (*Foeniculum vulgare* Mill., *Ligusticum striatum* DC., *Prunella vulgaris* L., *Chrysanthemum morifolium* Ramat., *Cinnamomum cassia* (Nees & T.Nees) J.Presl, and *Santalum album* L.) abrogated the increase in TNF-α levels (Figure 4). Of the 20 examined essential oils, eight including *Chrysanthemum morifolium* Ramat., *Cinnamomum cassia* (Nees & T.Nees) J.Presl, *Santalum album* L., *Perilla frutescens* (L.) Britton, *Syzygium aromaticum* (L.) Merr. & L.M. Perry, *Citrus reticulata* Blanco, *Atractylodes lancea* (Thunb.) DC., and *Myristica fragrans* Houtt. suppressed TNF-α or IL-6 production at a low dose of 0.1 µg/mL. Moreover, three essential oils (*Ligusticum striatum* DC., *Cinnamomum cassia* (Nees & T.Nees) J.Presl, and *Santalum album* L.) significantly decreased the levels of both the assessed inflammatory cytokines (Figure 4). At the investigated doses, no beneficial effects were observed for *Thuja orientalis* L., *Acorus gramineus* Sol., *Magnolia biondii* Pamp., *Zingiber officinale* Roscoe, *Nardostachys jatamansi* (D. Don) DC., *Angelica acutiloba* (Siebold & Zucc.) Kitag., and *Agastache rugosa* (Fisch. & C.A.Mey.) Kuntze.

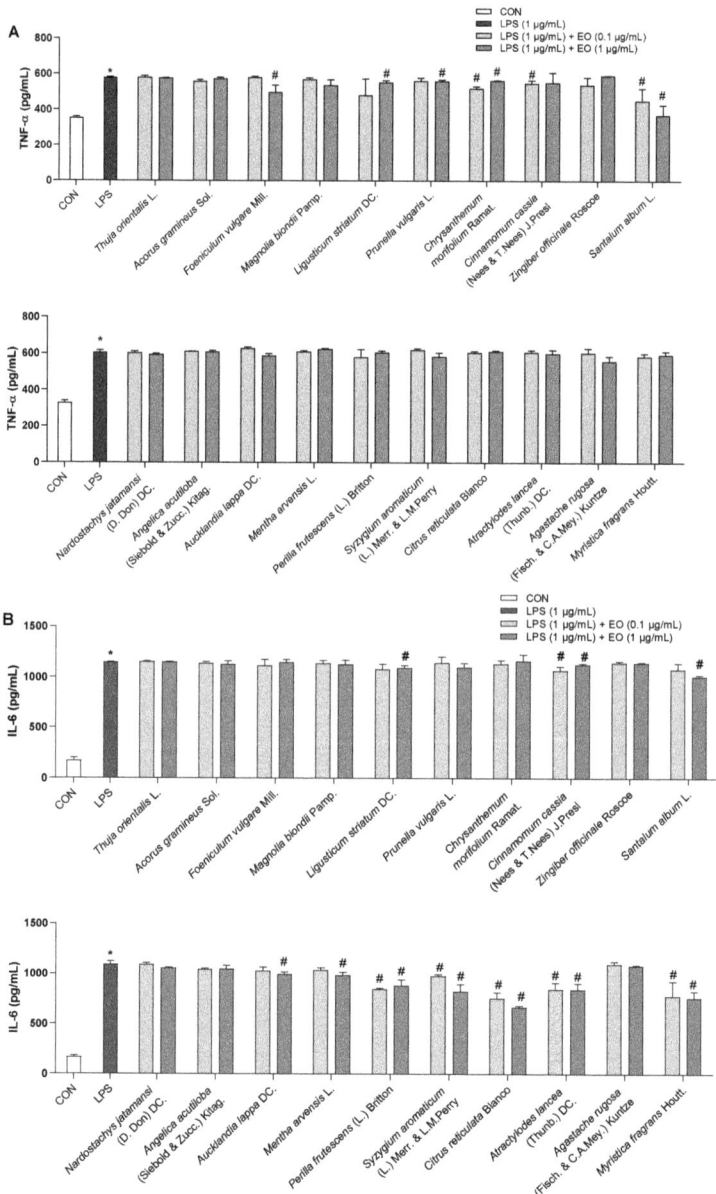

Figure 4. Effects of essential oils on LPS-induced neuroinflammation in BV2 cells. (**A**) TNF-α levels (pg/mL). (**B**) IL-6 levels (pg/mL). Results are presented as means ± SDs (n = 3 per experiment). * $p < 0.05$ vs. CON, # $p < 0.05$ vs. LPS-treated cells.

3.3. Rapid-Acting Effect of Essential Oils on Behavior Changes of Mice in the TST and EPM

Based on the in vitro results, 19 potential essential oils were used for the in vivo experiments. Thirty minutes after intranasal administration, the TST and EPM were conducted to investigate the effects of essential oils on the behavior of mice. During the TST, *Chrysanthemum morifolium* Ramat., *Zingiber officinale* Roscoe, *Santalum album* L., *Citrus reticulata* Blanco, *Atractylodes lancea* (Thunb.) DC., and *Myristica fragrans* Houtt. essential oil treatments exhibited antidepressant-like effects by decreasing the immobility time compared with the control mice (Figure 5). There was a reduction in the immobility time of mice in the TST after memantine treatment, while no statistically significant change was observed in the EPM (Figures 5 and 6). As shown in Figure 6, both *Chrysanthemum morifolium* Ramat. and *Myristica fragrans* Houtt. essential oils enhanced the percentage of distance covered in the open arms in the EPM test. In addition, *Myristica fragrans* Houtt. significantly increased the number of open arm entries, while *Chrysanthemum morifolium* Ramat. treatment increased the time of mice exploring the open arms, indicating antianxiety-like effects. In contrast, *Magnolia biondii* Pamp. exerted the opposite effect, significantly reducing exploration time in the open arms.

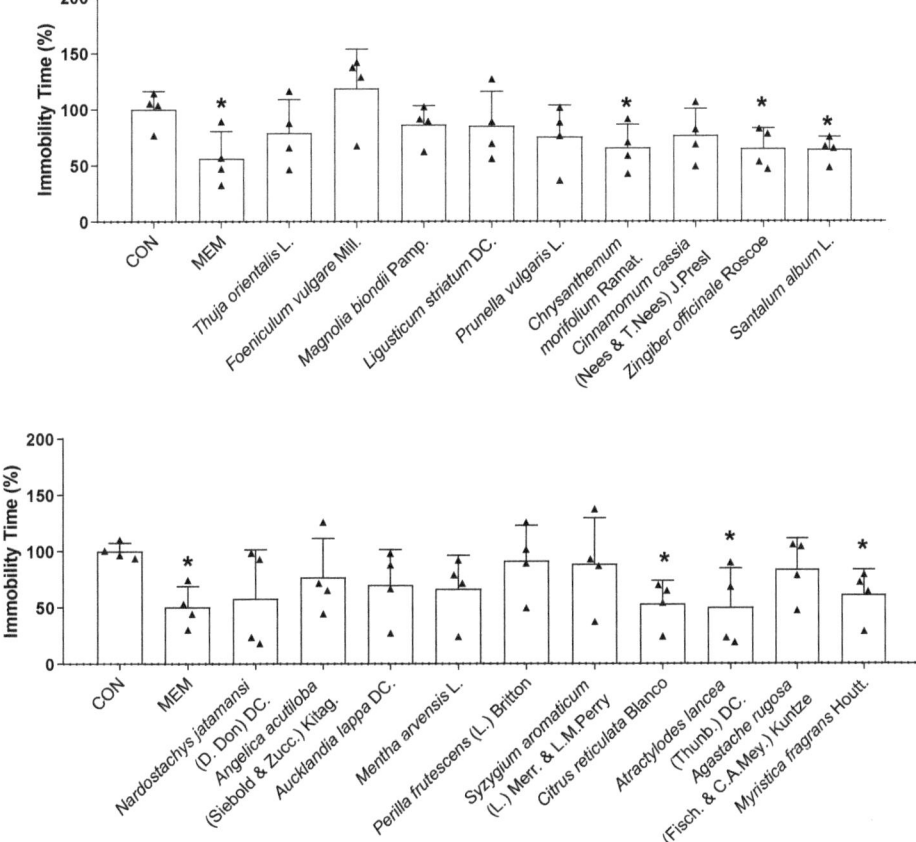

Figure 5. Effects of essential oils on the behavioral changes of mice in TST test. The immobility time in TST was recorded. Each black triangle indicates the value of each mouse subject in groups. Results are presented as means percentage relative to control ± SDs (n = 4 mice per group). * $p < 0.05$ vs. CON.

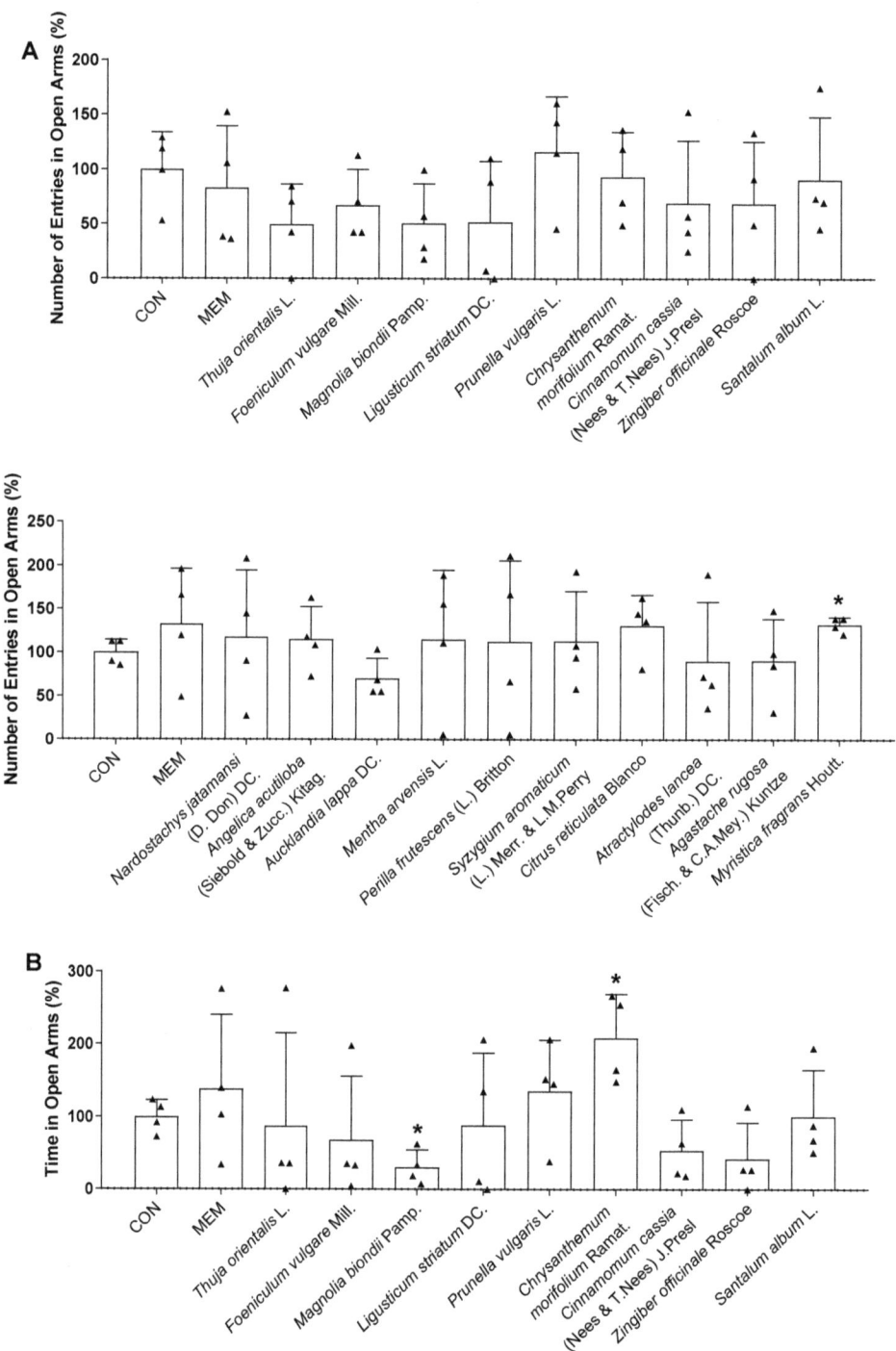

Figure 6. *Cont.*

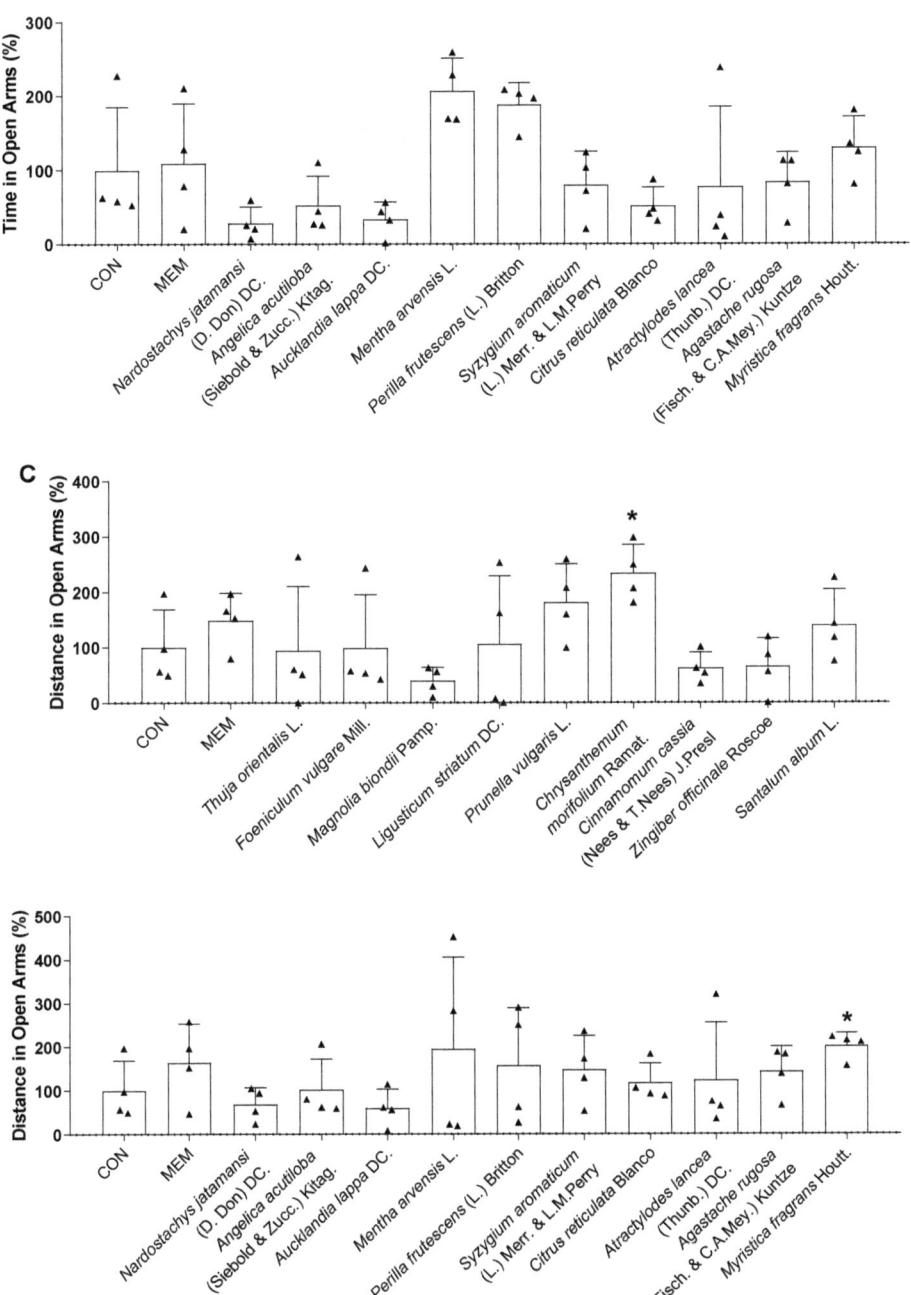

Figure 6. Effects of essential oils on the behavioral changes of mice in EPM test. The (**A**) number of entries, (**B**) time, and (**C**) distance in open arms were recorded. Each black triangle indicates the value of each mouse subject in groups. Results are presented as means percentage relative to control ± SDs (*n* = 4 mice per group). * $p < 0.05$ vs. CON.

3.4. Molecular Docking Analysis of Essential Oil Main Compounds

Molecular docking was conducted to investigate the five major compounds of the seven essential oils that modified depressant- or anxiety-related behaviors in animal tests (Table 1). After removing duplicates, 27 compounds remained (Table 2). The docking protocol was validated through a re-docking experiment using the native ligand. Root mean square deviation (RMSD) values of less than 2 Å were observed, suggesting that the ligand-receptor conformations had a high docking accuracy (Figure 7). The molecular docking of compounds against the GluN1, GluN2B, and GluA2 proteins obtained using Autodock Vina are presented in Table 3, with higher negative binding energies indicating better affinity between components. Among the 27 natural compounds, 24, 22, and 13 had docking scores of less than −6.0 kcal/mol toward GluN1, GluN2B, and GluA2, respectively, suggesting a highly stable complex. When compared with the reference compounds, four compounds, including atractylon, α-curcumene, α-farnesene, and selina-4(14),7(11)-dien-8-one, had lower energy binding than ketamine when interacting with all three proteins, while none had lower docking scores than ifenprodil and TAK-653. The 2D conformations are visualized in Figures 8–10.

Table 1. Main compounds of essential oils.

No.	Essential Oil	Main Compounds					Ref.
1	*Magnolia biondii* Pamp.	Camphor	*trans*-Caryophyllene	1,8-Cineole	α-Pinene	β-Pinene	[44–46]
2	*Chrysanthemum morifolium* Ramat.	α-Curcumene	α-Farnesene	*n*-Heptadecane	Linoleic Acid	Nonadecane	[47,48]
3	*Zingiber officinale* Roscoe	Camphene	1,8-Cineole	β-Myrcene	β-Phellandrene	α-Pinene	[49–51]
4	*Santalum album* L.	(Z)-*trans*-α-Bergamotol	(Z)-Lanceol	(E)-Nuciferol	(Z)-α-Santalol	(E)-β-Santalol	[52–54]
5	*Citrus reticulata* Blanco	Limonene	Linalool	β-Myrcene	α-Pinene	γ-Terpinene	[55–58]
6	*Atractylodes lancea* (Thunb.) DC.	Atractylodin	Atractylon	β-Eudesmol	Elemol	Selina-4(14),7(11)-dien-8-one	[59–61]
7	*Myristica fragrans* Houtt.	Limonene	β-Myrcene	α-Phellandrene	α-Pinene	β-Pinene	[62–64]

Table 2. List of ligands.

No.	Compound	Pubchem CID
	Reference compounds	
1	Ketamine	3821
2	Ifenprodil	3689
3	TAK-653	56655833
	Herbal compounds	
1	Atractylodin	5321047
2	Atractylon	3080635
3	(Z)-*trans*-α-Bergamotol	5368743
4	Camphene	6616
5	Camphor	2537
6	*trans*-Caryophyllene	5281515
7	1,8-Cineole	2758
8	α-Curcumene	92139
9	Elemol	92138
10	β-Eudesmol	91457
11	α-Farnesene	5281516
12	*n*-Heptadecane	12398
13	(Z)-Lanceol	15560069
14	Limonene	22311
15	Linalool	6549
16	Linoleic Acid	5280450

Table 2. Cont.

No.	Compound	Pubchem CID
17	β-Myrcene	31253
18	Nonadecane	12401
19	(E)-Nuciferol	6429177
20	α-Phellandrene	7460
21	β-Phellandrene	11142
22	α-Pinene	6654
23	β-Pinene	14896
24	(Z)-α-Santalol	11085337
25	(E)-β-Santalol	11031396
26	Selina-4(14),7(11)-dien-8-one	13986099
27	γ-Terpinene	7461

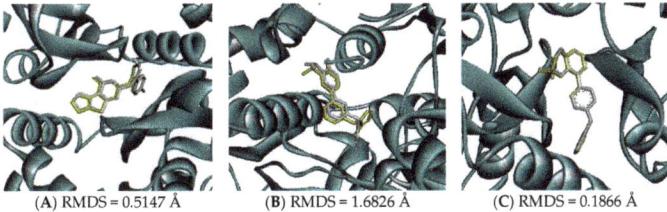

(A) RMDS = 0.5147 Å   (B) RMDS = 1.6826 Å   (C) RMDS = 0.1866 Å

Figure 7. Superimposed zoomed-in image of native ligand and redocked native ligand in the active site of (A) GluN1, (B) GluN2B, and (C) GluA2 (native ligand: gray color, redocked ligand: yellow color).

Table 3. Docking results of ligands towards GluN1, GluN2B, and GluA2 proteins.

No.	Ligand	Binding Energy (kcal/mol)		
		GluN1	GluN2B	GluA2
	Native ligand	−10.4	−10.7	−9.9
1	Ketamine	−8.2	−5.9	−4.9
2	Ifenprodil	−9.6	−9.7	−9.2
3	TAK-653	−8.6	−8.6	−9.2
4	Atractylodin	−7.2	−7.2	−6.0
5	Atractylon	−8.7	−8.8	−6.1
6	(Z)-trans-α-Bergamotol	−7.9	−7.0	−5.8
7	Camphene	−5.8	−5.3	−4.7
8	Camphor	−5.9	−4.6	−4.3
9	trans-Caryophyllene	−7.0	−6.4	−5.6
10	1,8-Cineole	−6.0	−5.6	−4.5
11	α-Curcumene	−8.8	−9.3	−7.0
12	Elemol	−7.2	−7.8	−6.4
13	β-Eudesmol	−7.0	−6.0	−6.2
14	α-Farnesene	−8.2	−8.4	−6.7
15	n-Heptadecane	−6.3	−6.6	−5.8
16	(Z)-Lanceol	−7.8	−8.1	−6.9
17	Limonene	−6.6	−7.5	−6.0
18	Linalool	−6.4	−6.7	−5.7
19	Linoleic Acid	−7.6	−7.2	−6.6
20	β-Myrcene	−6.4	−6.9	−5.0
21	Nonadecane	−6.8	−8.1	−6.9
22	(E)-Nuciferol	−8.1	−8.4	−6.9
23	α-Phellandrene	−6.7	−7.4	−6.1
24	β-Phellandrene	−6.4	−7.5	−6.1
25	α-Pinene	−6.1	−5.7	−4.6
26	β-Pinene	−6.1	−6.2	−4.4
27	(Z)-α-Santalol	−7.4	−6.4	−5.7
28	(E)-β-Santalol	−7.2	−5.5	−6.0
29	Selina-4(14),7(11)-dien-8-one	−8.8	−6.8	−7.6
30	γ-Terpinene	−7.0	−7.4	−5.9

The colors indicate binding energy values corresponding to binding affinity of ligands to the receptor subunits. Redder color: lower energy value, higher binding affinity; Whiter color: higher energy value, lower binding affinity.

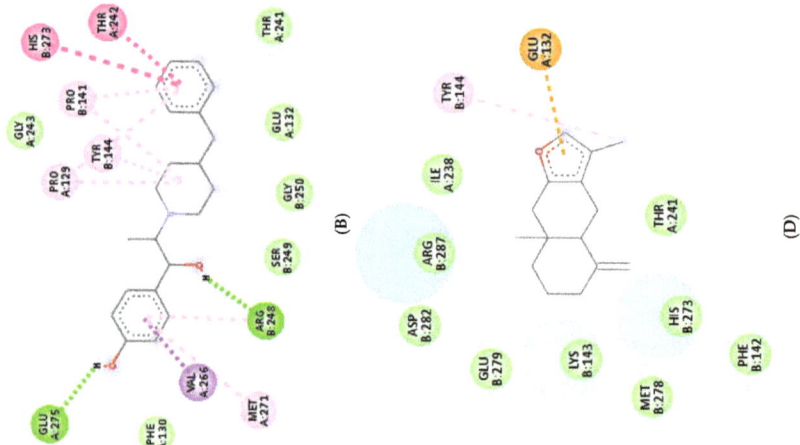

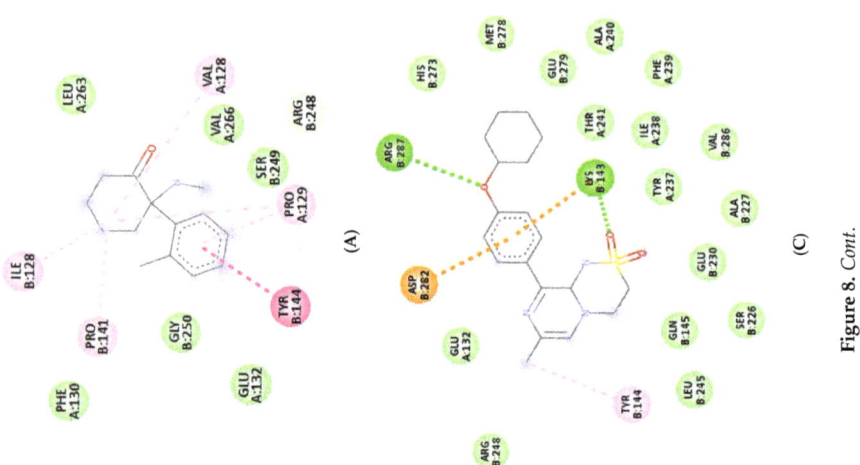

Figure 8. Cont.

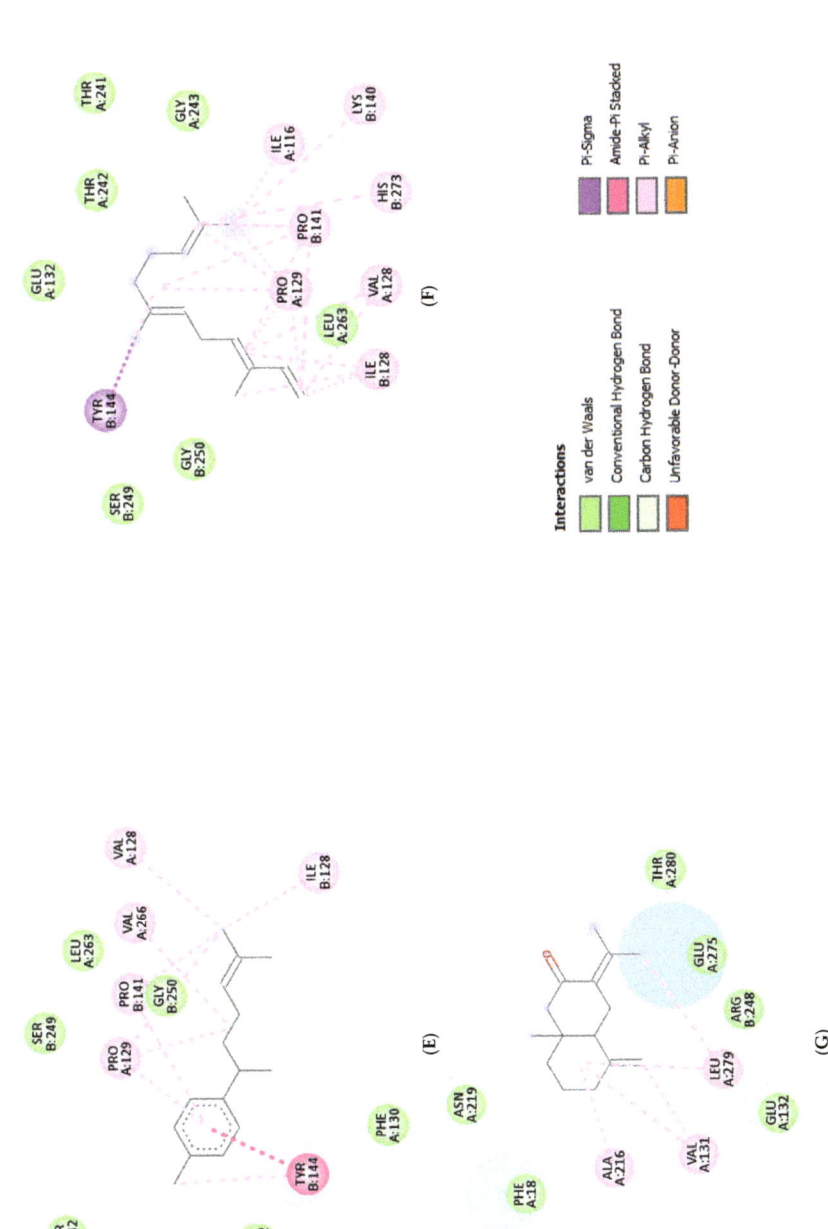

Figure 8. 2D interactions between (**A**) ketamine, (**B**) ifenprodil, (**C**) TAK-653, (**D**) atractylon, (**E**) α-curcumene, (**F**) α-farnesene, and (**G**) selina-4(14),7(11)-dien-8-one with GluN1 protein.

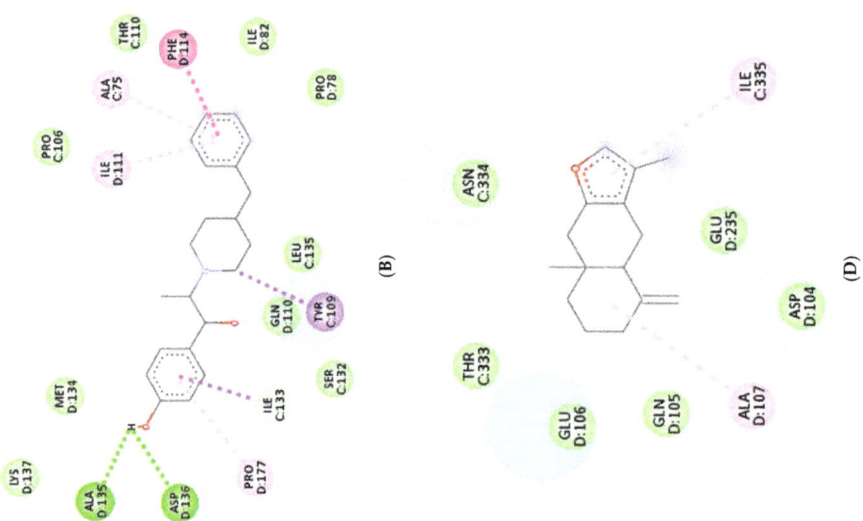

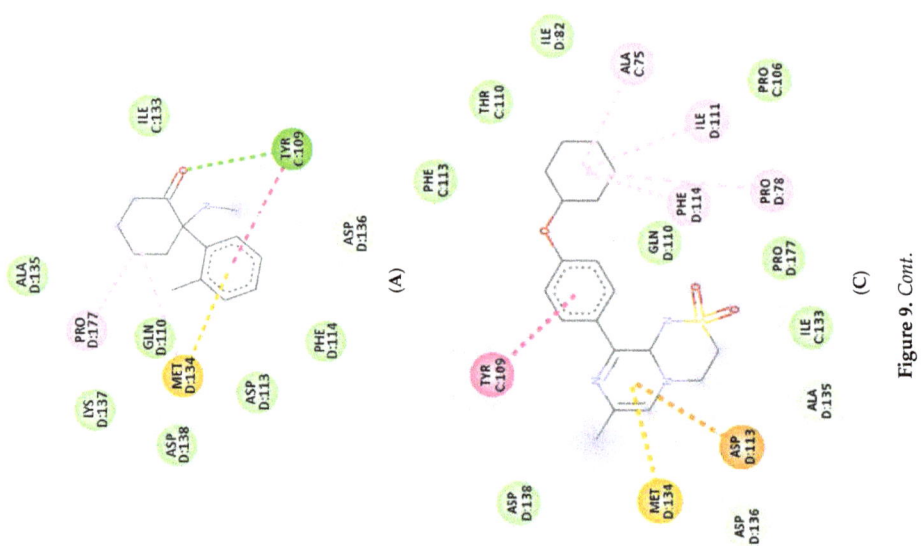

Figure 9. Cont.

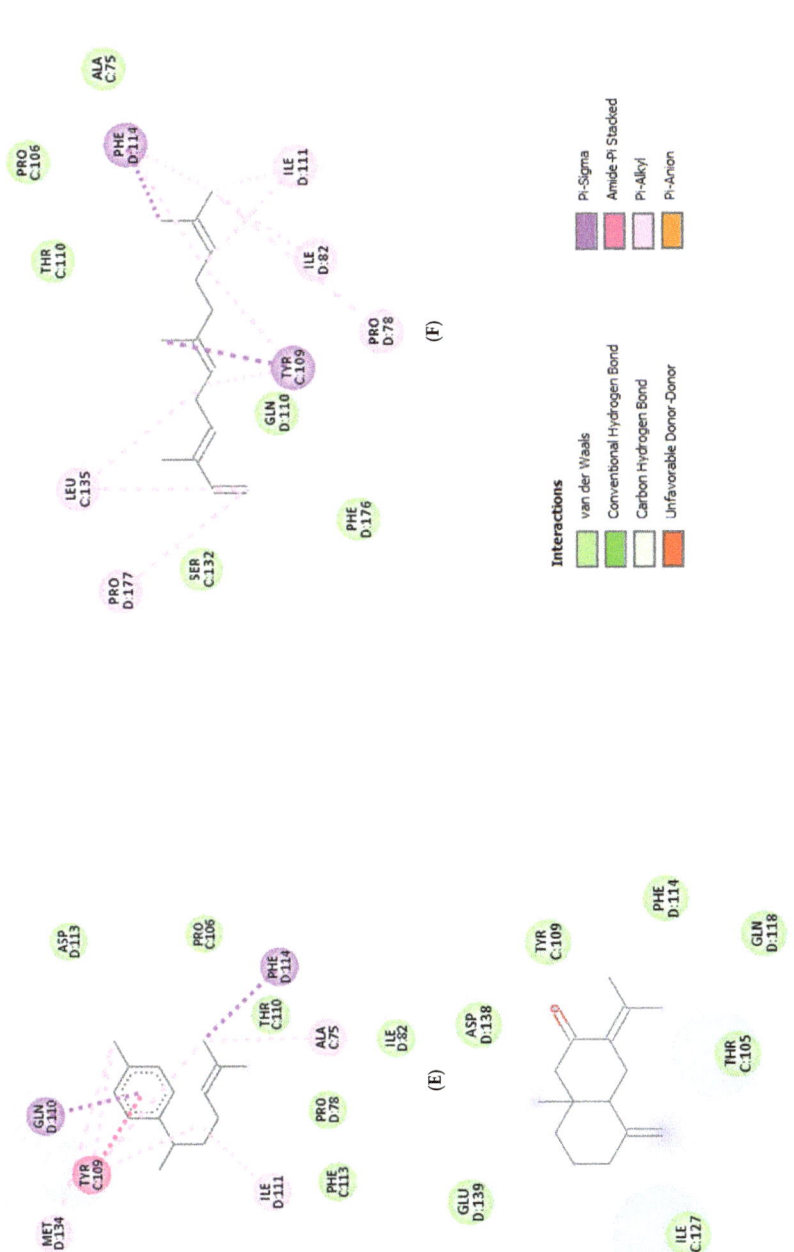

Figure 9. 2D interactions between (**A**) ketamine, (**B**) ifenprodil, (**C**) TAK-653, (**D**) atractylon, (**E**) α-curcumene, (**F**) α-farnesene, and (**G**) selina-4(14),7(11)-dien-8-one with GluN2B protein.

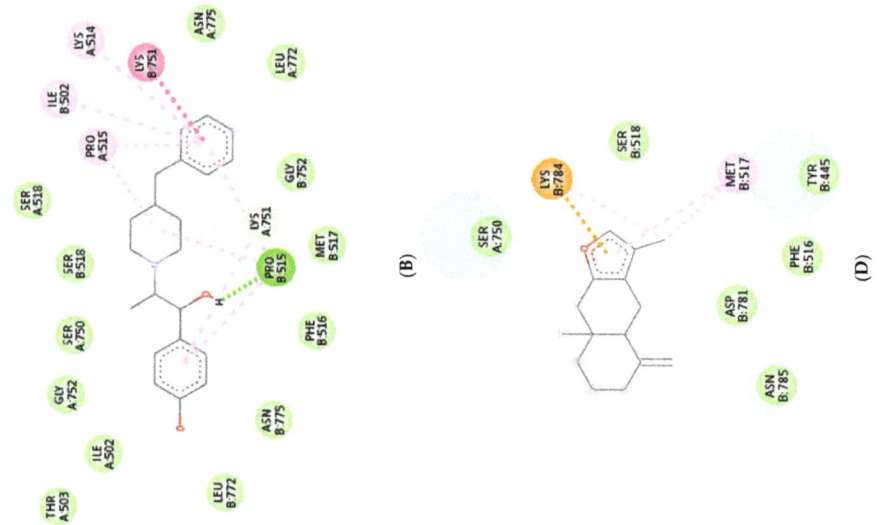

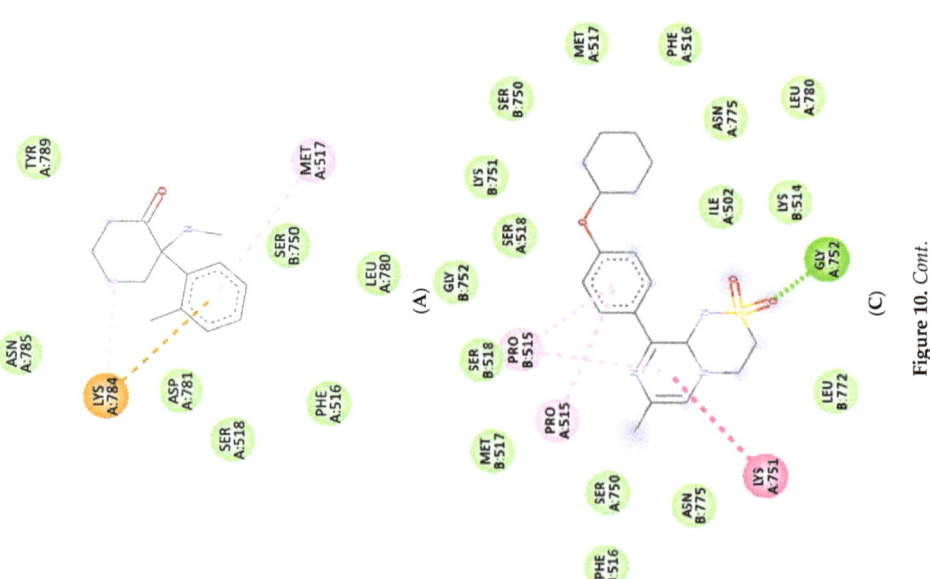

Figure 10. Cont.

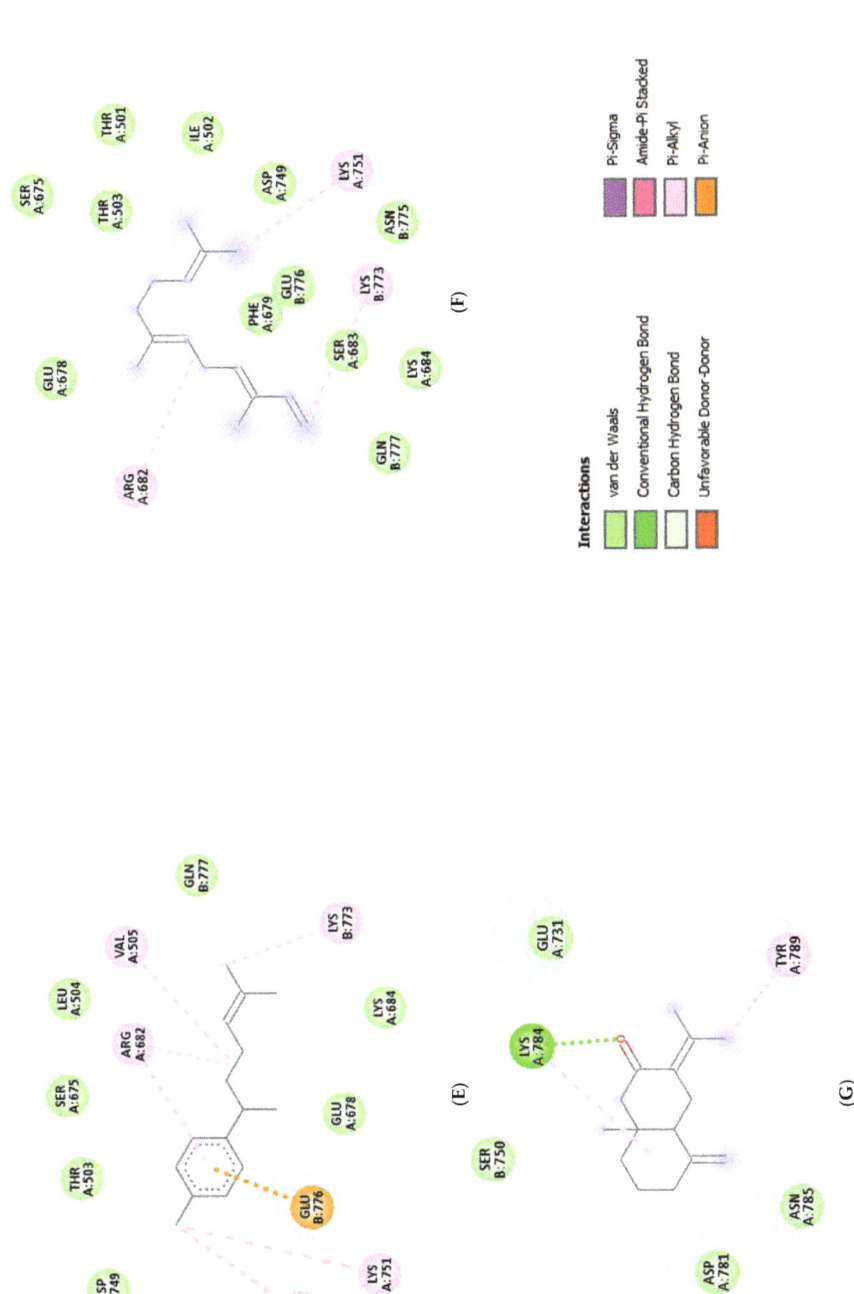

Figure 10. 2D interactions between (**A**) ketamine, (**B**) ifenprodil, (**C**) TAK-653, (**D**) atractylon, (**E**) α-curcumene, (**F**) α-farnesene, and (**G**) selina-4(14),7(11)-dien-8-one with GluA2 protein.

4. Discussion

Side effects and delayed onset of action are the limitations of current antidepressants. Ketamine was reported to alleviate depressive symptoms within hours post-treatment, but rapid-acting antidepressants have not yet made any other striking progress [65,66]. Essential oils possessing antianxiety and antidepressant properties with fewer side effects have been reported [67]. They mainly consist of small and lipophilic molecules, and therefore can quickly and easily bypass the BBB to target brain tissues, acting on the cerebral cortex, thalamus, and limbic system, indicating their potential application in alleviating symptoms of anxiety and depression in a rapid manner [21,22]. Additionally, recent studies have revealed the advantages of intranasal administration over other routes of administration [26]. Hence, the purpose of this study was to identify essential oils with rapid-acting antidepressant effects when administered intranasally. As expected, our results suggested that different essential oils exerted neuroprotective effects in vitro and rapid antidepressant-like effects in a normal mouse model (Table 4). In addition, the effects of essential oils were comparable to those of MEM, a common medication used to treat moderate-to-severe dementia, whose acute antidepressant-like effects have also been reported in previous studies [68,69].

Table 4. Summary of key research findings: neuroprotective, anti-neuroinflammatory effects in vitro and rapid-acting anti-anxiety and anti-depressant effects in vivo of 20 essential oils.

No.	Herb	In Vitro			In Vivo	
		Neuroprotective Dose (µg/mL)	Anti-Neuroinflammatory Dose (µg/mL)		Rapid Anti-Depressant Dose (mg/kg)	Rapid Anti-Anxiety Dose (mg/kg)
			TNF-α	IL-6		
1	*Thuja orientalis* L.	1	-	-	-	-
2	*Acorus gramineus* Sol.	-	-	-	-	-
3	*Foeniculum vulgare* Mill.	0.1, 1	1	-	-	-
4	*Magnolia biondii* Pamp.	1	-	-	-	-
5	*Ligusticum striatum* DC.	1	1	1	-	-
6	*Prunella vulgaris* L.	1	1	-	-	-
7	*Chrysanthemum morifolium* Ramat.	0.1, 1	0.1, 1	-	25	25
8	*Cinnamomum cassia* (Nees & T.Nees) J.Presl	1	0.1	0.1, 1	-	-
9	*Zingiber officinale* Roscoe	1	-	-	25	-
10	*Santalum album* L.	1	0.1, 1	1	25	-
11	*Nardostachys jatamansi* (D. Don) DC.	1	-	-	-	-
12	*Angelica acutiloba* (Siebold & Zucc.) Kitag.	0.1, 1	-	-	-	-
13	*Aucklandia lappa* DC.	0.1, 1	-	1	-	-
14	*Mentha arvensis* L.	1	-	1	-	-
15	*Perilla frutescens* (L.) Britton	1	-	0.1, 1	-	-
16	*Syzygium aromaticum* (L.) Merr. & L.M.Perry	0.1, 1	-	0.1, 1	-	-
17	*Citrus reticulata* Blanco	0.1, 1	-	0.1, 1	25	-
18	*Atractylodes lancea* (Thunb.) DC.	0.1, 1	-	0.1, 1	25	-
19	*Agastache rugosa* (Fisch. & C.A.Mey.) Kuntze.	1	-	-	-	-
20	*Myristica fragrans* Houtt.	0.1, 1	-	0.1, 1	25	25

Neuroinflammation is a common feature in patients with depression. Several studies have reported that inflammation in the brain and the associated over-release of pro-inflammatory cytokines TNF-α, IL-6, or IL-1β can lead to a loss of hippocampal neurogenesis, promoting depression-like behaviors [10]. The underlying mechanism may be related to microglial cells, which influence neuronal excitability and neurotransmission [70]. Under threats such as the LPS challenge, microglia are activated to undergo morphological changes and secrete pro-inflammatory cytokines [71]. These cytokines can decrease the levels of serotonin and norepinephrine, which are neurotransmitters involved in mood regulation [72]. In addition, pro-inflammatory cytokines can affect the function of the hippocampus, a brain region that is important for learning, memory, and mood regulation [12]. In the present study, we treated the murine microglial cell line BV2 with LPS and essential oils, with the hypothesis that essential oils that could reduce LPS-induced pro-inflammatory cytokines would have potential antidepressant effects. Essential oils such as *Chrysanthemum morifolium* Ramat., *Santalum album* L., *Citrus reticulata* Blanco, and *Atractylodes lancea* (Thunb.) DC., which inhibited TNF-α or IL-6 released from LPS-treated BV2 cells, significantly decreased the immobility time of mice in TST, suggesting their antidepressant effects occurred through inactivating glial cells and reducing neuroinflammation.

Depression is also accompanied by the overproduction of CORT, which affects numerous physiological processes in neurons and astrocytes, such as apoptosis and synaptic plasticity [73]. High concentrations of CORT can increase the production of reactive oxygen species (ROS) and pro-inflammatory cytokines, which can damage neuronal cells [74,75]. Additionally, through activating glucocorticoid receptors (GRs) in neurons, CORT can cause a cascade of apoptosis-related enzymes known as caspases that are responsible for initiating programmed cell death [76]. GRs are mainly distributed in the hippocampus, and CORT-induced GR overexpression can lead to structural changes such as hippocampal atrophy, loss of dendritic synapses, and synaptic plasticity alternation, resulting in the development of anxiety and depression [77–81]. In this study, PC12 cells, a classical neuronal cell line, were treated with CORT to mimic the features of depression, and essential oils that protect cells from CORT-induced toxicity may have the potential to treat depression. PC12 cell viability was evaluated using a WST assay based on mitochondrial succinate dehydrogenase activity, indicative of cellular energy capacity, compared to LDH leakage, indicative of apoptosis [82]. Our results showed that 19 of the 20 essential oils included in this study inhibited CORT-induced cell death and LDH leakage, indicating their potential in the treatment of depression, probably by decreasing neuronal apoptosis. In addition, a very small dose of essential oil (SDE extract), including 0.1 or 1 µg/mL, was sufficient to exhibit anti-inflammatory and neuroprotective effects. Previous studies using ethanol or methanol extracts of herbal materials normally required an effective dose of 10–100 µg/mL. This demonstrates one benefit of essential oils in drug development applications [83–86].

The TST is an important behavioral model that is widely used to screen for new antidepressants. In animals subjected to inescapable stress, immobility has been suggested as a key indicator of behavioral despair, reminiscent of depressive disorders in humans [37]. In the present study, a significant decrease in immobility time in treated mice was observed with six essential oils only 30 min after intranasal administration, indicating their fast antidepressant-like activity. This is the first time the rapid antidepressant effects of *Chrysanthemum morifolium* Ramat., *Zingiber officinale* Roscoe, *Santalum album* L., *Citrus reticulata* Blanco, *Atractylodes lancea* (Thunb.) DC., and *Myristica fragrans* Houtt. essential oils have been reported, particularly through intranasal administration. Although the antidepressant activity of nutmeg (*Myristica fragrans*) seeds has been reported in previous studies, its effect was observed after oral administration for three days [87,88].

The EPM is an extensively used model for the assessment of novel anxiolytic agents, based on the natural tendency of rodents to avoid open and elevated areas [38]. Because high levels of anxiety result in depression, and that approximately 85% of patients with depression have significant anxiety, anxiety is considered one of the symptoms of depression [89,90]. Among the two effective essential oils, *Chrysanthemum morifolium* Ramat. increased the time mice spent in the open arms, whereas *Myristica fragrans* Houtt. increased open-arm entries. Although no essential oils significantly elevated either parameter, increasing trends were observed. Moreover, mice treated with the two essential oils also showed notably higher total distances in the open arms than that demonstrated in the control group. Therefore, these essential oils might have exerted anti-anxiety effects to a certain extent, as evidenced by an increased exploration in the open elevated space, which contributed to the reduction of depression-like behaviors.

Ketamine and ifenprodil, an NMDAR antagonist and a GluN2B-selective NMDAR antagonist, respectively, have been proven to be rapid-acting antidepressant therapies in clinical and in vivo studies. Their mechanisms may be related to the de-inhibition of mTOR activity, which induces protein biosynthesis, leading to synaptic potentiation [33,91]. In addition, by blocking spontaneous NMDAR-mediated neurotransmission, ketamine can suppress eukaryotic elongation factor 2 (eEF2) kinase function, preventing eEF2 substrate phosphorylation and enhancing BDNF translation. Ketamine can also upregulate AMPAR, especially the GluA1 and GluA2 subunits, thereby enhancing synaptic strengthening and transmission [91,92]. TAK-653, an AMPAR potentiator, exerts antidepressant effects in vivo. It can also directly activate AMPAR, stimulating the mammalian target of rapamycin (mTOR) and BDNF signaling in vitro [36]. In 2015, a study revealed that ketamine conferred fast antidepressant effects in mice 30 min after intraperitoneal injection, favorably suppressing NMDAR subunits GluN1 and GluN2B functioning in the hippocampus [31]. Additionally, Li et al. suggested that ketamine exerts antidepressant effects by enhancing AMPAR expression [34]. Indeed, current concepts regarding glutamate receptors suggest that drugs that increase AMPAR signaling or decrease NMDAR function may be effective antidepressants. Therefore, we performed a molecular docking analysis of the main compounds from the essential oils toward GluN1, GluN2B, and GluA2 proteins using ketamine, ifenprodil, and TAK-653 as reference compounds.

Molecular docking is a computational technique that predicts the binding orientation and affinity of small molecules (compounds) to a target protein or macromolecule (receptor subunits). It provides insights into the mechanisms of drug action and allows researchers to identify potential drug candidates and optimize their binding properties before conducting costly and time-consuming experiments [93,94]. Besides, through simulating the binding interactions between molecules and targets, the technique may also suggest whether a candidate drug has similar actions to other reference compounds. Here, we showed that in comparison with ketamine (with docking scores of -8.2, -5.9, and -4.9 kcal/mol toward GluN1, GluN2B, and GluA2, respectively), four compounds including atractylon, α-curcumene, α-farnesene, and selina-4(14),7(11)-dien-8-one had much lower docking scores, indicating stronger binding to the targeted receptors. Hence, these compounds that are main components of *Atractylodes lancea* (Thunb.) DC. and *Chrysanthemum morifolium* Ramat. essential oils are of greater concern.

Atractylodes lancea (Thunb.) DC. is a type of Atractylodis Rhizoma, whose extract has been commonly used for the treatment of digestive disorders owing to its anti-inflammatory and gastroprotective effects [59]. *Atractylodes lancea* (Thunb.) DC. may also have the potential to treat depression. A previous study suggested that drugs inhibiting gastric acid secretion can be used to treat depressive symptoms and antidepressants can be an effective treatment for stress ulcers, indicating a similar mechanism of pathogenesis shared by the two ailments [95]. This is consistent with our results showing that *Atractylodes lancea* (Thunb.) DC. essential oil significantly reduced depression-like behaviors in mice in the TST. Furthermore, atractylon, one of the major constituents of this essential oil, was recently found to improve cognitive dysfunction in mice by inhibiting microglial activation and exerting anti-inflammatory activity in vitro through the inhibition of cyclooxygenase-2 (COX-2) and inducible nitric oxide synthase (iNOS) expression [96,97]. Such an action has been previously revealed to curb depressive symptoms by reducing neuroinflammation [12,72]. Compared with ketamine, atractylon has a lower binding energy for the three glutamate receptor subunits, indicating a stronger binding capacity than ketamine. Notably, atractylon can interact with GluN1 and GluA2 subunits through the same amino acids as that of ketamine, suggesting a similar mechanism of action for its rapid-acting antidepressant effect (Figures 8 and 10). Regarding selina-4(14),7(11)-dien-8-one, also a major component of *Atractylodes lancea* (Thunb.) DC., the pharmacological activity of this compound has not been reported to date. However, based on the molecular docking results, this compound was able to interact with the GluA2 subunit at sites similar to those of ketamine and ifenprodil (Figure 10). Hence, selina-4(14),7(11)-dien-8-one is also a compound with potential for the research and development of antidepressants.

Chrysanthemum morifolium Ramat. is a traditional herb widely used for the treatment of fever, headache, sore throat, and hypertension, due to the variety of flavonoids, anthocyanins, alkaloids, and phenolic acid components found in its extract [98]. Notably, neuroprotective and antioxidant effects, as well as its ability to reduce ROS levels and lipid peroxidation, have also been reported [99,100]. ROS and oxidative stress are known to cause dysfunction in neurotransmission and the HPA axis, reduced neuroplasticity, and neuroinflammation, all of which are involved in the pathogenesis of depression [101]. Hence, the antidepressant potential of *Chrysanthemum morifolium* Ramat. should not be overlooked. However, until now, only one previous study revealed the chronic antidepressant effect of *Chrysanthemum morifolium* on CORT-injected C57BL/6 mice, evidenced by significantly elevated sucrose consumption and serum serotonin levels [102]. Our results showed that *Chrysanthemum morifolium* Ramat. essential oil improved both anxiety-like and depression-like symptoms after only a single dose, suggesting an acute effect on depression. We predict that such an effect may originate from the two main compounds of the essential oil, α-curcumene, and α-farnesene, although only the anti-inflammatory effect of α-farnesene has been reported to date [103]. We found that the interaction of these two compounds with the glutamate receptor subunits were comparable to that of reference compounds. α-Curcumene and α-farnesene have binding energies for the three subunits surpassing that of ketamine, interact with GluN1 and GluN2B at many amino acids, similar to ketamine and ifenprodil, and form more bonds with the proteins than ketamine. This suggests that α-curcumene and α-farnesene not only bind well to NMDAR subunits but can also mimic the mechanisms by which ketamine and ifenprodil improve depression.

Myristica fragrans Houtt. or nutmeg is a well-characterized herb with various pharmacological properties such as antidiarrheal, antimicrobial, antifungal, antioxidant, cardioprotective, especially sedative and antidepressant effects [104]. However, to our best knowledge, this study is the first to report the neuroprotective effect in vitro as well as the rapid-acting antianxiety-like and antidepression-like effects in vivo of *Myristica fragrans* Houtt. essential oil via intranasal delivery. Unlike *Atractylodes lancea* (Thunb.) DC. and *Chrysanthemum morifolium* Ramat., fast actions of *Myristica fragrans* Houtt. appeared not to mainly exert via glutamate receptors since its main compounds such as limonene, β-myrcene, α-pinene, and β-pinene do not have a strong affinity towards GluN1 and GluA2 subunits. It should be noticed that not only glutamate receptors drive the rapid anxiolytic and antidepressant effects, but others might also do that function, for instance, gamma-aminobutyric acid B, or 5-hydroxytryptamine receptor 4 receptors [105–107]. A previous study showed that 3-day treatments of *Myristica fragrans* n-hexane extract reduced depression-like behaviors in mice by targeting the serotonergic and noradrenergic nervous systems [87,88]. Short-term inhalation of limonene has been found to restore chronic unpredictable mild stress-induced depression-like behavior by modulating the activity of the HPA axis, BDNF receptors, and monoamine neurotransmitter levels [23]. The acute anxiolytic effect of inhaled α-pinene after one day of treatment has also been reported, yet its underlying mechanism remains to be studied [108]. In short, though *Myristica fragrans* Houtt. essential oil is a potential material for rapid-acting antidepressant development, other mechanisms of action rather than glutamate pathway should be considered.

Notably, the rapid antidepressant-like effect of essential oils via intranasal administration is a novelty of this study. Nasal delivery has recently been shown to have advantages over other routes, such as oral administration or intraperitoneal injection. Since intranasal intervention directly transports exogenous materials from the nasal cavity to the brain, avoiding first-pass metabolism in the liver, it results in a fast onset of action and higher bioavailability of drugs [109,110]. In our study, intranasal administration of essential oils only 30 min prior to the behavioral test produced positive changes in the behavior of mice. We postulate that the olfactory bulb receives sensory information from the olfactory receptors in the lining of the nasal cavity and projects signals to certain brain regions, including the hippocampus and amygdala, which are involved in emotional processing and linked to the regulation of anxiety and depression [21,111]. In addition, compared to previous work, with the same herbal material but different forms of extract, essential oils delivered intranasally required a very small dosage but exerted their effects within a shorter time course [102]. Given these advantages, the use of essential oils for antidepressant development and its intranasal delivery are promising strategies and should be the focus of future research.

This study has some limitations that could be addressed in future research. First, the safety assessment of essential oils in mice administered intranasally was overlooked. Nasal delivery has been reported to be associated with irritation and dryness of the nasal mucosa, resulting in cracking, inflammation, and nosebleeds [112,113]. Hence, toxicity evaluation for the nasal mucosa and olfactory tissues is necessary before intranasal administration. The second limitation of this study was the tested dose (25 mg/kg), which was administered to mice for all 20 essential oils. Although we chose the dose based on previous studies [114–117], it should be noted that each essential oil has its own properties and characteristics; therefore, the effective doses and pathways in which they are absorbed or distributed are different. However, finding the right dose for each essential oil, including those that had never previously been studied or published, was relatively unfeasible. Thirdly, the compounds described in the molecular docking experiment were derived from a literature search, not a GC-MS analysis from our own samples. GC-MS analysis would be more appropriate for future in-depth research on each essential oil suggested in this paper. Finally, the resolution of the protein structure determines the accuracy of docking, yet there are currently no high-resolution data on other AMPAR subunits; hence, molecular docking could only be performed for the GluA2 subunit.

5. Conclusions

Chrysanthemum morifolium Ramat., *Zingiber officinale* Roscoe, *Santalum album* L., *Citrus reticulata* Blanco, *Atractylodes lancea* (Thunb.) DC., and *Myristica fragrans* Houtt. essential oils have been shown to possess neuroprotective or anti-neuroinflammatory effects in vitro and to exert rapid-acting antidepressant effects through intranasal delivery in mice. Notably, *Chrysanthemum morifolium* Ramat. and *Atractylodes lancea* (Thunb.) DC. essential oils and their volatile compounds, including atractylon, α-curcumene, α-farnesene, and selina-4(14),7(11)-dien-8-one, may be useful candidates for development as rapid-acting intranasal antidepressants through interactions with NMDARs and AMPARs. It is important for future work to validate the safety of these essential oils and compounds for intranasal delivery and the exact mechanism underlying their rapid-acting effects against depression. Additionally, they should be studied using a specific animal disease model.

Author Contributions: Conceptualization, I.-J.Y., K.N.T. and N.P.K.N.; methodology, K.N.T. and N.P.K.N.; software, K.N.T. and N.P.K.N.; formal analysis, K.N.T. and N.P.K.N.; writing—original draft preparation, K.N.T. and N.P.K.N.; writing—review and editing, I.-J.Y., H.-M.S. and L.T.H.N.; supervision, I.-J.Y., H.-M.S. and L.T.H.N.; project administration, I.-J.Y.; funding acquisition, I.-J.Y. All authors have read and agreed to the published version of the manuscript.

Funding: This research was funded by the Dongguk University Research Fund (2023) and the National Research Foundation (NRF-2021R1I1A2048979).

Institutional Review Board Statement: The study was conducted according to the guidelines of the Declaration of Helsinki and approved by the Institutional Review Board (or Ethics Committee) of the Institutional Animal Care and Use Committee of Dongguk University (protocol code IACUC-2021-15).

Informed Consent Statement: Not applicable.

Data Availability Statement: The data presented in this study are available in this article.

Conflicts of Interest: The authors declare no conflict of interest. The funders had no role in the design, execution, interpretation, or writing of the study.

References

1. Chand, S.P.; Arif, H. Depression. In *StatPearls*; StatPearls Publishing LLC.: Treasure Island, FL, USA, 2023. Available online: https://www.ncbi.nlm.nih.gov/books/NBK430847/ (accessed on 7 April 2023).
2. World Health Organization. *Depression*; World Health Organization: Geneva, Switzerland, 2021. Available online: https://www.who.int/news-room/fact-sheets/detail/depression (accessed on 7 April 2023).
3. Peng, S.; Zhou, Y.; Lu, M.; Wang, Q. Review of Herbal Medicines for the Treatment of Depression. *Nat. Prod. Commun.* 2022, 17, 1934578X221139082. [CrossRef]
4. Zhang, H.; Ren, Y.; Lv, M.; Xie, M.; Wang, K.; Yang, M.; Lv, C.; Li, X. Anti-depression effect and mechanism of Suanzaoren Decoction on mice with depression. *IOP Conf. Ser. Earth Environ. Sci.* 2021, 714, 022065. [CrossRef]
5. Borgogna, N.C.; Aita, S.L. Is the serotonin hypothesis dead? If so, how will clinical psychology respond? *Front. Psychol.* 2022, 13, 1027375. [CrossRef] [PubMed]
6. Moncrieff, J.; Cooper, R.E.; Stockmann, T.; Amendola, S.; Hengartner, M.P.; Horowitz, M.A. The serotonin theory of depression: A systematic umbrella review of the evidence. *Mol. Psychiatry* 2022. [CrossRef] [PubMed]
7. Fiksdal, A.; Hanlin, L.; Kuras, Y.; Gianferante, D.; Chen, X.; Thoma, M.V.; Rohleder, N. Associations between symptoms of depression and anxiety and cortisol responses to and recovery from acute stress. *Psychoneuroendocrinology* 2019, 102, 44–52. [CrossRef] [PubMed]
8. Pariante, C.M.; Lightman, S.L. The HPA axis in major depression: Classical theories and new developments. *Trends Neurosci.* 2008, 31, 464–468. [CrossRef]
9. Bendezú, J.J.; Calhoun, C.D.; Vinograd, M.; Patterson, M.W.; Rudolph, K.D.; Giletta, M.; Hastings, P.; Nock, M.K.; Slavich, G.M.; Prinstein, M.J. Exploring joint HPA-inflammatory stress response profiles in adolescent girls: Implications for developmental models of neuroendocrine dysregulation. *Dev. Psychobiol.* 2022, 64, e22247. [CrossRef]
10. Troubat, R.; Barone, P.; Leman, S.; Desmidt, T.; Cressant, A.; Atanasova, B.; Brizard, B.; El Hage, W.; Surget, A.; Belzung, C.; et al. Neuroinflammation and depression: A review. *Eur. J. Neurosci.* 2021, 53, 151–171. [CrossRef]
11. Mizoguchi, K.; Ishige, A.; Aburada, M.; Tabira, T. Chronic stress attenuates glucocorticoid negative feedback: Involvement of the prefrontal cortex and hippocampus. *Neuroscience* 2003, 119, 887–897. [CrossRef]
12. Seguin, J.A.; Brennan, J.; Mangano, E.; Hayley, S. Proinflammatory cytokines differentially influence adult hippocampal cell proliferation depending upon the route and chronicity of administration. *Neuropsychiatr. Dis. Treat.* 2009, 5, 5–14. [PubMed]
13. Feighner, J.P. Mechanism of action of antidepressant medications. *J. Clin. Psychiatry* 1999, 60 (Suppl. S4), 4–13. [PubMed]
14. Wang, S.M.; Han, C.; Bahk, W.M.; Lee, S.J.; Patkar, A.A.; Masand, P.S.; Pae, C.U. Addressing the Side Effects of Contemporary Antidepressant Drugs: A Comprehensive Review. *Chonnam Med. J.* 2018, 54, 101–112. [CrossRef] [PubMed]
15. Chamberlain, S.R.; Baldwin, D.S. Monoamine Oxidase Inhibitors (MAOIs) in Psychiatric Practice: How to Use them Safely and Effectively. *CNS Drugs* 2021, 35, 703–716. [CrossRef] [PubMed]
16. Commons, K.G.; Linnros, S.E. Delayed Antidepressant Efficacy and the Desensitization Hypothesis. *ACS Chem. Neurosci.* 2019, 10, 3048–3052. [CrossRef] [PubMed]
17. Machado-Vieira, R.; Salvadore, G.; Luckenbaugh, D.A.; Manji, H.K.; Zarate, C.A., Jr. Rapid onset of antidepressant action: A new paradigm in the research and treatment of major depressive disorder. *J. Clin. Psychiatry* 2008, 69, 946–958. [CrossRef]
18. Soares, G.A.B.E.; Bhattacharya, T.; Chakrabarti, T.; Tagde, P.; Cavalu, S. Exploring Pharmacological Mechanisms of Essential Oils on the Central Nervous System. *Plants* 2021, 11, 21. [CrossRef]
19. Liang, J.; Zhang, Y.; Chi, P.; Liu, H.; Jing, Z.; Cao, H.; Du, Y.; Zhao, Y.; Qin, X.; Zhang, W.; et al. Essential oils: Chemical constituents, potential neuropharmacological effects and aromatherapy—A review. *Pharmacol. Res.—Mod. Chin. Med.* 2023, 6, 100210. [CrossRef]
20. Hanif, M.A.; Nisar, S.; Khan, G.S.; Mushtaq, Z.; Zubair, M. Essential Oils. In *Essential Oil Research: Trends in Biosynthesis, Analytics, Industrial Applications and Biotechnological Production*; Malik, S., Ed.; Springer International Publishing: Cham, Switzerland, 2019; pp. 3–17. [CrossRef]
21. Fung, T.K.H.; Lau, B.W.M.; Ngai, S.P.C.; Tsang, H.W.H. Therapeutic Effect and Mechanisms of Essential Oils in Mood Disorders: Interaction between the Nervous and Respiratory Systems. *Int. J. Mol. Sci.* 2021, 22, 4844. [CrossRef]
22. Cui, J.; Li, M.; Wei, Y.; Li, H.; He, X.; Yang, Q.; Li, Z.; Duan, J.; Wu, Z.; Chen, Q.; et al. Inhalation Aromatherapy via Brain-Targeted Nasal Delivery: Natural Volatiles or Essential Oils on Mood Disorders. *Front. Pharmacol.* 2022, 13, 860043. [CrossRef]
23. Zhang, L.-L.; Yang, Z.-Y.; Fan, G.; Ren, J.-N.; Yin, K.-J.; Pan, S.-Y. Antidepressant-like Effect of *Citrus sinensis* (L.) Osbeck Essential Oil and Its Main Component Limonene on Mice. *J. Agric. Food Chem.* 2019, 67, 13817–13828. [CrossRef] [PubMed]
24. Sánchez-Vidaña, D.I.; Po, K.K.; Fung, T.K.; Chow, J.K.; Lau, W.K.; So, P.K.; Lau, B.W.; Tsang, H.W. Lavender essential oil ameliorates depression-like behavior and increases neurogenesis and dendritic complexity in rats. *Neurosci. Lett.* 2019, 701, 180–192. [CrossRef] [PubMed]
25. Chioca, L.R.; Ferro, M.M.; Baretta, I.P.; Oliveira, S.M.; Silva, C.R.; Ferreira, J.; Losso, E.M.; Andreatini, R. Anxiolytic-like effect of lavender essential oil inhalation in mice: Participation of serotonergic but not GABAA/benzodiazepine neurotransmission. *J. Ethnopharmacol.* 2013, 147, 412–418. [CrossRef] [PubMed]
26. Jin, Z.; Han, Y.; Zhang, D.; Li, Z.; Jing, Y.; Hu, B.; Sun, S. Application of Intranasal Administration in the Delivery of Antidepressant Active Ingredients. *Pharmaceutics* 2022, 14, 2070. [CrossRef]

27. Turner, P.V.; Brabb, T.; Pekow, C.; Vasbinder, M.A. Administration of substances to laboratory animals: Routes of administration and factors to consider. *J. Am. Assoc. Lab. Anim. Sci.* **2011**, *50*, 600–613. [PubMed]
28. Qi, X.J.; Liu, X.Y.; Tang, L.M.; Li, P.F.; Qiu, F.; Yang, A.H. Anti-depressant effect of curcumin-loaded guanidine-chitosan thermo-sensitive hydrogel by nasal delivery. *Pharm. Dev. Technol.* **2020**, *25*, 316–325. [CrossRef]
29. Wang, Q.-S.; Li, K.; Gao, L.-N.; Zhang, Y.; Lin, K.-M.; Cui, Y.-L. Intranasal delivery of berberine via in situ thermoresponsive hydrogel with non-invasive therapy exhibits better antidepressant-like effects. *Biomater. Sci.* **2020**, *8*, 2853–2865. [CrossRef]
30. Qi, X.-J.; Xu, D.; Tian, M.-L.; Zhou, J.-F.; Wang, Q.-S.; Cui, Y.-L. Thermosensitive hydrogel designed for improving the antidepressant activities of genipin via intranasal delivery. *Mater. Des.* **2021**, *206*, 109816. [CrossRef]
31. Xia, B.; Zhang, H.; Xue, W.; Tao, W.; Chen, C.; Wu, R.; Ren, L.; Tang, J.; Wu, H.; Cai, B.; et al. Instant and Lasting Down-Regulation of NR1 Expression in the Hippocampus is Associated Temporally with Antidepressant Activity after Acute Yueju. *Cell. Mol. Neurobiol.* **2016**, *36*, 1189–1196. [CrossRef]
32. Hall, B.J.; Ripley, B.; Ghosh, A. NR2B signaling regulates the development of synaptic AMPA receptor current. *J. Neurosci.* **2007**, *27*, 13446–13456. [CrossRef] [PubMed]
33. Yao, Y.; Ju, P.; Liu, H.; Wu, X.; Niu, Z.; Zhu, Y.; Zhang, C.; Fang, Y. Ifenprodil rapidly ameliorates depressive-like behaviors, activates mTOR signaling and modulates proinflammatory cytokines in the hippocampus of CUMS rats. *Psychopharmacology* **2020**, *237*, 1421–1433. [CrossRef]
34. Li, J.-M.; Liu, L.-L.; Su, W.-J.; Wang, B.; Zhang, T.; Zhang, Y.; Jiang, C.-L. Ketamine may exert antidepressant effects via suppressing NLRP3 inflammasome to upregulate AMPA receptors. *Neuropharmacology* **2019**, *146*, 149–153. [CrossRef] [PubMed]
35. Koike, H.; Iijima, M.; Chaki, S. Involvement of AMPA receptor in both the rapid and sustained antidepressant-like effects of ketamine in animal models of depression. *Behav. Brain Res.* **2011**, *224*, 107–111. [CrossRef] [PubMed]
36. Hara, H.; Suzuki, A.; Kunugi, A.; Tajima, Y.; Yamada, R.; Kimura, H. TAK-653, an AMPA receptor potentiator with minimal agonistic activity, produces an antidepressant-like effect with a favorable safety profile in rats. *Pharmacol. Biochem. Behav.* **2021**, *211*, 173289. [CrossRef]
37. Can, A.; Dao, D.T.; Terrillion, C.E.; Piantadosi, S.C.; Bhat, S.; Gould, T.D. The tail suspension test. *J. Vis. Exp.* **2012**, *59*, e3769. [CrossRef]
38. Hogg, S. A review of the validity and variability of the Elevated Plus-Maze as an animal model of anxiety. *Pharmacol. Biochem. Behav.* **1996**, *54*, 21–30. [CrossRef]
39. Joyce Gem, M.C.; Joanna, J.O.; Junie, B.B. In Silico Screening for Neuroreceptor Targets and Derivatization of Alkaloids from Phaeanthus Ophthalmicus. *Pharmacophore* **2022**, *13*, 27–43. [CrossRef]
40. Kaniakova, M.; Korabecny, J.; Holubova, K.; Kleteckova, L.; Chvojkova, M.; Hakenova, K.; Prchal, L.; Novak, M.; Dolezal, R.; Hepnarova, V.; et al. 7-phenoxytacrine is a dually acting drug with neuroprotective efficacy in vivo. *Biochem. Pharmacol.* **2021**, *186*, 114460. [CrossRef]
41. Wei, L.; Qi, X.; Yu, X.; Zheng, Y.; Luo, X.; Wei, Y.; Ni, P.; Zhao, L.; Wang, Q.; Ma, X.; et al. 3,4-Dihydrobenzo[e][1.2.3] oxathiazine 2,2-dioxide analogs act as potential AMPA receptor potentiators with antidepressant activity. *Eur. J. Med. Chem.* **2023**, *251*, 115252. [CrossRef] [PubMed]
42. Sweilam, S.H.; Alqarni, M.H.; Youssef, F.S. Antimicrobial Alkaloids from Marine-Derived Fungi as Drug Leads versus COVID-19 Infection: A Computational Approach to Explore their Anti-COVID-19 Activity and ADMET Properties. *Evid. Based Complement. Altern. Med.* **2022**, *2022*, 5403757. [CrossRef]
43. Ramadhan, D.S.F.; Siharis, F.; Abdurrahman, S.; Isrul, M.; Fakih, T.M. In silico analysis of marine natural product from sponge (*Clathria* Sp.) for their activity as inhibitor of SARS-CoV-2 Main Protease. *J. Biomol. Struct. Dyn.* **2022**, *40*, 11526–11532. [CrossRef]
44. Wu, W. GC-MS analysis of chemical components in essential oil from Flos magnoliae. *Zhong Yao Cai* **2000**, *23*, 538–541. [PubMed]
45. Hu, M.; Bai, M.; Ye, W.; Wang, Y.; Wu, H. Variations in Volatile Oil Yield and Composition of "Xin-yi" (*Magnolia biondii* Pamp. Flower Buds) at Different Growth Stages. *J. Oleo Sci.* **2018**, *67*, 779–787. [CrossRef]
46. Zeng, Z.; Xie, R.; Zhang, T.; Zhang, H.; Chen, J.Y. Analysis of volatile compositions of *Magnolia biondii* pamp by steam distillation and headspace solid phase micro-extraction. *J. Oleo Sci.* **2011**, *60*, 591–596. [CrossRef] [PubMed]
47. Kuang, C.L.; Lv, D.; Shen, G.H.; Li, S.S.; Luo, Q.Y.; Zhang, Z.Q. Chemical composition and antimicrobial activities of volatile oil extracted from *Chrysanthemum morifolium* Ramat. *J. Food Sci. Technol.* **2018**, *55*, 2786–2794. [CrossRef]
48. Peng, A.; Lin, L.; Zhao, M. Screening of key flavonoids and monoterpenoids for xanthine oxidase inhibitory activity-oriented quality control of *Chrysanthemum morifolium* Ramat. 'Boju' based on spectrum-effect relationship coupled with UPLC-TOF-MS and HS-SPME-GC/MS. *Food Res. Int.* **2020**, *137*, 109448. [CrossRef]
49. Li, X.; Ao, M.; Zhang, C.; Fan, S.; Chen, Z.; Yu, L. Zingiberis Rhizoma Recens: A Review of Its Traditional Uses, Phytochemistry, Pharmacology, and Toxicology. *Evid. Based Complement. Altern.* **2021**, *2021*, 6668990. [CrossRef]
50. Yu, D.-X.; Guo, S.; Wang, J.-M.; Yan, H.; Zhang, Z.-Y.; Yang, J.; Duan, J.-A. Comparison of Different Drying Methods on the Volatile Components of Ginger (*Zingiber officinale* Roscoe) by HS-GC-MS Coupled with Fast GC E-Nose. *Foods* **2022**, *11*, 1611. [CrossRef] [PubMed]
51. Gupta, S.; Pandotra, P.; Ram, G.; Anand, R.; Gupta, A.P.; Husain, K.; Bedi, Y.S.; Mallavarapu, G.R. Composition of a monoterpenoid-rich essential oil from the rhizome of *Zingiber officinale* from north western Himalayas. *Nat. Prod. Commun.* **2011**, *6*, 93–96. [CrossRef]

52. de Groot, A.C.; Schmidt, E. Essential Oils, Part VI: Sandalwood Oil, Ylang-Ylang Oil, and Jasmine Absolute. *Dermatitis* **2017**, *28*, 14–21. [CrossRef]
53. Braun, N.A.; Meier, M.; Pickenhagen, W. Isolation and Chiral GC Analysis of β-Bisabolols—Trace Constituents from the Essential Oil of *Santalum album* L. (Santalaceae). *J. Essent. Oil Res.* **2003**, *15*, 63–65. [CrossRef]
54. Mohankumar, A.; Kalaiselvi, D.; Levenson, C.; Shanmugam, G.; Thiruppathi, G.; Nivitha, S.; Sundararaj, P. Antioxidant and stress modulatory efficacy of essential oil extracted from plantation-grown *Santalum album* L. *Ind. Crop. Prod.* **2019**, *140*, 111623. [CrossRef]
55. Fahmy, N.M.; Elhady, S.S.; Bannan, D.F.; Malatani, R.T.; Gad, H.A. *Citrus reticulata* Leaves Essential Oil as an Antiaging Agent: A Comparative Study between Different Cultivars and Correlation with Their Chemical Compositions. *Plants* **2022**, *11*, 3335. [CrossRef] [PubMed]
56. Duan, L.; Guo, L.; Dou, L.-L.; Zhou, C.-L.; Xu, F.-G.; Zheng, G.-D.; Li, P.; Liu, E.H. Discrimination of *Citrus reticulata* Blanco and *Citrus reticulata* 'Chachi' by gas chromatograph-mass spectrometry based metabolomics approach. *Food Chem.* **2016**, *212*, 123–127. [CrossRef] [PubMed]
57. Chutia, M.; Deka Bhuyan, P.; Pathak, M.G.; Sarma, T.C.; Boruah, P. Antifungal activity and chemical composition of *Citrus reticulata* Blanco essential oil against phytopathogens from North East India. *LWT—Food Sci. Technol.* **2009**, *42*, 777–780. [CrossRef]
58. Lota, M.-L.; de Rocca Serra, D.; Tomi, F.; Joseph, C. Chemical variability of peel and leaf essential oils of mandarins from *Citrus reticulata* Blanco. *Biochem. Syst. Ecol.* **2000**, *28*, 61–78. [CrossRef]
59. Zhang, W.J.; Zhao, Z.Y.; Chang, L.K.; Cao, Y.; Wang, S.; Kang, C.Z.; Wang, H.Y.; Zhou, L.; Huang, L.Q.; Guo, L.P. Atractylodis Rhizoma: A review of its traditional uses, phytochemistry, pharmacology, toxicology and quality control. *J. Ethnopharmacol.* **2021**, *266*, 113415. [CrossRef]
60. Xu, R.; Lu, J.; Wu, J.; Yu, D.; Chu, S.; Guan, F.; Liu, W.; Hu, J.; Peng, H.; Zha, L. Comparative analysis in different organs and tissue-specific metabolite profiling of *Atractylodes lancea* from four regions by GC-MS and laser microdissection. *J. Sep. Sci.* **2022**, *45*, 1067–1079. [CrossRef]
61. Lei, H.; Yue, J.; Yin, X.Y.; Fan, W.; Tan, S.H.; Qin, L.; Zhao, Y.N.; Bai, J.H. HS-SPME coupled with GC-MS for elucidating differences between the volatile components in wild and cultivated Atractylodes chinensis. *Phytochem. Anal.* **2023**, *34*, 317–328. [CrossRef]
62. Ashokkumar, K.; Simal-Gandara, J.; Murugan, M.; Dhanya, M.K.; Pandian, A. Nutmeg (*Myristica fragrans* Houtt.) essential oil: A review on its composition, biological, and pharmacological activities. *Phytother. Res.* **2022**, *36*, 2839–2851. [CrossRef]
63. Gupta, A.D.; Bansal, V.K.; Babu, V.; Maithil, N. Chemistry, antioxidant and antimicrobial potential of nutmeg (*Myristica fragrans* Houtt*)*. *J. Genet. Eng. Biotechnol.* **2013**, *11*, 25–31. [CrossRef]
64. Ogunwande, I.A.; Olawore, N.O.; Adeleke, K.A.; Ekundayo, O. Chemical Composition of Essential Oil of *Myristica Fragrans* Houtt (Nutmeg) From Nigeria. *J. Essent. Oil Bear. Plants* **2003**, *6*, 21–26. [CrossRef]
65. Berman, R.M.; Cappiello, A.; Anand, A.; Oren, D.A.; Heninger, G.R.; Charney, D.S.; Krystal, J.H. Antidepressant effects of ketamine in depressed patients. *Biol. Psychiatry* **2000**, *47*, 351–354. [CrossRef]
66. Zarate, C.A., Jr.; Singh, J.B.; Carlson, P.J.; Brutsche, N.E.; Ameli, R.; Luckenbaugh, D.A.; Charney, D.S.; Manji, H.K. A randomized trial of an N-methyl-D-aspartate antagonist in treatment-resistant major depression. *Arch. Gen. Psychiatry* **2006**, *63*, 856–864. [CrossRef] [PubMed]
67. de Sousa, D.; Hocayen, P.D.A.S.; Andrade, L.N.; Andreatini, R. A Systematic Review of the Anxiolytic-Like Effects of Essential Oils in Animal Models. *Molecules* **2015**, *20*, 18620–18660. [CrossRef]
68. Almeida, R.C.; Souza, D.G.; Soletti, R.C.; López, M.G.; Rodrigues, A.L.; Gabilan, N.H. Involvement of PKA, MAPK/ERK and CaMKII, but not PKC in the acute antidepressant-like effect of memantine in mice. *Neurosci. Lett.* **2006**, *395*, 93–97. [CrossRef] [PubMed]
69. McShane, R.; Westby, M.J.; Roberts, E.; Minakaran, N.; Schneider, L.; Farrimond, L.E.; Maayan, N.; Ware, J.; Debarros, J. Memantine for dementia. *Cochrane Database Syst. Rev.* **2019**, *3*, Cd003154. [CrossRef]
70. Pascual, O.; Ben Achour, S.; Rostaing, P.; Triller, A.; Bessis, A. Microglia activation triggers astrocyte-mediated modulation of excitatory neurotransmission. *Proc. Natl. Acad. Sci. USA* **2012**, *109*, E197–E205. [CrossRef] [PubMed]
71. Nakamura, Y.; Si, Q.S.; Kataoka, K. Lipopolysaccharide-induced microglial activation in culture: Temporal profiles of morphological change and release of cytokines and nitric oxide. *Neurosci. Res.* **1999**, *35*, 95–100. [CrossRef]
72. Dunn, A.J.; Wang, J.; Ando, T. Effects of cytokines on cerebral neurotransmission. Comparison with the effects of stress. *Adv. Exp. Med. Biol.* **1999**, *461*, 117–127. [CrossRef]
73. Zhao, Z.; Zhang, L.; Guo, X.D.; Cao, L.L.; Xue, T.F.; Zhao, X.J.; Yang, D.D.; Yang, J.; Ji, J.; Huang, J.Y.; et al. Rosiglitazone Exerts an Anti-depressive Effect in Unpredictable Chronic Mild-Stress-Induced Depressive Mice by Maintaining Essential Neuron Autophagy and Inhibiting Excessive Astrocytic Apoptosis. *Front. Mol. Neurosci.* **2017**, *10*, 293. [CrossRef] [PubMed]
74. Mo, F.; Tang, Y.; Du, P.; Shen, Z.; Yang, J.; Cai, M.; Zhang, Y.; Li, H.; Shen, H. GPR39 protects against corticosterone-induced neuronal injury in hippocampal cells through the CREB-BDNF signaling pathway. *J. Affect. Disord.* **2020**, *272*, 474–484. [CrossRef] [PubMed]
75. Jin, W.; Xu, X.; Chen, X.; Qi, W.; Lu, J.; Yan, X.; Zhao, D.; Cong, D.; Li, X.; Sun, L. Protective effect of pig brain polypeptides against corticosterone-induced oxidative stress, inflammatory response, and apoptosis in PC12 cells. *Biomed. Pharmacother.* **2019**, *115*, 108890. [CrossRef] [PubMed]

76. Gruver-Yates, A.L.; Cidlowski, J.A. Tissue-specific actions of glucocorticoids on apoptosis: A double-edged sword. *Cells* **2013**, *2*, 202–223. [CrossRef]
77. Zhang, S.Q.; Cao, L.L.; Liang, Y.Y.; Wang, P. The Molecular Mechanism of Chronic High-Dose Corticosterone-Induced Aggravation of Cognitive Impairment in APP/PS1 Transgenic Mice. *Front. Mol. Neurosci.* **2020**, *13*, 613421. [CrossRef]
78. Wang, Q.; Van Heerikhuize, J.; Aronica, E.; Kawata, M.; Seress, L.; Joels, M.; Swaab, D.F.; Lucassen, P.J. Glucocorticoid receptor protein expression in human hippocampus; stability with age. *Neurobiol. Aging* **2013**, *34*, 1662–1673. [CrossRef] [PubMed]
79. Gradin, V.B.; Pomi, A. The role of hippocampal atrophy in depression: A neurocomputational approach. *J. Biol. Phys.* **2008**, *34*, 107–120. [CrossRef]
80. Hao, Y.; Shabanpoor, A.; Metz, G.A. Stress and corticosterone alter synaptic plasticity in a rat model of Parkinson's disease. *Neurosci. Lett.* **2017**, *651*, 79–87. [CrossRef]
81. Xu, L.; Holscher, C.; Anwyl, R.; Rowan, M.J. Glucocorticoid receptor and protein/RNA synthesis-dependent mechanisms underlie the control of synaptic plasticity by stress. *Proc. Natl. Acad. Sci. USA* **1998**, *95*, 3204–3208. [CrossRef]
82. Kumar, P.; Nagarajan, A.; Uchil, P.D. Analysis of Cell Viability by the Lactate Dehydrogenase Assay. *Cold Spring Harb. Protoc.* **2018**, *2018*. [CrossRef]
83. Park, Y.-k.; Chung, Y.S.; Kim, Y.S.; Kwon, O.Y.; Joh, T.H. Inhibition of gene expression and production of iNOS and TNF-α in LPS-stimulated microglia by methanol extract of Phellodendri cortex. *Int. Immunopharmacol.* **2007**, *7*, 955–962. [CrossRef]
84. Lee, S.H.; Lee, J.H.; Oh, E.Y.; Kim, G.Y.; Choi, B.T.; Kim, C.; Choi, Y.H. Ethanol extract of Cnidium officinale exhibits anti-inflammatory effects in BV2 microglial cells by suppressing NF-κB nuclear translocation and the activation of the PI3K/Akt signaling pathway. *Int. J. Mol. Med.* **2013**, *32*, 876–882. [CrossRef]
85. Wu, F.; Li, H.; Zhao, L.; Li, X.; You, J.; Jiang, Q.; Li, S.; Jin, L.; Xu, Y. Protective effects of aqueous extract from Acanthopanax senticosus against corticosterone-induced neurotoxicity in PC12 cells. *J. Ethnopharmacol.* **2013**, *148*, 861–868. [CrossRef] [PubMed]
86. Yu, Z.; Jin, W.; Cui, Y.; Ao, M.; Liu, H.; Xu, H.; Yu, L. Protective effects of macamides from Lepidium meyenii Walp. against corticosterone-induced neurotoxicity in PC12 cells. *RSC Adv.* **2019**, *9*, 23096–23108. [CrossRef]
87. Dhingra, D.; Sharma, A. Antidepressant-like activity of n-hexane extract of nutmeg (*Myristica fragrans*) seeds in mice. *J. Med. Food* **2006**, *9*, 84–89. [CrossRef] [PubMed]
88. Iwata, N.; Kobayashi, D.; Kawashiri, T.; Kubota, T.; Kawano, K.; Yamamuro, Y.; Miyagi, A.; Deguchi, Y.; Chijimatsu, T.; Shimazoe, T. Mechanisms and Safety of Antidepressant-Like Effect of Nutmeg in Mice. *Biol. Pharm. Bull.* **2022**, *45*, 738–742. [CrossRef]
89. Muris, P.; Merckelbach, H.; Schmidt, H.; Gadet, B.; Bogie, N. Anxiety and depression as correlates of self-reported behavioural inhibition in normal adolescents. *Behav. Res. Ther.* **2001**, *39*, 1051–1061. [CrossRef]
90. Tiller, J.W. Depression and anxiety. *Med. J. Aust.* **2013**, *199*, S28–S31. [CrossRef] [PubMed]
91. Zanos, P.; Gould, T.D. Mechanisms of ketamine action as an antidepressant. *Mol. Psychiatry* **2018**, *23*, 801–811. [CrossRef]
92. Sanacora, G.; Schatzberg, A.F. Ketamine: Promising Path or False Prophecy in the Development of Novel Therapeutics for Mood Disorders? *Neuropsychopharmacology* **2015**, *40*, 259–267. [CrossRef] [PubMed]
93. Shamsi, A.; Shahwan, M.; Khan, M.S.; Husain, F.M.; Alhumaydhi, F.A.; Aljohani, A.S.M.; Rehman, M.T.; Hassan, M.I.; Islam, A. Elucidating the Interaction of Human Ferritin with Quercetin and Naringenin: Implication of Natural Products in Neurodegenerative Diseases: Molecular Docking and Dynamics Simulation Insight. *ACS Omega* **2021**, *6*, 7922–7930. [CrossRef]
94. Khan, A.; Mohammad, T.; Shamsi, A.; Hussain, A.; Alajmi, M.F.; Husain, S.A.; Iqbal, M.A.; Hassan, M.I. Identification of plant-based hexokinase 2 inhibitors: Combined molecular docking and dynamics simulation studies. *J. Biomol. Struct. Dyn.* **2022**, *40*, 10319–10331. [CrossRef] [PubMed]
95. Zhang, S.; Xu, Z.; Gao, Y.; Wu, Y.; Li, Z.; Liu, H.; Zhang, C. Bidirectional crosstalk between stress-induced gastric ulcer and depression under chronic stress. *PLoS ONE* **2012**, *7*, e51148. [CrossRef]
96. Lin, Y.; Liu, X.; Tan, D.; Jiang, Z. Atractylon treatment prevents sleep-disordered breathing-induced cognitive dysfunction by suppression of chronic intermittent hypoxia-induced M1 microglial activation. *Biosci. Rep.* **2020**, *40*, BSR20192800. [CrossRef] [PubMed]
97. Chen, L.G.; Jan, Y.S.; Tsai, P.W.; Norimoto, H.; Michihara, S.; Murayama, C.; Wang, C.C. Anti-inflammatory and Antinociceptive Constituents of Atractylodes japonica Koidzumi. *J. Agric. Food Chem.* **2016**, *64*, 2254–2262. [CrossRef]
98. Lin, L.-Z.; Harnly, J.M. Identification of the phenolic components of chrysanthemum flower (*Chrysanthemum morifolium* Ramat). *Food Chem.* **2010**, *120*, 319–326. [CrossRef]
99. Duh, P.-D.; Tu, Y.-Y.; Yen, G.-C. Antioxidant Activity of Water Extract of Harng Jyur (*Chrysanthemum morifolium* Ramat). *LWT—Food Sci. Technol.* **1999**, *32*, 269–277. [CrossRef]
100. Yuan, H.; Jiang, S.; Liu, Y.; Daniyal, M.; Jian, Y.; Peng, C.; Shen, J.; Liu, S.; Wang, W. The flower head of *Chrysanthemum morifolium* Ramat. (Juhua): A paradigm of flowers serving as Chinese dietary herbal medicine. *J. Ethnopharmacol.* **2020**, *261*, 113043. [CrossRef]
101. Ibi, M.; Yabe-Nishimura, C. Chapter 1—The role of reactive oxygen species in the pathogenic pathways of depression. In *Oxidative Stress and Dietary Antioxidants in Neurological Diseases*; Martin, C.R., Preedy, V.R., Eds.; Academic Press: Cambridge, MA, USA, 2020; pp. 3–16. [CrossRef]
102. Liu, T.; Zhou, N.; Xu, R.; Cao, Y.; Zhang, Y.; Liu, Z.; Zheng, X.; Feng, W. A metabolomic study on the anti-depressive effects of two active components from *Chrysanthemum morifolium*. *Artif. Cells Nanomed. Biotechnol.* **2020**, *48*, 718–727. [CrossRef] [PubMed]

103. Schepetkin, I.A.; Özek, G.; Özek, T.; Kirpotina, L.N.; Khlebnikov, A.I.; Klein, R.A.; Quinn, M.T. Neutrophil Immunomodulatory Activity of Farnesene, a Component of Artemisia dracunculus Essential Oils. *Pharmaceuticals* **2022**, *15*, 642. [CrossRef]
104. Ha, M.T.; Vu, N.K.; Tran, T.H.; Kim, J.A.; Woo, M.H.; Min, B.S. Phytochemical and pharmacological properties of *Myristica fragrans* Houtt.: An updated review. *Arch. Pharmacal Res.* **2020**, *43*, 1067–1092. [CrossRef]
105. Workman, E.R.; Niere, F.; Raab-Graham, K.F. mTORC1-dependent protein synthesis underlying rapid antidepressant effect requires GABABR signaling. *Neuropharmacology* **2013**, *73*, 192–203. [CrossRef] [PubMed]
106. Mendez-David, I.; David, D.J.; Darcet, F.; Wu, M.V.; Kerdine-Römer, S.; Gardier, A.M.; Hen, R. Rapid Anxiolytic Effects of a 5-HT4 Receptor Agonist Are Mediated by a Neurogenesis-Independent Mechanism. *Neuropsychopharmacology* **2014**, *39*, 1366–1378. [CrossRef]
107. Faye, C.; Hen, R.; Guiard, B.P.; Denny, C.A.; Gardier, A.M.; Mendez-David, I.; David, D.J. Rapid Anxiolytic Effects of RS67333, a Serotonin Type 4 Receptor Agonist, and Diazepam, a Benzodiazepine, Are Mediated by Projections from the Prefrontal Cortex to the Dorsal Raphe Nucleus. *Biol. Psychiatry* **2020**, *87*, 514–525. [CrossRef] [PubMed]
108. Satou, T.; Kasuya, H.; Maeda, K.; Koike, K. Daily inhalation of α-pinene in mice: Effects on behavior and organ accumulation. *Phytother. Res.* **2014**, *28*, 1284–1287. [CrossRef] [PubMed]
109. Shringarpure, M.; Gharat, S.; Momin, M.; Omri, A. Management of epileptic disorders using nanotechnology-based strategies for nose-to-brain drug delivery. *Expert Opin. Drug Deliv.* **2021**, *18*, 169–185. [CrossRef]
110. Long, Y.; Yang, Q.; Xiang, Y.; Zhang, Y.; Wan, J.; Liu, S.; Li, N.; Peng, W. Nose to brain drug delivery—A promising strategy for active components from herbal medicine for treating cerebral ischemia reperfusion. *Pharmacol. Res.* **2020**, *159*, 104795. [CrossRef]
111. Walf, A.A.; Frye, C.A. A Review and Update of Mechanisms of Estrogen in the Hippocampus and Amygdala for Anxiety and Depression Behavior. *Neuropsychopharmacology* **2006**, *31*, 1097–1111. [CrossRef]
112. Meltzer, E.O. Formulation considerations of intranasal corticosteroids for the treatment of allergic rhinitis. *Ann. Allergy Asthma Immunol.* **2007**, *98*, 12–21. [CrossRef] [PubMed]
113. Caimmi, D.; Neukirch, C.; Louis, R.; Malard, O.; Thabut, G.; Demoly, P. Effect of the Use of Intranasal Spray of Essential Oils in Patients with Perennial Allergic Rhinitis: A Prospective Study. *Int. Arch. Allergy Immunol.* **2021**, *182*, 182–189. [CrossRef]
114. Vale, T.G.; Matos, F.J.A.; de Lima, T.C.M.; Viana, G.S.B. Behavioral effects of essential oils from *Lippia alba* (Mill.) N.E. Brown chemotypes. *J. Ethnopharmacol.* **1999**, *67*, 127–133. [CrossRef]
115. Guo, J.; Duan, J.A.; Tang, Y.; Jia, N.; Li, X.; Zhang, J. Fast onset of action and the analgesic and sedative efficacy of essential oil from Rhizoma Chuanxiong after nasal administration. *Pharmazie* **2010**, *65*, 296–299. [PubMed]
116. Guo, J.; Duan, J.A.; Tang, Y.; Li, Y. Sedative and anticonvulsant activities of styrax after oral and intranasal administration in mice. *Pharm. Biol.* **2011**, *49*, 1034–1038. [CrossRef] [PubMed]
117. Can, Ö.D.; Demir Özkay, Ü.; Kıyan, H.T.; Demirci, B. Psychopharmacological profile of Chamomile (*Matricaria recutita* L.) essential oil in mice. *Phytomedicine* **2012**, *19*, 306–310. [CrossRef] [PubMed]

Disclaimer/Publisher's Note: The statements, opinions and data contained in all publications are solely those of the individual author(s) and contributor(s) and not of MDPI and/or the editor(s). MDPI and/or the editor(s) disclaim responsibility for any injury to people or property resulting from any ideas, methods, instructions or products referred to in the content.

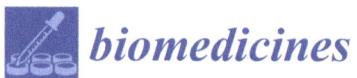

Article

Stimulated Parotid Saliva Is a Better Method for Depression Prediction

Yangyang Cui [1,2,3], Hankun Zhang [1,2,3], Song Wang [3,*], Junzhe Lu [3], Jinmei He [3], Lanlan Liu [3] and Weiqiang Liu [1,2,3,*]

1. Tsinghua Shenzhen International Graduate School, Tsinghua University, Shenzhen 518055, China
2. Department of Mechanical Engineering, Tsinghua University, Beijing 100084, China
3. Biomechanics and Biotechnology Lab, Research Institute of Tsinghua University in Shenzhen, Shenzhen 518057, China
* Correspondence: wangs@tsinghua-sz.org (S.W.); weiqliu@hotmail.com (W.L.); Tel.: +86-0755-26558633 (S.W.); +86-0755-26551376 (W.L.)

Abstract: Background: Saliva cortisol is considered to be a biomarker of depression prediction. However, saliva collection methods can affect the saliva cortisol level. Objective: This study aims to determine the ideal saliva collection method and explore the application value of saliva cortisol in depression prediction. Methods: 30 depressed patients and 30 healthy controls were instructed to collect saliva samples in the morning with six collection methods. Simultaneous venous blood was collected. Enzyme-linked immunosorbent assay was used to determine the cortisol level. The 24-observerrated Hamilton depression rating scale (HAMD-24) was used to assess the severity of depression. Results: The significant differences in saliva cortisol levels depend on the saliva collection methods. The level of unstimulated whole saliva cortisol was most correlated with blood (r = 0.91). The stimulated parotid saliva cortisol can better predict depression. The area under the curve was 0.89. In addition, the saliva cortisol level of the depression patients was significantly higher than the healthy controls. The correlation between the cortisol level and the HAMD-24 score was highly significant. The higher the saliva cortisol level, the higher the HAMD-24 score. Conclusions: All the above findings point to an exciting opportunity for non-invasive monitoring of cortisol through saliva.

Keywords: saliva; cortisol; biomarker; depression; prediction; level; collection; methods; correction; blood

Citation: Cui, Y.; Zhang, H.; Wang, S.; Lu, J.; He, J.; Liu, L.; Liu, W. Stimulated Parotid Saliva Is a Better Method for Depression Prediction. *Biomedicines* 2022, 10, 2220. https://doi.org/10.3390/biomedicines10092220

Academic Editor: Masaru Tanaka and Simone Battaglia

Received: 12 August 2022
Accepted: 6 September 2022
Published: 7 September 2022

Publisher's Note: MDPI stays neutral with regard to jurisdictional claims in published maps and institutional affiliations.

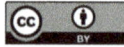

Copyright: © 2022 by the authors. Licensee MDPI, Basel, Switzerland. This article is an open access article distributed under the terms and conditions of the Creative Commons Attribution (CC BY) license (https://creativecommons.org/licenses/by/4.0/).

1. Introduction

Depression is a mental illness characterized by a long period of sadness with several social and psychiatric factors that have been identified as the main cause of suicide [1,2]. Moreover, its lifetime prevalence rate is as high as 16% [3]. Despite the high prevalence and significant morbidity of depression in the population, the exact physical causes of depression remain unknown [4]. Some studies pointed out that the factors that should draw attention to the study of depression, especially related to depression and stress, may include, but are not limited to, the pathogenic involvement of diet and microbiota, stress and mitochondrial impairment, aging and comorbidity, and cognitive and motor function [5–7]. Among them, stress has been proved to be one of the underlying causes of depression [8]. Further research on the biological pathways related to stress in people with depression may help to understand the causes of stress related to depression [9,10].

The hypothalamic-pituitary-adrenal (HPA) axis is one of the potential neurobiological pathways of depression, and the HPA axis reflects the regulation of stress by the neuroendocrine system [11,12]. Cortisol is the main component of the glucocorticoid secreted by the adrenal cortex. Its level fluctuates with the circadian rhythm of the HPA axis. It can reflect the function of the HPA axis [13,14]. For most biotypes, cortisol levels are at their highest in the morning, which can reflect the function of the adrenal cortex, usually around

9 a.m. [15]. Saliva has been proven to have high correlation values to cortisol levels in blood with a non-invasive in situ collection method, so it is more lucrative for cortisol determination compared with blood [16,17]. In clinical practice, about 80% of the cortisol in the blood is combined with cortieosteroid-binding globulin (CBG), and the rest is in a free state [18]. It is only the free fraction that is biologically active and can activate signaling pathways via glucocorticoid hormone receptors in cells [19]. Since saliva does not contain CBG, saliva cortisol can well reflect the level of free cortisol with biological activity in the blood [20]. Moreover, saliva contains biomarkers, which, like blood, can reflect changes in human physiological functions. Thus, saliva can be an ideal alternative to blood [21]. Therefore, it has been widely used in mental and psychological research [22]. Previous studies have found that the saliva cortisol level of patients with depression is higher than that of healthy people [23,24], but some researchers hold the opposite conclusion [25,26] or believe that there is no difference [27]. In addition, a number of studies have shown that saliva sampling methods have an impact on the content of cortisol in saliva, and there is no parallel comparison between these saliva cortisol measurements and serum cortisol values [28,29].

So, in this study, participants included 30 depressed patients and 30 healthy controls who were instructed to collect saliva samples in the morning when waking up. They used six collection methods, including unstimulated and stimulated whole saliva (UWS, SWS), unstimulated and stimulated sublingual/submandibular saliva (USS, SSS), and unstimulated and stimulated parotid saliva (UPS, SPS). Simultaneous venous blood sampling was collected. Enzyme-linked immunosorbent assay was used to determine the level of cortisol. The 24-observer-rated Hamilton depression rating scale (HAMD-24) was used to assess the severity of depression in the study participants. The differences in saliva cortisol levels between depression patients and healthy controls were compared, and the relationship between the severity of depression and saliva cortisol levels was analyzed. Moreover, the value of saliva cortisol in the diagnosis of depression and the receiver operating characteristic (ROC) method in the diagnosis of depression were analyzed.

2. Materials and Methods

2.1. Participants and Study Design

In this study, 60 participants were included, which were divided into two groups: the patient group (N = 30) and the control group (N = 30). The patient group meets the diagnostic criteria and meets the tenth edition «The International Statistical Classification of Diseases and Related Health Problems 10th Revision» (ICD-10) [30]; selection criteria: 18 to 65 years old with no history of psychotropic medication and diagnosed by two associate chief physicians. A total of 30 healthy controls from the physical examination center during the same period were selected as the control group. Selection criteria: 18 to 65 years old, regardless of sex. On the day of saliva collection, two psychiatrists assessed all participants with HAMD-24, and the total score of the scale reflects the severity of depression. A total score of <8 points, no depression; a total score of 8–20 points, may have mild depression; a total score of 20–35 points, mild to moderate depression; total score >35 points, severe depression [31]. All study participants signed an informed consent form. The collection of human blood and saliva samples was approved by the local ethics committee at Tsinghua University.

2.2. Laboratory Tests

Before the collection, the participants were told to pay close attention to the collection: no drinking within 12 h before the collection, no eating within 1 h, and no brushing or drinking water within 10 min. The collection time was 7:30–9:30 in the morning. For each participant, samples of the parotid gland, mandibular/sublingual gland, and whole saliva were collected with and without stimulation (as shown in Figure 1). The swabs included acid stimulated and untreated swabs, so the different swabs in the parotid, sublingual/submandibular, and whole mouth were represented by UWS, SWS, UPS, SPS, USS, and SSS, respectively, where the saliva collection method was the same as in our previous studies [32,33]. All the saliva samples were collected in the same clinical room and at the same time, between 7:30 and 9:30 in the morning. To prevent the degradation of sensitive peptides, all samples were collected in prechilled polypropylene tubes on ice. The total amount of saliva collected by all methods is 5 mL. In the end, it was routinely transported to the laboratory, transferred to a centrifuge tube, centrifuged, and the supernatant was taken and stored at −20 °C for later use. After the last saliva sample was collected, venous blood samples were collected from all participants. The sample was gently mixed for 1 min and then immediately placed on ice for 30 min. The sample was then centrifuged at 1000 r for 15 min at 4 °C, and the upper 2/3 aliquot of plasma was stored at −80 °C until analysis. Saliva cortisol levels were determined using a particular enzyme-linked immunosorbent test (ELISA, Beijing Furui Runkang Biotechnology Co., Ltd., Beijing, China).

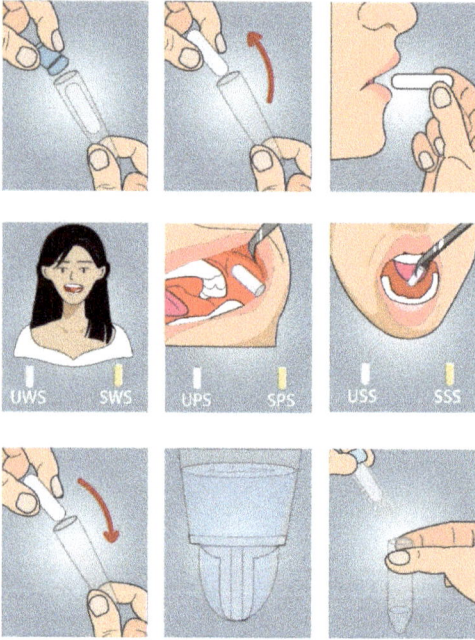

Figure 1. Six methods for collecting saliva samples, UWS/SWS: the swab in the test tube was taken out and put in the mouth to chew for 3 min; UPS/SPS: the swab was placed near the left parotid duct, and it was taken out after 3 min; USS/SSS: the swab was put under the tongue, and it was taken out after 3 min.

2.3. Statistical Analyses

Statistical analyses were carried out using GraphPad Prism 8.0 (GraphPad Software, San Diego, CA, USA, www.graphpad.com). In order to facilitate comparisons between groups, the data χ^2 were reported as relative numbers. Measurement data were transformed into a normal distribution and presented as mean standard deviation ($\bar{x} \pm s$), and a t-test was employed to make group comparisons. To determine if the data are normally distributed, we utilized the Shapiro–Wilk test. When describing data that were not normally distributed, minimum and maximum values were used, whereas when describing data that was regularly distributed, the standard normal distribution statistic, ($\bar{x} \pm s$), was used. Because the saliva cortisol level of the control group was normally distributed while the saliva cortisol level of the patient group was non-normally distributed, the saliva cortisol level of the two groups was compared using the Wilcoxon rank sum test. The correlation between saliva cortisol and HAMD-24 score was analyzed by Spearman rank correlation analysis. The saliva cortisol of the participants of different genders and ages in each group was compared using a t-test of two independent samples. In this study, the ROC method was used to comprehensively evaluate the diagnostic value of saliva cortisol testing for depression. $p < 0.05$ indicated that the difference was statistically significant.

3. Results

3.1. Sample Characteristics

The 30 participants in the depression group included 12 males (40%) and 18 females (60%), with an average age of (43.5 ± 5.2) years; the 30 participants in the healthy control group included 16 males (53.3%) and 14 females (46.7%), with an average age of (40.1 ± 4.7) years. As shown in Table 1, there was no significant difference in sex (t = 0.613, p = 0.367) and age (t = 0.173, p = 0.467) between the two groups.

Table 1. Sample characteristics of the studied groups.

Sample Characteristics	Depression Group	Healthy Controls	p
Age	43.5 ± 5.2	40.1 ± 4.7	0.467
HAMD-24 scores	25.7 ± 10.3	3.9 ± 1.8	<0.001

The distribution of HAMD-24 scores in the patient group ranged from 9 to 48 points. A total of 10 patients with a total score of 8–20 points, which was mild depression; 15 patients with a total score of 20–35, which were mild to moderate depression. There were 5 patients with a total score of >35 points, which meant severe depression. The scores of HAMD-24 in the control group were all <8 points, showing a non-normal distribution, and the median (25% and 75%) points were 3 (0, 5). Figure 2 shows the distribution of male and female age and HAMD-24 scores.

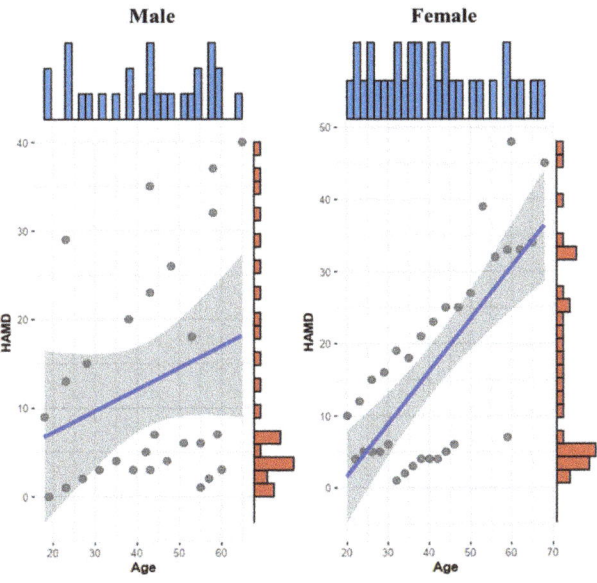

Figure 2. Male and female age and HAMD-24 score distribution chart.

3.2. Saliva Cortisol

Additionally, the patient group had greater saliva cortisol levels (average levels) than the control group in all six saliva samples (as shown in Table 2), with the highest level of SWS cortisol and the lowest level of UPS cortisol, as illustrated in Figure 3.

Table 2. The average levels of saliva cortisol for each group (depressed patient/control and stimulated/unstimulated).

Cortisol Levels (nmol/L)	UWS	SWS	UPS	SPS	USS	SSS
Patients (N = 30)	14.87 ± 6.22	16.91 ± 6.91 **	13.39 ± 5.60	16.13 ± 6.61	14.12 ± 5.91	15.37 ± 6.29
Controls (N = 30)	10.69 ± 4.07	12.25 ± 4.53	9.62 ± 3.67 *	11.71 ± 4.33	10.15 ± 3.87	11.15 ± 4.11

** Maximum level of saliva cortisol. * Minimum level saliva cortisol.

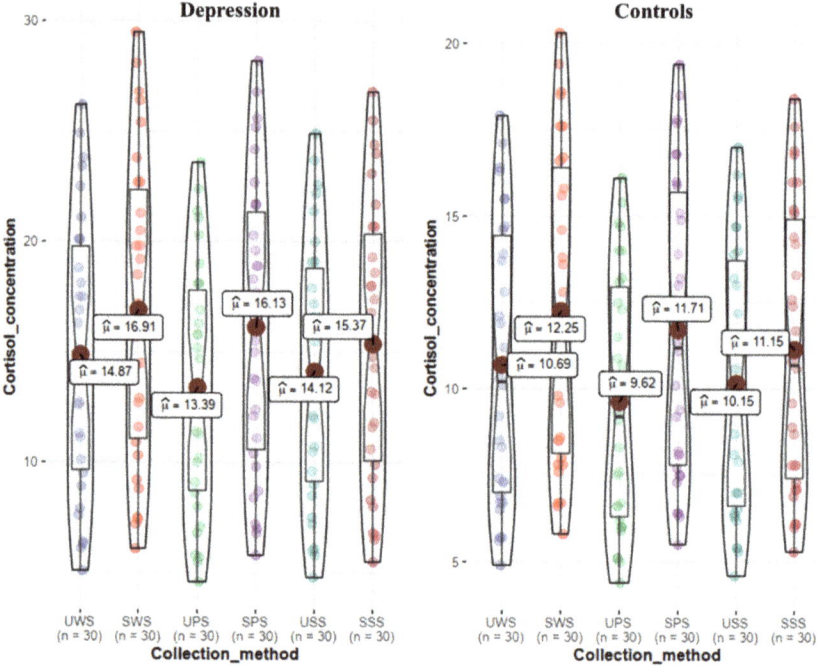

Figure 3. Saliva cortisol levels in the patient group and the control group.

The frequency distribution of saliva cortisol levels in the two groups showed that the saliva cortisol levels in the patient group showed a non-normal distribution, and the median (25% and 75%) of different saliva collection methods were different, and the overall distribution range was 6.5–29.4 nmol/L. The saliva cortisol level of the control group showed a non-normal distribution, as shown in Figure 3. The distribution range was 4.8–20.2 nmol/L. Using the Wilcoxon rank sum test to compare the saliva cortisol levels of the two groups, the saliva cortisol level of the patient group was significantly higher than that of the control group, and the difference was statistically significant ($p < 0.001$). The higher the saliva cortisol level, the higher the HAMD-24 score ($r = 0.812$, $p < 0.001$). There is a slight correlation between cortisol level and age ($r = 0.353$, $p = 0.017$). There was a slight correlation between cortisol level and sex ($p = 0.031$).

3.3. Blood and Saliva Cortisol Correlation

In this section, six methods (UWS, SWS, USS, SSS, UPS, and SPS) were used for the collection of saliva. The correlation between each saliva sample and blood cortisol was analyzed. Figure 4 shows the correlation between the six saliva collection methods and blood cortisol. It can be seen that the saliva cortisol level obtained by the six saliva collection methods has a very strong correlation with blood cortisol. The UWS was the closest to the blood cortisol level ($r = 0.91$). It can also be found that the cortisol level of the patient group was correlated with the blood cortisol level, which was higher than that of the control group. Moreover, there was no significant correlation between the irritating saliva collection method and the nonirritating collection method.

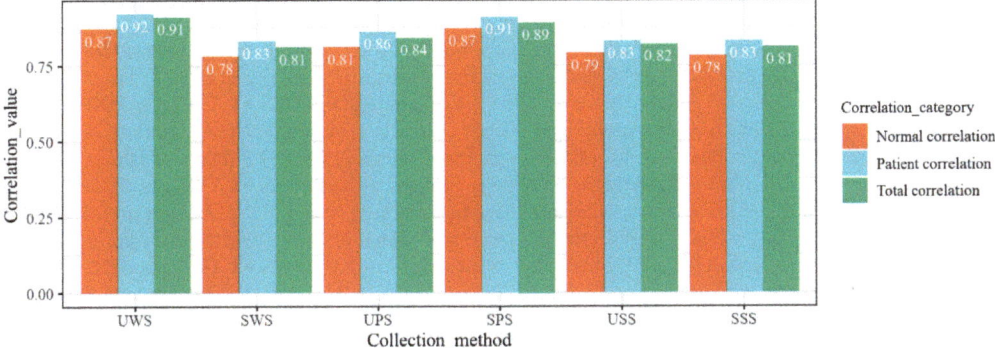

Figure 4. Correlation between six collection methods and blood cortisol.

3.4. Validation of Diagnostic Performance by ROC Curve

According to the ROC curve, the best cut-off value of SPS cortisol level for diagnosing depression was 15.9 nmol/L, with the highest sensitivity and specificity, which were 66.66% and 96.66%, respectively, and the area under the curve (AUC) = 0.89. Next was blood cortisol, with an AUC of 0.86. UWS ranked third with an AUC of 0.85, as shown in Figure 5. In addition, in our study, we found the increased prevalence of depression was related to saliva cortisol $\geq$ 15.9 nmol/L, the AUC reached 0.75, and the diagnostic performance was classified as good.

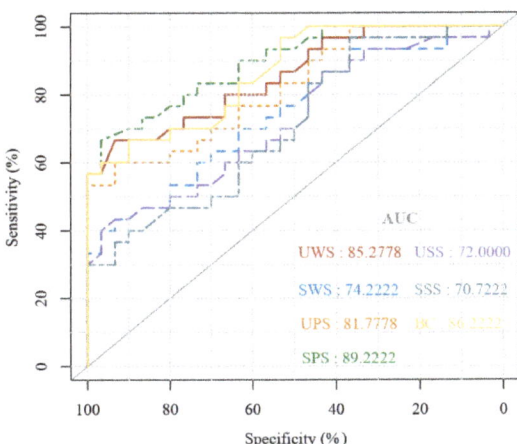

Figure 5. The ROC curve of cortisol in the diagnosis of depression.

4. Discussion

Early detection of depression is crucial because only an early diagnosis can provide long-term symptom alleviation [34]. As a result, strategies for identifying the illness in the early stages are badly needed [35,36]. Six saliva collection methods were employed in this study on 30 healthy controls and 30 depressed patients in the morning to determine the ideal saliva collection method. The saliva cortisol levels of these participants were measured using an enzyme-linked immunosorbent assay. We needed to be able to detect saliva cortisol levels using a simple and reliable method. This study also found that the effectiveness of saliva as a diagnostic biological fluid was dependent on the consistency of collection procedures in order to deliver the most accurate and helpful results. The methods used to collect saliva have a considerable impact on cortisol levels and correlation. As a result, standardizing a saliva collection process is crucial for mitigating the impact of variability in saliva composition within and between individuals.

Saliva is frequently misunderstood as a single fluid [37]; instead, saliva is typically divided into single gland saliva and mixed saliva. Parotid saliva, submandibular saliva, and sublingual saliva are examples of single gland saliva [38,39]. The proportionate contribution of different glands to the total saliva sample varies depending on the collection method, level of stimulation, age, and even time of day [40]. Because saliva secretion varies, different methodologies may be required for researching its components or their potential relevance as markers of specific physiological states [41]. Although there is a substantial body of literature on the diagnostic potential of saliva, there is no standardized method for obtaining saliva samples. Different sampling methods are frequently used in different studies, and many studies do not or rarely describe patient preparation or sampling procedures [42,43]. Furthermore, without a complete clinical assessment, participants' characteristics are frequently insufficient. The majority of saliva cortisol research publications concentrate on analyzing the whole saliva since it is easily acquired by spitting it into a test tube or letting it flow from the mouth [44,45]. Few people are aware of ductal saliva, which is produced by several salivary glands. Furthermore, a cohort with meticulous characterization and clinical assessment was used to compare the cortisol expression of whole saliva and glandular saliva. The results show that different collection procedures produce significant disparities in saliva cortisol snapshots [46]. The findings of this study also show that different saliva collecting procedures produce significant changes in snapshots of saliva biomarkers for depression.

Alternative saliva collection methods would be appropriate for collecting saliva in a clinical situation. It was critical that we could detect saliva cortisol levels using a simple and reliable procedure. We measured saliva cortisol levels using six saliva collection methods in this study: UWS, SWS, USS, SSS, SPS, and UPS. Different saliva collection procedures have a significant impact on cortisol levels and correlation. Second, while the unstimulated approach of directly collecting saliva is practical and easy for patients to accept, the amount of saliva collected is insufficient to meet the needs of detection [47]. Because the effect of stimulation methods on salivary cortisol is unknown, we conducted the first study to compare six different saliva collection methods and investigate the relationship between saliva cortisol and blood cortisol level. The main conclusions derived from this work were summarized as follows: The UWS cortisol level was strongly associated with the blood cortisol level, but the SPS cortisol level can be better used to predict depression. In participants with depression and without depression, there was a slight correlation between cortisol levels and age, and females had a higher prevalence of depression than men. It was found that the saliva cortisol level of depressed patients was higher than that of healthy controls. The higher the saliva cortisol level, the higher the HAMD-24 score. It has been proved that saliva cortisol testing as an auxiliary method for the diagnosis of depression can help identify patients at risk of depression for early prevention strategies.

The HAMD-24 score of the patient group was normally distributed, with a mean ± standard deviation of (25 ± 10) points and a distribution range of 9 to 48 points. The depression patient group covered mild, moderate, and severe conditions. Among the 30 people selected in the patient group, 18 were female, and 12 were male, which was consistent with the higher incidence of depression in females than in males [48,49]. The average age of the patient group was (43.5 ± 5.2) years, which was also in line with the higher incidence of depression and menopause [50,51]. This may be because females show greater activation of the HPA axis than males, and the loss of estrogen during menopause shows the greatest HPA axis dysregulation [52,53]. The distribution of HAMD-24 scores in the control group ranged from 0 to 7, and none of them had depressive symptoms. The higher the saliva cortisol level, the higher of HAMD-24 score, indicating that the saliva cortisol level in the morning can reflect the severity of depression in people with depression, which was consistent with conclusions of previous studies [54,55]. This study found that the saliva cortisol level of females was different from that of males, and the difference was statistically significant ($p < 0.05$), suggesting that the difference in saliva cortisol may be related to sex in patients with depression. The saliva cortisol level in the group of female patients with depression may be higher than that in males, and it needs to be further verified by multiple trials. In the control group, there was no difference between the saliva cortisol levels of females and males, and the difference was not statistically significant ($p > 0.05$), which was inconsistent with the results reported by some larger cortisol studies. It is considered that the sample of participants in this study is small, and the saliva cortisol difference that may exist between the sexes has not been found.

Cortisol is a hormone related to the HPA axis [56]. It has a strong circadian rhythm. Its level reaches its highest peak within 1 h in the morning and then decreases rapidly [57,58], so this study strictly followed the collection time during the specimen collection process to ensure the accuracy of data. This study compared six different saliva collection methods and explored the relationship between saliva cortisol and blood cortisol levels. It was found that the unstimulated whole saliva cortisol level was most correlated with the blood cortisol level, which can accurately reflect the level of blood cortisol. It further suggests that saliva cortisol can be used as a measure of stress response to assist in the diagnosis of depression.

At the same time, this study found that the level of nonirritating saliva cortisol was continuously lower than that of stimulating saliva cortisol, which is consistent with the results reported in previous studies [59–61]. Poll [62] also recently demonstrated that the collection method affects the measurement accuracy of cortisol in saliva. The ROC analysis method combines sensitivity and specificity for analysis and is an ideal method for the comprehensive and accurate evaluation of diagnostic tests [63,64]. The ROC analysis method was used to evaluate the diagnostic value of saliva cortisol detection for depression, and the calculated AUC was 0.765 (95% confidence interval: 0.679–0.838). According to the evaluation criteria of Swets [65], when the AUC = 0.5, the diagnosis is completely ineffective; when the AUC is less than 0.5, it is not in line with the actual situation; it is generally believed that $0.5 < AUC \leq 0.7$ indicates low diagnostic value. It is only for reference in practical applications; $0.7 < AUC \leq 0.9$ indicates a certain degree of accuracy and can be used in clinical diagnosis, with a medium diagnostic value; $AUC > 0.9$ indicates a relatively high diagnostic value, which can be used in clinical diagnosis as an important diagnostic basis [66,67]. In the results of this study, the AUC was 0.89, close to 0.9, so we think that saliva cortisol testing can be considered an auxiliary method for the clinical diagnosis of depression, and its diagnostic value is moderate. In addition, the collection of saliva cortisol in this study allows for non-invasive collection at regular intervals, which can be stably collected for several days before the experiment, so that the HPA axis in the free state can be effectively evaluated [68,69]. The assessment of cortisol in saliva has proven effective and reliable in reflecting the respective unbound hormones in the blood [70,71]. Therefore, in this study, we assessed the level of cortisol through saliva samples. In addition, compared with the enzyme-linked immunosorbent assay, saliva cortisol is determined by chemiluminescence immunoassay, which has higher sensitivity and specificity [72].

However, this study has shortcomings. First of all, it is difficult to determine the causal relationship between only one assessment of saliva cortisol and current depression symptoms. Secondly, this study lacks a concurrent evaluation of the HPA axis function, and there is no information about saliva gene expression. In addition, the exclusion criteria do not include corticosteroid therapy for somatic diseases that may affect the HPA axis function. Finally, saliva cortisol secretion presents a circadian rhythm. This study used morning saliva cortisol for research and analysis. Although previous studies support that the morning cortisol level is the highest and the best time for measurement, it is necessary to perform multiple time-point research so as to fully understand the role of saliva cortisol in the diagnosis of depression. Due to the limited number of data points, further research is necessary, including validity testing, retesting, and multi-factorial testing, even if this study offers the best performance for the early detection of depressed patients. Finally, there are still many issues in this study that need to be resolved and further investigated. For instance, the proximity of the submandibular and sublingual glands makes it challenging to categorically distinguish the saliva from both glands. For this reason, saliva was taken from both glands in the current investigation. The distinction between sublingual and submandibular saliva is another area that requires more investigation. In order to make the diagnosis of depression in saliva more accurate, numerous risk variables (such as living environment, work environment, etc. [73]) should also be taken into consideration.

5. Conclusions

This study found that the levels of cortisol in saliva are highly correlated with those found in the blood. Moreover, the significant difference in saliva cortisol level depends on the saliva collection method, the level of UWS cortisol was most correlated with blood level; however, the SPS cortisol can better predict depression. In addition, this study found that the saliva cortisol level of the patients with depression was significantly higher than the patients without depression. Moreover, the correlation between the cortisol level and the HAMD-24 score was highly significant. The higher the saliva cortisol level, the higher the HAMD-24 score. Finally, it was found that cortisol level has a slight correlation with age and sex. This study demonstrated that early morning saliva cortisol has excellent diagnostic characteristics and, as such, is a robust, convenient test for screening and diagnosis of depression, which can help people with depression be aware of their negative thoughts and early prevention of them.

Author Contributions: Y.C.: Writing-original draft, Data curation, Methodology, Project administration; H.Z.: Data curation, Formal analysis, Methodology, Software; S.W.: Writing-review &editing, Funding acquisition, Investigation, Supervision; J.L.: Data curation, Formal analysis, Methodology, Validation; J.H.: Data curation, Formal analysis, Methodology, Visualization; L.L.: Data curation, Formal analysis, Methodology; W.L.: Funding acquisition, Investigation, Resources, Supervision. All authors have read and agreed to the published version of the manuscript.

Funding: This project was supported by the Guangdong Basic and Applied Basic Research Foundation (Grant No. 2020B1515120082), the Innovation Commission of Science and Technology of Shen-zhen Municipality (Grant No. JCYJ20190807144001746, Grant No. JCYJ20200109150605937, Grant No. JSGG20191129114422849).

Institutional Review Board Statement: Not applicable.

Informed Consent Statement: All study participants signed an informed consent form, and the collection of human blood and saliva samples was approved by the local ethics committee at Tsinghua University.

Data Availability Statement: The study did not report any data.

Conflicts of Interest: The authors declare no conflict of interest.

References

1. Kim, B.J.; Kihl, T. Suicidal ideation associated with depression and social support: A survey-based analysis of older adults in South Korea. *BMC Psychiatry* **2021**, *21*, 2520. [CrossRef]
2. Kalin, N.H. Anxiety, depression, and suicide in youth. *Am. J. Psychiatry* **2021**, *178*, 275–279. [CrossRef]
3. Ronald, C.K.; Patricia, B.; Olga, D.; Robert, J.; Kathleen, R.M.; Ellen, E.W. Lifetime prevalence and age of-onset distributions of dsmiv disorders in the national comorbidity survey replication. *Arch. Gen. Psychiatry* **2005**, *62*, 593–602.
4. Wu, Y.; Zhang, C.; Liu, H.; Duan, C.; Li, C.; Fan, J.; Huang, H.F. Perinatal depressive and anxiety symptoms of pregnant women during the coronavirus disease 2019 outbreak in China. *Am. J. Obstet. Gynecol.* **2020**, *223*, 240.e1–240.e9. [CrossRef] [PubMed]
5. Kovtun, A.S.; Averina, O.V.; Angelova, I.Y.; Yunes, R.A.; Zorkina, Y.A.; Morozova, A.Y.; Pavlichenko, A.V.; Syunyakov, T.S.; Karpenko, O.A.; Kostyuk, G.P.; et al. Alterations of the Composition and Neurometabolic Profile of Human Gut Microbiota in Major Depressive Disorder. *Biomedicines* **2022**, *10*, 2162. [CrossRef]
6. Brasso, C.; Bellino, S.; Blua, C.; Bozzatello, P.; Rocca, P. The Impact of SARS-CoV-2 Infection on Youth Mental Health: A Narrative Review. *Biomedicines* **2022**, *10*, 772. [CrossRef]

7. Kim, I.-B.; Lee, J.-H.; Park, S.-C. The Relationship between Stress, Inflammation, and Depression. *Biomedicines* **2022**, *10*, 1929. [CrossRef]
8. Shen, F.; Song, Z.; Xie, P.; Li, L.; Wang, B.; Peng, D.; Zhu, G. Polygonatum sibiricum polysaccharide prevents depression-like behaviors by reducing oxidative stress, inflammation, and cellular and synaptic damage. *J. Ethnopharmacol.* **2021**, *275*, 114164. [CrossRef]
9. Kandola, A.; Ashdown-Franks, G.; Hendrikse, J.; Sabiston, C.M.; Stubbs, B. Physical activity and depression: Towards understanding the antidepressant mechanisms of physical activity. *Neurosci. Biobehav. Rev.* **2019**, *107*, 525–539. [CrossRef] [PubMed]
10. Lin, D.; Wang, L.; Yan, S.; Zhang, Q.; Zhang, J.H.; Shao, A. The role of oxidative stress in common risk factors and mechanisms of cardio-cerebrovascular ischemia and depression. *Oxid. Med. Cell. Longev.* **2019**, *2019*, 2491927. [CrossRef] [PubMed]
11. Adam, E.K.; Quinn, M.E.; Tavernier, R.; McQuillan, M.T.; Dahlke, K.A.; Gilbert, K.E. Diurnal cortisol slopes and mental and physical health outcomes: A systematic review and meta-analysis. *Psychoneuroendocrinology* **2017**, *83*, 25–41. [CrossRef] [PubMed]
12. Hostinar, C.E.; Gunnar, M.R. Future directions in the study of social relationships as regulators of the HPA axis across development. In *Future Work in Clinical Child and Adolescent Psychology*; Routledge: London, UK, 2018; pp. 333–344.
13. Jones, C.; Gwenin, C. Cortisol level dysregulation and its prevalence—Is it nature's alarm clock? *Physiol. Rep.* **2021**, *8*, e14644. [CrossRef]
14. Kinlein, S.A.; Karatsoreos, I.N. The hypothalamic-pituitary-adrenal axis as a substrate for stress resilience: Interactions with the circadian clock. *Front. Neuroendocrinol.* **2020**, *56*, 100819. [CrossRef]
15. Høifødt, R.S.; Wang, C.E.; Eisemann, M.; Figenschau, Y.; Halvorsen, M. Cortisol levels and cognitive profile in major depression: A comparison of currently and previously depressed patients. *Psychoneuroendocrinology* **2019**, *99*, 57–65. [CrossRef]
16. Rickert, D.; Simon, R.; von Fersen, L.; Baumgartner, K.; Bertsch, T.; Kirschbaum, C.; Erhard, M. Saliva and Blood Cortisol Measurement in Bottlenose Dolphins (*Tursiops truncatus*): Methodology, Application, and Limitations. *Animals* **2022**, *12*, 22. [CrossRef] [PubMed]
17. Weaver, S.J.; Hynd, P.I.; Ralph, C.R.; Edwards, J.H.; Burnard, C.L.; Narayan, E.; Tilbrook, A.J. Chronic elevation of plasma cortisol causes differential expression of predominating glucocorticoid in plasma, saliva, fecal, and wool matrices in sheep. *Domest. Anim. Endocrinol.* **2021**, *74*, 106503. [CrossRef]
18. Therriault, D.H.; Wheeler, D.H. Symposium: Binding of upids by proteins conducted Ly the American Oil Chemists' Society at its 37tn pall meeting, Minneapolis, Minnesota September 30–October 2, 1963. *J. Am. Oil Chem. Soc.* **1964**, *41*, 481–490. [CrossRef]
19. Bhake, R.; Russell, G.M.; Kershaw, Y.; Stevens, K.; Zaccardi, F.; Warburton, V.E.; Lightman, S.L. Continuous free cortisol profiles in healthy men: Validation of microdialysis method. *J. Clin. Endocrinol. Metab.* **2020**, *105*, e1749–e1761. [CrossRef] [PubMed]
20. Bechert, U.; Hixon, S.; Schmitt, D. Diurnal variation in serum concentrations of cortisol in captive African (*Loxodonta africana*) and Asian (*Elephas maximus*) elephants. *Zoo Biol.* **2021**, *40*, 458–471. [CrossRef]
21. Cui, Y.; Yang, M.; Zhu, J.; Zhang, H.; Duan, Z.; Wang, S.; Liu, W. Developments in diagnostic applications of saliva in Human Organ Diseases. *Med. Nov. Technol. Devices* **2022**, *13*, 100115. [CrossRef]
22. Bellosta, B.M.; Carmen, B.G.M.; Rodríguez, A.M. Brief mindfulness session improves mood and increases salivary oxytocin in psychology students. *Stress Health* **2020**, *36*, 469–477. [CrossRef] [PubMed]
23. Furtado, G.E.; Letieri, R.V.; Silva-Caldo, A.; Trombeta, J.C.; Monteiro, C.; Rodrigues, R.N.; Ferreira, J.P. Combined Chair-Based Exercises Improve Functional Fitness, Mental Well-Being, Salivary Steroid Balance, and Anti-microbial Activity in Pre-frail Older Women. *Front. Psychol.* **2021**, *12*, 577. [CrossRef]
24. Van Cappellen, P.; Edwards, M.E.; Fredrickson, B.L. Upward spirals of positive emotions and religious behaviors. *Curr. Opin. Psychol.* **2021**, *40*, 92–98. [CrossRef] [PubMed]
25. Khan, Q.U. Relationship of Salivary Cortisol level with severe depression and family history. *Cureus* **2020**, *12*, e11548. [CrossRef]
26. Krishnaveni, P.; Ganesh, V. Electron transfer studies of a conventional redox probe in human sweat and saliva bio-mimicking conditions. *Sci. Rep.* **2021**, *11*, 7663. [CrossRef] [PubMed]
27. Frenk, P.; Nancy, A.N.; Johannes, B. Levels and variability of daily life cortisol secretion in major depression. *Psychiatry Res.* **2004**, *126*, 1–13.
28. Kovács, L.; Kézér, F.L.; Bodó, S.; Ruff, F.; Palme, R.; Szenci, O. Salivary cortisol as a non-invasive approach to assess stress in dystocic dairy calves. *Sci. Rep.* **2021**, *11*, 6200. [CrossRef]
29. Moghadam, F.M.; Bigdeli, M.; Tamayol, A.; Shin, S.R. TISS nanobiosensor for salivary cortisol measurement by aptamer Ag nanocluster SAIE supraparticle structure. *Sens. Actuators B Chem.* **2021**, *344*, 130160. [CrossRef]
30. World Health Organization. Icd-10: International statistical classification of diseases and related health problems: Tenth revision. *Acta Chir. Iugosl.* **2010**, *56*, 65–69.
31. Pan, S.; Liu, Z.W.; Shi, S.; Ma, X.; Song, W.Q.; Guan, G.C.; Lv, Y. Hamilton rating scale for depression-24 (HAM-D24) as a novel predictor for diabetic microvascular complications in type 2 diabetes mellitus patients. *Psychiatry Res.* **2017**, *258*, 177–183. [CrossRef] [PubMed]
32. Cui, Y.; Zhang, H.; Zhu, J.; Peng, L.; Duan, Z.; Liu, T.; Liu, W. Unstimulated Parotid Saliva Is a Better Method for Blood Glucose Prediction. *Appl. Sci.* **2021**, *11*, 11367. [CrossRef]
33. Cui, Y.; Zhang, H.; Zhu, J.; Liao, Z.; Wang, S.; Liu, W. Correlations of Salivary and Blood Glucose Levels among Six Saliva Collection Methods. *Int. J. Environ. Res. Public Health* **2022**, *19*, 4122. [CrossRef] [PubMed]
34. Krakauer, E.L.; Kane, K.; Kwete, X.; Afshan, G.; Bazzett-Matabele, L.; Bien-Aimé, D.D.; Borges, L.F.; Byrne-Martelli, S.; Connor, S.; Correa, R.; et al. Essential package of palliative care for women with cervical cancer: Responding to the suffering of a highly vulnerable population. *JCO Glob. Oncol.* **2021**, *7*, 873–885. [CrossRef] [PubMed]

35. Adhikari, S.P.; Meng, S.; Wu, Y.J.; Mao, Y.P.; Ye, R.X.; Wang, Q.Z.; Zhou, H. Epidemiology, causes, clinical manifestation and diagnosis, prevention and control of coronavirus disease (COVID-19) during the early outbreak period: A scoping review. *Infect. Dis. Poverty* **2020**, *9*, 29. [CrossRef] [PubMed]
36. Laxminarayan, R.; Duse, A.; Wattal, C.; Zaidi, A.K.; Wertheim, H.F.; Sumpradit, N.; Cars, O. Antibiotic resistance—The need for global solutions. *Lancet Infect. Dis.* **2013**, *13*, 1057–1098. [CrossRef]
37. Jackson, K.R.; Layne, T.; Dent, D.A.; Tsuei, A.; Li, J.; Haverstick, D.M.; Landers, J.P. A novel loop-mediated isothermal amplification method for identification of four body fluids with smartphone detection. *Forensic Sci. Int. Genet.* **2020**, *45*, 102195. [CrossRef]
38. Pedersen, A.M.; Bardow, A.; Jensen, S.B.; Nauntofte, B. Saliva and gastrointestinal functions of taste, mastication, swallowing and digestion. *Oral Dis.* **2002**, *8*, 117–129. [CrossRef]
39. Pedersen, A.M.L.; Sørensen, C.E.; Proctor, G.B.; Carpenter, G.H. Salivary functions in mastication, taste and textural perception, swallowing and initial digestion. *Oral Dis.* **2018**, *24*, 1399–1416. [CrossRef] [PubMed]
40. Sim, D.; Brothers, M.C.; Slocik, J.M.; Islam, A.E.; Maruyama, B.; Grigsby, C.C.; Kim, S.S. Biomarkers and detection Platforms for human health and performance monitoring: A Review. *Adv. Sci.* **2022**, *9*, 2104426. [CrossRef] [PubMed]
41. Synnott, A.; Howes, D. From measurement to meaning. Anthropologies of the body. *Anthropos* **1992**, *87*, 147–166.
42. Elo, S.; Kääriäinen, M.; Kanste, O.; Pölkki, T.; Utriainen, K.; Kyngäs, H. Qualitative content analysis: A focus on trustworthiness. *SAGE Open* **2014**, *4*, 2158244014522633. [CrossRef]
43. Moser, A.; Korstjens, I. Series: Practical guidance to qualitative research. Part 3: Sampling, data collection and analysis. *Eur. J. Gen. Pract.* **2018**, *24*, 9–18. [CrossRef]
44. Bhattarai, K.R.; Kim, H.R.; Chae, H.J. Compliance with saliva collection protocol in healthy volunteers: Strategies for managing risk and errors. *Int. J. Med. Sci.* **2018**, *15*, 823. [CrossRef] [PubMed]
45. Szefler, S.J.; Wenzel, S.; Brown, R.; Erzurum, S.C.; Fahy, J.V.; Hamilton, R.G.; Minnicozzi, M. Asthma outcomes: Biomarkers. *J. Allergy Clin. Immunol.* **2012**, *129*, S9–S23. [CrossRef] [PubMed]
46. Cui, Y.; Zhang, H.; Zhu, J.; Liao, Z.; Wang, S.; Liu, W. Investigation of Whole and Glandular Saliva as a Biomarker for Alzheimer's Disease Diagnosis. *Brain Sci.* **2022**, *12*, 595. [CrossRef]
47. Jasim, H.; Olausson, P.; Hedenberg-Magnusson, B.; Ernberg, M.; Ghafouri, B. The proteomic profile of whole and glandular saliva in healthy pain-free subjects. *Sci. Rep.* **2016**, *6*, 39073. [CrossRef] [PubMed]
48. Hibbert, M.P.; Brett, C.E.; Porcellato, L.A.; Hope, V.D. Image and performance enhancing drug use among men who have sex with men and women who have sex with women in the UK. *Int. J. Drug Policy* **2021**, *95*, 102933. [CrossRef] [PubMed]
49. Dostanic, N.; Djikanovic, B.; Jovanovic, M.; Stamenkovic, Z.; Đeric, A. The association between family violence, depression and anxiety among women whose partners have been treated for alcohol dependence. *J. Fam. Violence* **2022**, *37*, 313–324. [CrossRef]
50. Garay, R.P.; Charpeaud, T.; Logan, S.; Hannaert, P.; Garay, R.G.; Llorca, P.M.; Shorey, S. Pharmacotherapeutic approaches to treating depression during the perimenopause. *Expert Opin. Pharmacother.* **2019**, *20*, 1837–1845. [CrossRef]
51. Lee, J.; Han, Y.; Cho, H.H.; Kim, M.R. Sleep disorders and menopause. *J. Menopausal Med.* **2019**, *25*, 83–87. [CrossRef] [PubMed]
52. Murack, M.; Chandrasegaram, R.; Smith, K.B.; Ah-Yen, E.G.; Rheaume, É.; Malette-Guyon, É.; Ismail, N. Chronic sleep disruption induces depression-like behavior in adolescent male and female mice and sensitization of the hypothalamic-pituitary-adrenal axis in adolescent female mice. *Behav. Brain Res.* **2021**, *399*, 113001. [CrossRef]
53. Ahmad, M.H.; Fatima, M.; Mondal, A.C. Role of hypothalamic-pituitary-adrenal axis, hypothalamic-pituitary-gonadal axis and insulin signaling in the pathophysiology of Alzheimer's disease. *Neuropsychobiology* **2019**, *77*, 197–205. [CrossRef]
54. Ceruso, A.; Martínez-Cengotitabengoa, M.; Peters-Corbett, A.; Diaz-Gutierrez, M.J.; Martinez-Cengotitabengoa, M. Alterations of the HPA axis observed in patients with major depressive disorder and their relation to early life stress: A systematic review. *Neuropsychobiology* **2020**, *79*, 417–427. [CrossRef] [PubMed]
55. Sung, J.; Woo, J.M.; Kim, W.; Lim, S.K.; Chung, E.J. The effect of cognitive behavior therapy-based "forest therapy" program on blood pressure, salivary cortisol level, and quality of life in elderly hypertensive patients. *Clin. Exp. Hypertens.* **2012**, *34*, 1–7. [CrossRef] [PubMed]
56. Muehlhan, M.; Höcker, A.; Miller, R.; Trautmann, S.; Wiedemann, K.; Lotzin, A.; Schäfer, I. HPA axis stress reactivity and hair cortisol concentrations in recently detoxified alcoholics and healthy controls with and without childhood maltreatment. *Addict. Biol.* **2020**, *25*, e12681. [CrossRef] [PubMed]
57. Jia, Y.; Liu, L.; Sheng, C.; Cheng, Z.; Cui, L.; Li, M.; Chen, L. Increased serum levels of cortisol and inflammatory cytokines in people with depression. *J. Nerv. Ment. Dis.* **2019**, *207*, 271–276. [CrossRef]
58. Lages, A.D.S.; Frade, J.G.; Oliveira, D.; Paiva, I.; Oliveira, P.; Rebelo-Marques, A.; Carrilho, F. Late-night salivary cortisol: Cut-off definition and diagnostic accuracy for cushing's syndrome in a portuguese population. *Acta Med. Port.* **2019**, *32*, 381–387. [CrossRef] [PubMed]
59. Libanori, A.; Chen, G.; Zhao, X.; Zhou, Y.; Chen, J. Smart textiles for personalized healthcare. *Nat. Electron.* **2022**, *5*, 142–156. [CrossRef]
60. Li, D.; Yao, K.; Gao, Z.; Liu, Y.; Yu, X. Recent progress of skin-integrated electronics for intelligent sensing. *Light Adv. Manuf.* **2021**, *2*, 39–58. [CrossRef]
61. Ye, S.; Feng, S.; Huang, L.; Bian, S. Recent progress in wearable biosensors: From healthcare monitoring to sports analytics. *Biosensors* **2020**, *10*, 205. [CrossRef] [PubMed]

62. Poll, E.M.; Kreitschmann-Andermahr, I.; Langejuergen, Y.; Stanzel, S.; Gilsbach, J.M.; Gressner, A.; Yagmur, E. Saliva collection method affects predictability of serum cortisol. *Clin. Chim. Acta* **2007**, *382*, 15–19. [CrossRef]
63. Hajian-Tilaki, K. Receiver operating characteristic (ROC) curve analysis for medical diagnostic test evaluation. *Casp. J. Intern. Med.* **2013**, *4*, 627.
64. Obuchowski, N.A.; Bullen, J.A. Receiver operating characteristic (ROC) curves: Review of methods with applications in diagnostic medicine. *Phys. Med. Biol.* **2018**, *63*, 07TR01. [CrossRef]
65. Cai, J.; Luo, J.; Wang, S.; Yang, S. Feature selection in machine learning: A new perspective. *Neurocomputing* **2018**, *300*, 70–79. [CrossRef]
66. Mayberg, M.; Reintjes, S.; Patel, A.; Moloney, K.; Mercado, J.; Carlson, A.; Broyles, F. Dynamics of postoperative serum cortisol after transsphenoidal surgery for Cushing's disease: Implications for immediate reoperation and remission. *J. Neurosurg.* **2017**, *129*, 1268–1277. [CrossRef] [PubMed]
67. Yadan, Z.; Jian, W.; Yifu, L.; Haiying, L.; Jie, L.; Hairui, L. Solving the inverse problem based on UPEMD for electrocardiographic imaging. *Biomed. Signal Processing Control* **2022**, *76*, 103665. [CrossRef]
68. Bashiri, H.; Houwing, D.J.; Homberg, J.R.; Salari, A.A. The combination of fluoxetine and environmental enrichment reduces postpartum stress-related behaviors through the oxytocinergic system and HPA axis in mice. *Sci. Rep.* **2021**, *11*, 8518. [CrossRef] [PubMed]
69. Del Toro-Barbosa, M.; Hurtado-Romero, A.; Garcia-Amezquita, L.E.; García-Cayuela, T. Psychobiotics: Mechanisms of action, evaluation methods and effectiveness in applications with food products. *Nutrients* **2020**, *12*, 3896. [CrossRef] [PubMed]
70. Gevaerd, A.; Watanabe, E.Y.; Belli, C.; Marcolino-Junior, L.H.; Bergamini, M.F. A complete lab-made point of care device for non-immunological electrochemical determination of cortisol levels in salivary samples. *Sens. Actuators B Chem.* **2021**, *332*, 129532. [CrossRef]
71. Remer, T.; Maser, G.C.; Wudy, S.A. Glucocorticoid measurements in health and disease-metabolic implications and the potential of 24-h urine analyses. *Mini Rev. Med. Chem.* **2008**, *8*, 153–170. [CrossRef] [PubMed]
72. Liu, R.; Ye, X.; Cui, T. Recent progress of biomarker detection sensors. *Research* **2020**, *2020*, 7949037. [CrossRef]
73. Willi, J.; Süss, H.; Grub, J.; Ehlert, U. Biopsychosocial predictors of depressive symptoms in the perimenopause—Findings from the Swiss Perimenopause Study. *Menopause* **2021**, *28*, 247–254. [CrossRef]

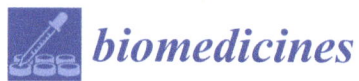 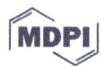

Review

Biomarkers of Neurodegeneration in Post-Traumatic Stress Disorder: An Integrative Review

Ravi Philip Rajkumar

Department of Psychiatry, Jawaharlal Institute of Postgraduate Medical Education and Research (JIPMER), Puducherry 605006, India; jd0422@jipmer.ac.in; Tel.: +91-413-229-6280

Abstract: Post-Traumatic Stress Disorder (PTSD) is a chronic psychiatric disorder that occurs following exposure to traumatic events. Recent evidence suggests that PTSD may be a risk factor for the development of subsequent neurodegenerative disorders, including Alzheimer's dementia and Parkinson's disease. Identification of biomarkers known to be associated with neurodegeneration in patients with PTSD would shed light on the pathophysiological mechanisms linking these disorders and would also help in the development of preventive strategies for neurodegenerative disorders in PTSD. With this background, the PubMed and Scopus databases were searched for studies designed to identify biomarkers that could be associated with an increased risk of neurodegenerative disorders in patients with PTSD. Out of a total of 342 citations retrieved, 29 studies were identified for inclusion in the review. The results of these studies suggest that biomarkers such as cerebral cortical thinning, disrupted white matter integrity, specific genetic polymorphisms, immune-inflammatory alterations, vitamin D deficiency, metabolic syndrome, and objectively documented parasomnias are significantly associated with PTSD and may predict an increased risk of subsequent neurodegenerative disorders. The biological mechanisms underlying these changes, and the interactions between them, are also explored. Though requiring replication, these findings highlight a number of biological pathways that plausibly link PTSD with neurodegenerative disorders and suggest potentially valuable avenues for prevention and early intervention.

Keywords: post-traumatic stress disorder; dementia; Parkinson's disease; β-amyloid; inflammation; hippocampus; white matter integrity; genetics

Citation: Rajkumar, R.P. Biomarkers of Neurodegeneration in Post-Traumatic Stress Disorder: An Integrative Review. *Biomedicines* **2023**, *11*, 1465. https://doi.org/10.3390/biomedicines11051465

Academic Editor: Simone Battaglia

Received: 10 April 2023
Revised: 11 May 2023
Accepted: 15 May 2023
Published: 17 May 2023

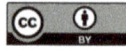

Copyright: © 2023 by the author. Licensee MDPI, Basel, Switzerland. This article is an open access article distributed under the terms and conditions of the Creative Commons Attribution (CC BY) license (https://creativecommons.org/licenses/by/4.0/).

1. Introduction

Post-Traumatic Stress Disorder (PTSD) is a chronic mental illness characterized by symptoms of increased vigilance and arousal, intrusive re-experiencing, avoidance behavior, and changes in effect and cognition lasting more than a month and following direct or indirect exposure to a traumatic stressor. Such stressors typically involve a risk of death, significant injury, or sexual violence [1,2]. It is estimated that PTSD affects around 5–10% of the world's population, with an approximate 2:1 female-to-male ratio [3]. In countries and regions characterized by high levels of traumatic stress or civil unrest, the prevalence of PTSD is estimated to be much higher, affecting over 25% of the population [4]. Though the course of PTSD is heterogeneous, it tends to be chronic and persistent in many individuals. Standard treatments for PTSD include both psychological approaches, such as cognitive and group therapy, and pharmacological agents, such as selective serotonin reuptake inhibitors. However, a substantial proportion of patients do not respond fully to these treatments: short-term response rates have been estimated to be around 35–40% for psychotherapies [5] and 50–60% for pharmacotherapies [6]. A meta-analysis of remission rates for PTSD over a period of three or more years found that only 44% of patients could be considered "non-cases"; in other words, more than half remained symptomatic over this period [7]. PTSD is associated with significant levels of disability [8], impaired quality of life [9], high levels of comorbidity with psychiatric and substance use disorders [10,11], increased rates of several chronic medical illnesses [12,13], and an increased risk of suicide [14].

The processes involved in the pathogenesis of PTSD are complex, involving interactions between genetic vulnerability, exposure to stress or trauma in early life, and the nature and severity of the specific trauma exposure triggering the disorder [15–20]. These interactions may, in turn, be moderated by protective factors, which can be either individual or social [21]. Neuroimaging studies have identified several structural and functional alterations in the brains of individuals with PTSD, involving connections between cortical and limbic regions associated with cognition and emotion [22]. PTSD has also been associated with significant alterations in several key biochemical processes, particularly those related to hypothalamic–pituitary–adrenal (HPA) axis functioning, immune regulation, systemic inflammation, and oxidative stress [23–25]. As these changes may be associated with an increased risk of certain medical conditions, some researchers have labeled PTSD a systemic disorder [26]. More recent research has highlighted the fundamental cellular and electrophysiological changes associated with these disruptions [27–31], their behavioral correlates [32,33], and the mechanisms through which they influence the links between neural, immune, endocrine, and cardiovascular functioning [34]. This research has also identified novel pharmacological strategies for the prevention and management of PTSD, which may offer significant advantages over existing treatment approaches [35,36].

In addition to the comorbidities and complications listed above, several recent studies have suggested that PTSD may be a risk factor for the development of subsequent neurodegenerative disorders and, more specifically, for dementia. This association was initially documented in military veterans with a history of combat-related trauma [37]. It was subsequently found that PTSD was associated with an approximately 1.5 to 2-fold increase in the risk of dementia in both military and civilian populations [38], and this finding has been confirmed in large cohort studies involving both these groups [39,40]. Some researchers have also reported a longitudinal association between PTSD and the risk of Parkinson's disease in both civilian and military populations [41,42]. These associations have led to speculations about the mechanisms linking PTSD with neurodegeneration, such as accelerated aging [43], increased systemic inflammation [44], and stress-related neurotoxicity affecting key brain regions [45]. However, other authors have emphasized the need for caution in assuming a direct causal link between PTSD and neurodegenerative disorders. These authors have pointed out a possible bi-directional relationship between PTSD and dementia [46] and the need to distinguish between correlation and causation, particularly in the presence of confounding factors [47].

In this context, the identification of specific biological markers known to be associated with neurodegeneration in patients with PTSD would be of significant value. Such markers would allow researchers to confirm the hypothesis of a causal relationship between PTSD and neurodegeneration, to identify the specific mechanisms mediating this association, and to develop preventive or early intervention strategies for patients who are in the pre-symptomatic or prodromal phase of neurodegeneration [48]. The aims of the current review are:

(a) to summarize the existing research on biological markers associated with neurodegenerative disorders in individuals suffering from PTSD;
(b) to critically examine the contributions of possible confounding factors;
(c) to synthesize this information in a manner that would be useful to future researchers in this field.

2. Study Selection and Search Strategy

The current review was a scoping review of the existing research on biological markers associated with neurodegeneration in patients with a diagnosis of PTSD. For the purpose of this review, the definition of "biomarker" provided by the United States Food and Drug Administration-National Institutes of Health (FDA-NIH) Biomarker Working Group was used: "A defined characteristic that is measured as an indicator of normal biological processes, pathogenic processes or responses to an exposure or intervention". Biomarkers "can be derived from molecular, histologic, radiographic, or physiologic characteristics" and are objective in nature, as opposed to clinical outcomes obtained through interviews or external observations of patients [49]. Given the heterogeneity of the available literature and the integrative nature of this review, all potential biomarkers were considered for inclusion. As a result, a formal systematic review or meta-analysis was not undertaken. Instead, a scoping review methodology was adopted in accordance with the PRISMA-ScR guidelines [50].

The criteria used to select studies for inclusion in this review were as follows:
- The study population should consist of patients with a diagnosis of PTSD, established using standard diagnostic criteria or rating scales, with or without a control or comparator group;
- Study participants should not currently fulfill the criteria for dementia or other neurodegenerative disorders;
- The study should measure one or more biomarkers that are actually or potentially linked to neurodegeneration, and this should be stated by the authors in the study methodology or protocol;
- Only human studies were included to ensure the specificity of any identified biomarkers for human subjects with PTSD;
- Only original research was included.

The PubMed and Scopus literature databases were searched using the key words "post-traumatic stress disorder" (OR its variants "post-traumatic stress disorder" and "PTSD") AND either "neurodegeneration" (OR its variant "neurodegenerative") OR "dementia" OR "Alzheimer's disease (OR its variant "Alzheimer's dementia") OR "Parkinson's disease", AND various terms used to identify studies of biological markers: the broad terms "biological marker" and "biomarker" (OR their plural forms), OR "genetic" (OR variants) OR "immune" (OR variants) OR "inflammation" (OR variants) OR "amyloid" OR "tau protein" OR "endocrine" (OR variants such as "neuroendocrine") OR "imaging" OR "MRI" OR "fMRI" OR "PET" OR "SPECT" OR "DTI" (OR their expansions, such as "magnetic resonance imaging" OR "positron emission tomography"). A complete list of the search strings used for the PubMed search, along with numerical results for the results retrieved, has been uploaded in Supplementary Table S1.

Through this process, a total of 342 citations were retrieved. After the removal of duplicate citations, the titles and abstracts of 252 citations were screened. Publication types other than original research in humans (n = 164) were excluded at this stage. In the next stage of the literature search, the full texts of the remaining 88 papers were checked to see if they fulfilled the review inclusion criteria. At this stage, 60 papers were excluded either because they did not measure biomarkers or because they did not include study participants with PTSD. Finally, the reference lists of the remaining 28 papers were searched for relevant research that might have been missed, and one further study was identified by this method. The current review thus covered a total of twenty-nine original studies of potential biomarkers of neurodegeneration in subjects diagnosed with PTSD [51–79].

The above process is depicted graphically in Figure 1.

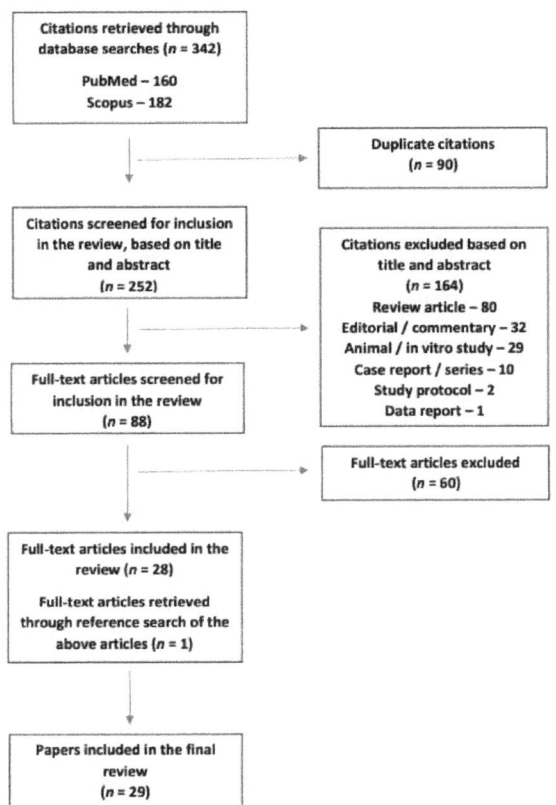

Figure 1. Flow diagram of the review process, based on PRISMA-ScR guidelines.

3. Characteristics of the Included Studies

A complete list of the studies included in this review is provided in Table 1. From a preliminary review of each study's methodology, it was found that they fell into five broad categories: brain imaging studies ($n = 16$), genetic, epigenetic, and gene expression studies ($n = 8$), biochemical marker studies ($n = 9$), immune-inflammatory marker studies ($n = 4$) and sleep-related marker studies ($n = 5$). The sum of these numbers is greater than 29 because twelve studies used more than one modality or examined the interaction between two or more biomarkers. Of the 29 studies included, 18 were conducted on military veterans and 11 on civilians; 4 of the civilian studies involved World Trade Center responders. Of the 18 studies involving military personnel, 8 studies included subjects with a history of mild to moderate traumatic brain injury (TBI) but with no diagnosis of dementia or other marked cognitive impairment related to their injury. All the studies that fulfilled the inclusion criteria for this review were from high-income countries in North America or Europe. Except for one study published in 2001, all the papers included in this review were published between 2014 and 2023.

Table 1. Details of all studies included in the current review.

Scheme	Modality	Study Population	Design	Biomarker(s) Studied	Results
		Brain imaging studies			
Chao et al., 2014 [51]	Structural MRI	Military veterans with PTSD as per DSM-IV criteria (n = 55)	Cross-sectional; association	Hippocampal volume as test region; caudate nucleus volume as a control region	Duration of PTSD significantly and negatively correlated with right hippocampal volume, even after adjusting for confounders. No association between PTSD duration and left hippocampal or caudate volumes.
Mueller et al., 2015 [52]	Structural MRI	Military veterans with (n = 40) and without (n = 45) significant PTSD symptoms as measured using CAPS	Cross-sectional; case-control	Cortical and hippocampal volumes; structural connectivity of the prefrontal-limbic network	PTSD significantly associated with reduced rostral cingulate and insular cortical thickness but no hippocampal volume loss. Evidence of reduced prefrontal-limbic structural connectivity in PTSD.
Main et al., 2017 [53]	DTI	Military veterans (n = 109); 71.6% PTSD as per DSM-IV criteria; 57.8% mild TBI; 9.2% moderate TBI	Cross-sectional; association	FA and diffusivity of white matter fiber tracts	Altered parameters in left cingulum and inferior frontal-occipital fasciculus and right anterior thalamic tract specifically associated with TBI. Altered white matter parameters in right cingulum and inferior longitudinal fasciculus and left anterior thalamic radiation associated with PTSD.
Basavaraju et al., 2021 [54]	Structural MRI	Older adults (age $\geq$ 50 years) with a history of trauma exposure with (n = 55) and without (n = 36) PTSD	Cross-sectional; case-control	Cortical volume	Significant reduction of right parahippocampal cortical volume, but not other cortical regions, in PTSD.
Olivé et al., 2021 [55]	Functional MRI	Patients with PTSD (n = 103; 38 with dissociative subtype of PTSD); healthy controls (n = 46)	Cross-sectional; case-control	Variability of BOLD signal in basal forebrain regions	Increased BOLD signal variability in extended amygdala and nucleus accumbens in dissociative PTSD compared to both PTSD and controls.
Brown et al., 2022 [56]	Structural MRI	Military veterans (n = 254); 59.8% PTSD as per DSM-IV-TR criteria; 34.4% severe PTSD; (CAPS $\geq$ 60); 45.7% mild TBI	Longitudinal (2-year follow-up) with group comparisons (severe vs. non-severe PTSD)	Changes in cortical thickness, area, and volume	Severe PTSD associated with reduced cortical thickness, area, and volume, especially in frontal regions. More marked reductions in severe PTSD with mild TBI.

Table 1. Cont.

Scheme	Modality	Study Population	Design	Biomarker(s) Studied	Results
Brain imaging studies					
Kritikos et al., 2022 [57]	DTI	World Trade Center responders (n = 99); 48.4% cognitive impairment not amounting to dementia; 47.5% PTSD as per DSM-IV criteria	Cross-sectional; association	Whole-brain FA of white matter tracts	Reduced FA in fornix, cingulum, forceps minor, and right uncinate fasciculus in subjects with PTSD and cognitive impairment. Reduced FA in superior thalamic radiation and cerebellum in PTSD regardless of cognitive impairment.
Genetic, epigenetic, and gene expression studies					
Kuan et al., 2019 [58]	Peripheral blood transcriptome	World Trade Center responders with (n = 20) and without (n = 19) PTSD as per DSM-IV criteria	Cross-sectional; case-control	Transcriptome-wide analysis of gene expression in four peripheral blood immune cell subtypes	*FKBP5* and *PI4KAP1* upregulated across all cell types in PTSD. *REST* and *SEPT4* upregulated in monocytes in PTSD.
Sragovich et al., 2021 [59]	Somatic mutation	Military veterans with (n = 27) and without (n = 55) PTSD as per DSM-IV criteria	Cross-sectional; case-control	Rates of somatic mutations based on peripheral blood samples	Increased number of mutations related to cytoskeletal genes and inflammation in PTSD.
Wolf et al., 2021 [60]	Post-mortem gene expression	Post-mortem cortical brain tissue from military veterans (n = 97); 43.3% PTSD as per DSM-5 criteria; 30.9% alcohol use disorder	Post-mortem; association	DNA methylation-based estimates of cellular age in relation to chronological age (DNAm age residuals); gene expression in cortical tissue.	Specific interaction effects with age residuals identified for four genes (*SNORA73B*, *COL6A3*, *GCNT1*, and *GPRIN3*) specific to PTSD.
Biochemical marker studies					
Clouston et al., 2019 [61]	Plasma assay	World Trade Center responders with (n = 17) and without (n = 17) probable PTSD as per PCL-17	Cross-sectional; case-control	Plasma total amyloid-beta, amyloid-beta 42/40 ratio, total tau, and NfL	PTSD associated with lower plasma amyloid-beta and higher amyloid-beta 42/40 ratio.
Cimino et al., 2022 [62]	Serum assay	Adults, age ≥ 50, with a history of trauma exposure with (n = 44) and without (n = 26) subsequent PTSD as per DSM-5 criteria	Cross-sectional; case-control	Serum amyloid-beta 42 and 40 levels and ratio; serum total tau	No significant differences in amyloid-beta levels, ratios, or total tau levels between groups.
Immune-inflammatory marker studies					
Zhang et al., 2022 [63]	Serum assay	Residents living near the World Trade Center; 43.2% probable PTSD as per PCL; 50.3% dust cloud exposure	Cross-sectional; association	Serum CRP	Total CRP level and "high" CRP (>3 mg/L) both associated with PTSD. PCL score was a significant predictor of serum CRP.

Table 1. Cont.

Scheme	Modality	Study Population	Design	Biomarker(s) Studied	Results
Sleep-related marker studies					
Elliott et al., 2018 [64]	Polysomnography, self-report	Military veterans with a history of TBI ($n = 130$); 37.7% PTSD as per DSM-5 criteria	Cross-sectional; association	Sleep EEG/EMG; self-reported sleep disturbance; sensory (noise and light) sensitivity	Sleep disturbance and sensory sensitivity associated with PTSD in veterans with TBI.
Elliott et al., 2020 [65]	Polysomnography	Military veterans ($n = 394$); 28.6% probable PTSD as per PCL-5; 19.2% mild TBI	Cross-sectional; association	RSBD and other parasomnias	Increased rates of RSBD both in veterans with mild TBI and PTSD and in those with PTSD alone.
Feemster et al., 2022 [66]	Polysomnography	Patients with PTSD ($n = 36$), idiopathic RSBD ($n = 18$), and healthy controls ($n = 51$)	Cross-sectional; case-control	REM sleep with atonia	Higher REM sleep with atonia associated with PTSD independent of dream enactment behavior.
Liu et al., 2023 [67]	Self-report	Adults from fifteen countries ($n = 21,870$) during the COVID-19 pandemic; 3% COVID-19 positive; PTSD symptoms assessed using abbreviated PCL	Cross-sectional; association	Dream enactment behavior, weekly and lifetime	Screening positive for PTSD associated with a 1.2 to 1.4-fold increase in dream enactment behavior.
Multi-modality studies					
Baker et al., 2001 [68]	Plasma and CSF assays	Combat veterans ($n = 11$) with PTSD as per DSM-IV criteria; matched healthy controls ($n = 8$)	Cross-sectional; case-control	CSF levels of CRH, IL-6, norepinephrine; plasma levels of IL-6, ACTH, cortisol and norepinephrine	Increased CSF IL-6 in PTSD. Positive correlation between plasma IL-6 and norepinephrine in PTSD, but not in controls.
Mohlenhoff et al., 2014 [69]	Self-report (sleep); structural MRI (brain imaging)	Military veterans ($n = 136$); 7% PTSD as per DSM-IV criteria	Cross-sectional; association	Self-reported sleep disturbance; hippocampal volume	No association between PTSD and hippocampal volume. Possible association between sleep disturbance and left hippocampal volume.
Miller et al., 2015 [70]	Genetic association; structural MRI	Military veterans ($n = 146$); PTSD symptoms measured as a continuous variable using CAPS	Cross-sectional; interaction	Oxidative stress-related genes (ALOX12 and ALOX15); prefrontal cortex thickness	PTSD symptom severity negatively correlated with right, but not left, prefrontal volume. Two SNPs of ALOX12 moderated association between PTSD and right prefrontal volume.
O'Donovan et al., 2015 [71]	Serum assays; structural MRI	Military veterans with ($n = 73$) and without ($n = 132$) PTSD as per DSM-IV criteria	Cross-sectional; interaction	Serum IL-6 and sTNF-RII; hippocampal volume	sTNF-RII level negatively correlated with hippocampal volume regardless of PTSD diagnosis. PTSD severity associated with increased sTNF-RII and decreased IL-6.

Table 1. Cont.

Scheme	Modality	Study Population	Design	Biomarker(s) Studied	Results
		Multi-modality studies			
Wolf et al., 2016 [72]	Plasma assays; structural MRI	Military veterans (n = 346); 77.2% PTSD as per DSM-IV criteria	Cross-sectional; interaction	Prevalence of metabolic syndrome as per NCEP-ATP III criteria; cortical thickness	Metabolic syndrome and its criteria more common in veterans with PTSD. Metabolic syndrome found to significantly mediate the association between PTSD and reduced cortical volume in precuneus, temporal cortex, rostral anterior cingulate cortex, and postcentral gyrus.
Hayes et al., 2017 [73]	Polygenic risk score; structural MRI	Military veterans (n = 160); 70% PTSD as per DSM-IV criteria; 65.6% mild TBI	Cross-sectional; interaction	Polygenic risk score for Alzheimer's disease; cortical thickness	No significant association between cortical thickness and PTSD, either alone or in association with TBI or polygenic risk score.
Hayes et al., 2018 [74]	Genetic association; structural and functional MRI	Military veterans (n = 165); 66.7% mild TBI; 43% PTSD as per DSM-IV-TR criteria	Cross-sectional; interaction	BDNF genotype (9 SNPs); hippocampal volume; default mode network functional connectivity	No direct effect of PTSD on right or left hippocampal volume. TBI associated with reduced hippocampal volumes. Significant interaction between BDNF rs1157659 and TBI on hippocampal volume. No BDNF by PTSD interaction.
Kang et al., 2020 [75]	Peripheral blood and urine assays; structural MRI	Military veterans with (n = 102) and without (n = 113) PTSD as per DSM-IV criteria	Cross-sectional; interaction	Leukocyte telomere length; urinary catecholamines; amygdala volume	Shorter telomere length and increased amygdala volume associated with PTSD only in veterans exposed to high levels of trauma. Telomere shortening associated with increased urinary norepinephrine.
Terock et al., 2020 [76]	Genetic association; serum assay	1653 adults with a history of trauma exposure; 3.8% PTSD as per DSM-IV criteria	Cross-sectional; interaction	Serum total vitamin D; two specific SNPs of the GC gene	Lower serum vitamin D associated with PTSD. Vitamin D deficiency more frequent in those with PTSD. CC genotype of rs4588 associated with lower risk of PTSD. T allele of rs7041 associated with increased risk of PTSD.
Guedes et al., 2021 [77]	Extracellular vesicle assay	Military veterans (n = 144); 31.3% PTSD as per PCL-5 screening; 80.6% mild TBI	Cross-sectional; association	Extracellular vesicle levels of 798 miRNAs; extracellular vesicle and plasma levels of NfL, amyloid-beta 42 and 40, tau, IL-10, IL-6, TNF-α, and VEGF	Elevated extracellular vesicle levels of NfL in patients with mTBI and PTSD. Significant association between miR-139-5p and PTSD symptom severity.

Table 1. Cont.

Scheme	Modality	Study Population	Design	Biomarker(s) Studied	Results
		Multi-modality studies			
Weiner et al., 2022 [78]	CSF assay; structural MRI; PET	Military veterans (n = 289); 60.6% PTSD as per DSM-IV criteria; 47.8% moderate to severe TBI	Longitudinal (5-year follow-up) with group comparisons	CSF amyloid-beta 42, total tau, and p-tau181; PET measures of amyloid-beta and tau; cortical, hippocampal, and amygdala volume	No significant association of PTSD with biochemical or imaging markers, either cross-sectionally or at follow-up
Kritikos et al., 2023 [79]	Plasma assay; structural MRI	World Trade Center responders (n = 1173); 11.2% probable PTSD as per PCL-C; 16.4% mild cognitive impairment; 4.3% possible dementia	Cross-sectional; interaction	Plasma amyloid-beta 40/42 ratio, p-tau 181, NfL; hippocampal volume (only in 75 participants)	Significant intercorrelation between amyloid-beta 40/42, p-tau181, and NfL. PTSD associated with elevated amyloid-beta 40/42 ratio. Amyloid-beta 40/42 and p-tau 181 associated with reduced hippocampal volume.

Note: Italics indicate gene names as per standard naming conventions. Abbreviations: ACTH, adrenocorticotrophic hormone; *ALOX12*, arachidonate 12-lipoxygenase gene; *ALOX15*, arachidonate 15-lipoxygenase gene; *BDNF*, brain-derived neurotrophic factor gene; BOLD, blood oxygen-level dependent; CAPS, Clinician-Administered PTSD Scale; *COL6A3*, collagen alpha-3 gene; CRH; corticotrophin-releasing hormone; CRP, C-reactive protein; CSF, cerebrospinal fluid; DSM, Diagnostic and Statistical Manual of Mental Disorders; DTI, diffusion tensor imaging; EEG, electroencephalogram; EMG; electromyogram; FA, fractional anisotropy; *FKBP5*, FK506 binding protein gene; GC, vitamin D-binding protein gene; *GCNT1*, glucosaminyl (N-acetyl) transferase 1 gene; *GPRIN3*, GPRIN family member 3 gene; IL, interleukin; miRNA, microRNA; MRI, magnetic resonance imaging; NCEP-ATP III, National Cholesterol Education Program—Adult Treatment Panel III; NfL, neurofilament light; PET, positron emission tomography; PCL, Post-traumatic Disorder Checklist; *PI4KAP1*, phosphatidylinositol 4-kinase alpha pseudogene 1; PTSD, post-traumatic stress disorder; REM, rapid-eye movement sleep; *REST*, RE1-silencing transcription factor gene; RSBD, REM sleep behaviour disorder; *SEPT4*, septin 4 gene; *SNORA73B*, small nucleolar RNA, H/ACA box 73B gene; SNP, single nucleotide polymorphism; TBI, traumatic brain injury; TNF, tumor necrosis factor; VEGF, vascular endothelial growth factor.

4. Brain Imaging Studies

Both structural and functional imaging have been used to identify potential markers of neurodegeneration in subjects with PTSD. Structurally, PTSD has been associated with reduced volumes of specific cortical brain regions, including the rostral anterior cingulate cortex, insula, and right parahippocampal cortex [52,54]. Severe PTSD has been associated with a general reduction in overall cortical thickness, particularly in frontal regions [56] and, more specifically, in the right frontal lobe [70]. A longer duration of PTSD has been associated with reduced right hippocampal volume [51]. However, negative findings regarding an association between PTSD and hippocampal volume have also been reported by several researchers [52,69,74]. An overall reduction in structural gray matter connectivity between the prefrontal cortex and amygdala has also been observed in PTSD [52]. In contrast to these findings of volume loss, a single study has reported an increased amygdalar volume in veterans with PTSD, but only in those with a history of exposure to severe trauma [75].

Two studies have examined changes in white matter tract integrity in relation to PTSD. The first, which was conducted in veterans, found evidence of altered fractional anisotropy (FA) and diffusivity in the right cingulum, right inferior longitudinal fasciculus, and left anterior thalamic radiation; these changes were distinct from those associated with traumatic brain injury in the study sample [53]. The second, which involved civilians with trauma exposure related to the World Trade Center (WTC) terrorist attack, found reduced FA in the superior thalamic radiations and cerebellum in those with PTSD; in the subgroup of subjects with PTSD and mild cognitive impairment, further reductions in FA were reported in several other regions, including the fornix and right uncinate fasciculus [57]. Overall, structural imaging studies suggest that PTSD is associated with structural brain changes affecting cortical and limbic regions and white matter tracts, with some evidence of a right-sided predominance.

There are relatively few studies of functional imaging changes putatively linked to neurodegeneration in PTSD. In a study of civilians, increased variability of the BOLD signal, a measure of regional brain activity, was observed in patients with the dissociative subtype of PTSD compared to both other patients with PTSD and healthy controls [55]. A study of veterans did not report any specific functional MRI changes in patients with PTSD; however, two-thirds of the subjects also had a history of TBI [74]. A single study used positron emission tomography (PET) to estimate levels of amyloid beta and tau protein in veterans over a period of five years but did not find any significant association between PTSD and changes in these imaging markers [78].

5. Genetic, Epigenetic, and Gene Expression-Related Markers

Three association studies examined the associations between functional polymorphisms of specific genes and possible neurodegeneration related to PTSD. The first study examined the effects of functional polymorphisms of the *ALOX12* and *ALOX15* genes, which are related to oxidative stress, on PTSD-related reductions in brain volume. In this study, two specific single nucleotide polymorphisms (SNPs) of *ALOX12*—rs1042357 and rs10852889—appeared to mediate the association between PTSD symptom severity and reductions in right prefrontal cortical thickness [70]. The second study evaluated nine SNPs of the *BDNF* gene, a key regulator of neural plasticity, in relation to hippocampal volume changes in veterans with mild TBI and/or PTSD. In this study, a single SNP (rs1157659) interacted with TBI to reduce hippocampal volume; however, there was neither a direct effect of PTSD nor a genotype x PTSD effect on this outcome [74]. The third study examined the effects of two SNPs of the vitamin D-binding protein (*GC*) gene. In this study, PTSD was associated with lower serum vitamin D levels; of the two SNPs studied, homozygotes for the C allele of rs4588 were at a lower risk of PTSD, while carriers of the T allele of rs7041 were at a higher risk of this disorder [76].

In a study involving a small number of WTC responders with or without PTSD, peripheral blood gene expression was examined in four white cell subtypes. It was found that the expression of *FKBP5*, involved in hypothalamic-pituitary-axis functioning and the stress response, as well as the pseudogene *PI4KAP1*, were increased in all cell types in PTSD. Two further genes, *REST* and *SEPT4*, were upregulated in the monocytes of individuals with PTSD [58]. In a study of military veterans, an increased number of somatic mutations were observed in veterans with a diagnosis of PTSD. These mutations appeared to be linked to cytoskeletal and inflammation-related genes [59]. Finally, a post-mortem study of gene expression in the brains of veterans found four genes (*SNORA73B*, *COL6A3*, *GCNT1*, and *GPRIN3*) whose expression was associated with a lifetime diagnosis of PTSD [60].

To test for the possibility of functional interactions between the proteins encoded by these genes, all the above genes of interest were entered into the STRING database [80]. Two genes (*SNORA73B* and *PI4KAP1*) were excluded by the database as they did not encode any known functional product. Of the remaining nine genes analyzed, possible functional interactions were identified between three: *FKBP5*, *BDNF*, and *REST*. This is illustrated in Figure 2 below.

A single study examined the possible association between microRNAs (miRNAs) and PTSD. In this study, levels of 798 miRNAs were assessed. Of these, only miR-139-5p was significantly associated with PTSD symptom severity [77]. This particular miRNA is of significance as its expression has been found to differ significantly between patients with Alzheimer's disease and healthy controls [81].

In addition to these results, a single study examined the association between PTSD and telomere length, a putative marker of cellular aging, in military personnel. In this study, PTSD was associated with a shortened telomere length only in veterans with a history of exposure to severe trauma; this finding was also associated with an increased volume of the amygdala and increased urinary norepinephrine [75].

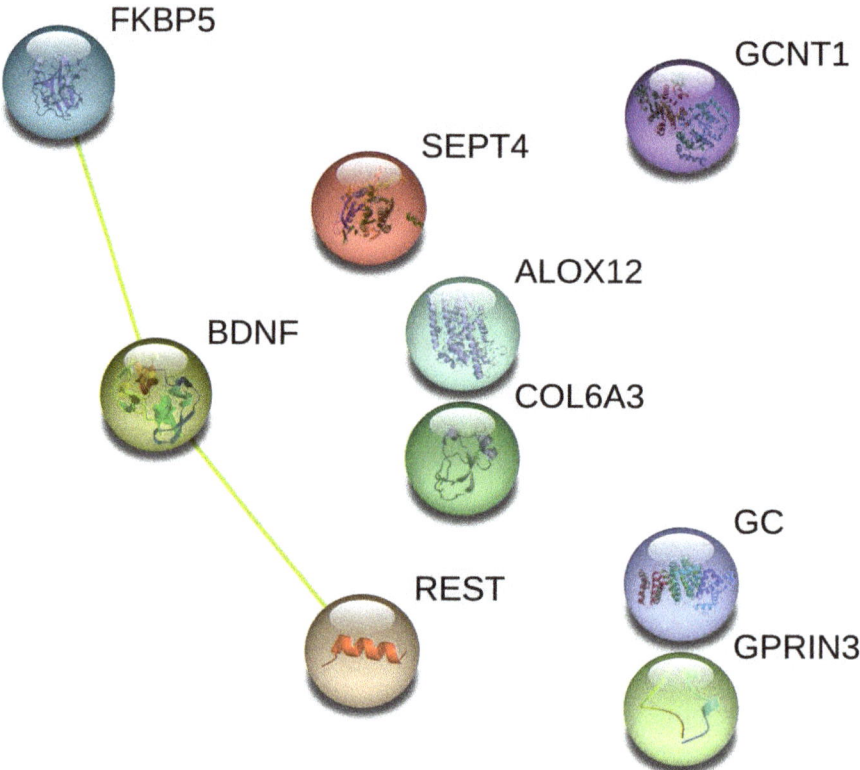

Figure 2. Protein–protein interactions for the products of genes linked to PTSD and neurodegeneration.

6. Biochemical Marker Studies

The biomarkers most frequently studied in this context are those putatively associated with dementia, such as levels of amyloid-beta (Aβ) or tau protein. In a study involving 34 WTC responders, PTSD was associated with both lower plasma Aβ and a lower Aβ 42/40 ratio [61], while a larger study (n = 1173) involving WTC responders also found a lower Aβ 42/40 ratio in those with PTSD, as well as an association between this parameter and hippocampal volume reduction. However, in a study of trauma-exposed adults with and without PTSD, no significant differences in Aβ or tau levels were observed between groups [62]. An assay of extracellular vesicle levels of Aβ and tau in military veterans found no association between these markers and a diagnosis of PTSD [77]. A similar negative association between Aβ and tau levels and PTSD was observed in the cerebrospinal fluid of veterans, though 60% of these subjects also had a history of TBI [78]. Neurofilament light (NfL), a marker of neural axonal damage, was found to be elevated in patients with a history of PTSD and mild TBI in a single study [77]. However, two other studies did not observe a significant association between PTSD and NfL levels [61,79].

Among other biochemical markers possibly related to neurodegeneration, PTSD has been associated with reduced serum total vitamin D [76] and an increased risk of a metabolic syndrome characterized by elevated plasma glucose and dyslipidemia [75]. In the latter study, metabolic syndrome appeared to mediate the association between a diagnosis of PTSD and reduced volumes of specific regions of the frontal, temporal, and parietal cortices [75].

7. Immune and Inflammatory Marker Studies

Four studies have examined the relationship between PTSD and elevated levels of immune or inflammatory markers linked to neurodegeneration. In the earliest study in this population, CSF and plasma levels of interleukin-6 (IL-6) were examined in relation to levels of norepinephrine and adrenocortical hormones. CSF IL-6 was significantly higher in veterans with PTSD than in controls, and plasma IL-6 was positively correlated with norepinephrine only in PTSD cases [68]. In a study of individuals living near the WTC at the time of the 2001 attack, 43.2% fulfilled the criteria for PTSD. These individuals had significantly elevated levels of C-reactive protein (CRP), and CRP levels were positively correlated with PTSD symptom severity [63]. In contrast, two studies of military veterans yielded divergent results. In the first, PTSD severity was negatively correlated with IL-6 levels but positively associated with levels of soluble tumor necrosis factor-alpha receptor (sTNF-RII). sTNF-RII levels were negatively correlated with hippocampal volume, but this association was independent of PTSD diagnostic status [71]. In the second, no significant association was observed between PTSD and plasma levels of IL-10, IL-6, or TNF-α.

8. Sleep-Related Studies

Sleep-related behavioral and electrophysiological markers associated with neurodegeneration have been evaluated in relation to PTSD in five studies. Three of these involved military veterans; among these studies, two also included subjects with TBI. The first of these found an association between reduced sleep and reduced left hippocampal volume, but this was not related to a PTSD diagnosis [69]. The second, in which all participants had a history of mild TBI, found that PTSD was associated with self-reported sleep disturbances [64]. The third, which included only some subjects with TBI, found a significant association between PTSD and REM sleep behavior disorder (RSBD), considered a forerunner of neurodegeneration, both in subjects with and without TBI [65].

A polysomnographic study comparing patients with PTSD to those with idiopathic RSBD and healthy controls found a higher rate of REM sleep with atonia, as measured by electromyography, in those with PTSD [66]. A larger study based on self-report data, including over 20,000 adults in the context of the COVID-19 pandemic, found a significant positive association between self-reported PTSD symptoms and dream enactment behavior, which is a symptom of RSBD [67].

9. Integration of Existing Results on Biomarkers of Neurodegeneration in PTSD

A list of possible biomarkers associated with neurodegeneration in patients with PTSD, based on the existing literature, is provided in Table 2 below.

From the above results, it can be observed that even after discarding negative results, there are several potential biological markers of neurodegeneration in post-traumatic stress disorder. Neuroimaging studies have found that PTSD is associated with evidence of significant volume reductions in cortical regions—particularly in the right hemisphere—as well as reduced white matter integrity. In addition, there is some evidence to suggest that this disorder is associated with impaired grey matter structural connectivity between prefrontal and limbic regions. There is a significant overlap between these findings and those obtained in studies of patients with neurodegenerative disorders, particularly Alzheimer's disease (AD). For example, progressive reductions in cortical thickness, implicating many of the same regions identified in patients with PTSD, have been identified both in patients with early evidence of Alzheimer's pathology [82] and in patients with an established diagnosis of AD [83]. Similarly, disruptions of white matter integrity have also been documented across the spectrum of severity of AD [84,85]. Many of these alterations involve regions that have been identified in studies of individuals with PTSD, such as the fornix, uncinate fasciculus, and inferior longitudinal fasciculus [53,57]. Altered basal forebrain functioning has also been documented in both mild cognitive impairment and AD [86]; this is similar to findings reported in patients with the dissociative subtype of PTSD [55]. Though these associations are by themselves insufficient to establish a causal link, they suggest that PTSD may be associated with structural brain changes that differ from those of AD in degree rather than in kind.

Table 2. Possible biomarkers linking post-traumatic stress disorder and neurodegeneration.

Biomarker Type	Level of Evidence
Brain imaging	
Reduced cortical thickness	++
Reduced volume of specific right cortical regions	++
Reduced white matter tract integrity	++
Reduced structural grey matter connectivity	+
Reduced right hippocampal volume	±
Increased amygdalar volume	?
Increased BOLD variability in the basal forebrain	?
Genetic and epigenetic	
Association between ALOX12 SNPs and reduced right prefrontal volume	+
Association between GC SNPs and PTSD risk	+
Upregulation of FKBP5, REST, SEPT4 in leukocytes	+
miR-139-5p	+
Reduced telomere length	?
Post-mortem expression of COL6A3, GCNT1, GPRIN3 in brain	?
Biochemical	
Reduced serum total vitamin D	+
Increased rate of metabolic syndrome	+
Elevated peripheral NfL	±
Reduced peripheral Aβ 42/40 ratio	±
Immune-inflammatory	
Serum CRP	+
Serum sTNF-RII	+
CSF IL-6	+
Sleep-related	
Increased rates of RSBD or dream enactment behavior	++
Increased REM sleep with atonia	+

Key: ++, positive evidence from more than one study; +, positive evidence from a single study; ±, conflicting results; ?, positive results only in sub-group analyses or results of uncertain significance.

Attempts to establish an association between biochemical markers of AD pathology, such as amyloid-beta and tau, have yielded inconsistent results in patients with PTSD. However, there is some evidence of indirect biochemical links between PTSD and neurodegenerative disorders. First, PTSD has been associated with an increased risk of metabolic syndrome, which is an established risk factor both for vascular dementia [87] and for disease onset and progression in AD [88,89]. Second, PTSD has been associated with low serum vitamin D, as well as with functional polymorphisms of the Gc protein that binds vitamin D and influences its levels. Vitamin D deficiency is associated with a modest but significant increase in the risk of dementia [90], as well as reductions in gray and white matter volumes [91], and there has been recent interest in vitamin D supplementation as a preventive measure against neurocognitive disorders [92]. Though both these findings require replication, they represent plausible pathways that could mediate the association between PTSD and neurodegeneration.

Immune and inflammatory mechanisms have been implicated in the progression of several neurodegenerative disorders, including AD [93], frontotemporal dementia [94], and Parkinson's disease [95]. PTSD has been consistently associated with increases in certain markers of systemic inflammation [24,96], though it is not known to what extent these correlate with central nervous system inflammatory activity. In the current review, these findings were replicated in the context of possible links with neurodegeneration, with results specifically implicating CRP, IL-6, and soluble TNF-α receptor II. Of these three inflammatory markers, CRP has been associated with progression to dementia even after adjustment for confounding factors [97], while IL-6 has been specifically associated with vascular dementia [98].

Among the genetic markers associated with features of neurodegeneration in PTSD in this review, four are of particular interest, and there is evidence linking them to neurodegenerative disorders in three cases. Methylation of *ALOX12* has been associated with carotid artery intimal thickness, which is a risk factor for stroke and vascular dementia [99]. Septin-4, the protein encoded by the *SEPT4* gene, has been identified in the alpha-synuclein-positive cytoplasmic inclusion bodies seen in Parkinson's and related diseases [100]. In a study comparing patients with AD and healthy controls, the expression of miR-139-5p was found to differ significantly between the two groups, suggesting a possible role for this specific microRNA in neurodegeneration [81,101]. Finally, on the basis of animal studies, it has been suggested that stress-induced changes in the methylation of *FKBP5* might contribute to late-life AD [102]. Thus, there are plausible mechanisms linking genetic markers associated with PTSD to specific types of neurodegenerative disorders.

REM sleep behavior disorder (RSBD) has been associated with an increase in the subsequent risk of neurodegenerative disorders, and more specifically of synucleinopathies such as Parkinson's disease and dementia with Lewy bodies [103]. There is consistent evidence of an increase in RSBD, its symptoms, and its electrophysiological correlates in patients with PTSD [104]. Despite the consistency of this association, relatively little is known about the neurobiological mechanisms linking these two disorders and their implications for progression to a subsequent neurodegenerative disorder [105]. It has been suggested by some researchers that RSBD-like phenomena in PTSD have a distinctive pathophysiology characterized by hyperarousal and increased adrenergic activity rather than neurodegeneration [106]. If this hypothesis is correct, then symptoms of RSBD in PTSD may not necessarily increase the subsequent risk of dementia or Parkinson's disease; however, it requires verification through both neurobiological and longitudinal clinical research.

The figure below (Figure 3) shows how these diverse findings can potentially be integrated. Innate genetic vulnerability, as well as epigenetic changes related to early life stressors and other environmental exposures, interact with exposure to one or more traumatic events, leading to the syndrome of PTSD. The biochemical, neurophysiological, and immune-inflammatory changes associated with PTSD can have an adverse impact on brain structure and function either directly or indirectly through atherogenesis and reduced cerebral blood flow. These changes may not be sufficient to lead to neurodegeneration in themselves, but they may interact with or amplify other risk factors, such as an innate genetic vulnerability towards neurodegenerative disorders, traumatic brain injury, or lifestyle factors. The outcomes of this process are likely to be heterogeneous, ranging from no or mild cognitive impairment to the clinical syndromes of AD, vascular dementia, or Parkinson's disease.

A key question that arises in this regard is whether the associations depicted in Figure 3 are of a correlational or a causal nature. In other words, does the syndrome of PTSD itself lead to pathophysiological processes that increase the risk of neurodegeneration, or are both disorders related to an inherent vulnerability or diathesis? This question is difficult to answer based on current evidence. Some authors believe that there is at least provisional evidence of a causal link between PTSD and subsequent neurodegenerative disorders [43,45], while others favor a simple correlation based on shared genetic or environmental risk factors [44,47]. There is some evidence to support the latter view. For example, it has been found that increased systemic inflammation may precede PTSD and predispose to it rather than represent a consequence of this disorder [107]. Longitudinal studies of both civilian and military populations involving measurements of specific biomarkers prior to as well as following exposure to traumatic stress are required to answer this question. However, such studies may be difficult to conduct in the former group.

Another issue that arises in this context is the specificity of the association, whether correlational or causal, between PTSD and neurodegeneration. Is it non-specific in nature, applying to a wide range or spectrum of neurodegenerative disorders, or is it specific to certain conditions, such as AD? Alternately, are there distinct pathways (for example, oxidative stress-induced atherogenesis in vascular dementia or RSBD-like sleep pathologies in Parkinson's disease) that mediate the association between PTSD and distinct types of neurodegenerative disorder? Research in this field is still in an early stage, and it is likely that more information on the specificity and consistency of these associations will be obtained in subsequent decades.

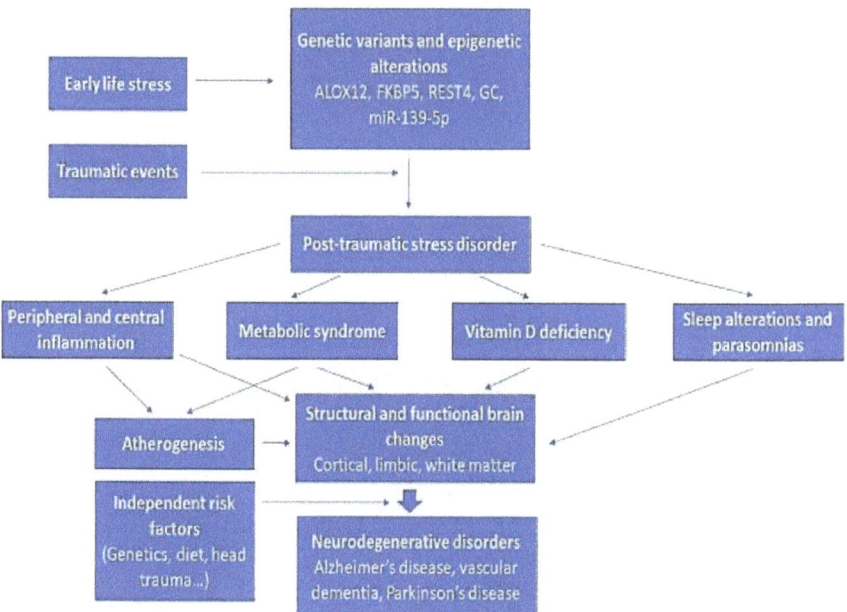

Figure 3. Integration of various risk factors linking post-traumatic stress disorder and neurodegenerative disorders.

10. Limitations of the Existing Data

Despite the promising nature of the leads obtained through the current body of research, certain key limitations of existing studies deserve mention. First, the majority of studies have been conducted in Western countries, and it is not clear to what extent they can be generalized to other countries or cultures. Significant inter-ethnic and cross-national variations in the occurrence of PTSD following trauma exposure have been reported in large-scale studies. The reasons for these variations are not clear, but they may reflect innate differences in genetic vulnerability, as well as differences in environmental factors such as diet and social support [108,109]. Second, most of the published research on biomarkers has involved either military personnel or individuals affected by a single specific traumatic exposure, namely the WTC terrorist attacks. It is not clear if similar results would be obtained in individuals who develop PTSD in response to more commonly encountered forms of trauma, such as motor vehicle accidents or sexual assault [110]. Third, most positive findings reported in this review have not yet been replicated. Fourth, many studies of military veterans have included subjects with head trauma, which is an independent risk factor for dementia [111]. Fifth, the majority of studies have been cross-sectional in nature; therefore, it is not possible to draw clear inferences regarding a causal link between PTSD and neurodegenerative disorders based on their results. Finally, there is some evidence that the link between PTSD and certain neurodegenerative disorders may be non-specific and may extend to other stress-related disorders, such as acute stress disorder and adjustment disorder [40,112]. This facet requires further exploration in longitudinal studies.

11. Conclusions

Research on the links between PTSD and neurodegenerative disorders is a young and rapidly evolving field: 97% of the literature included in this review has been published in the last decade. There is significant evidence that several biological markers, including structural changes in cerebral gray and white matter, increased levels of pro-inflammatory markers, genetic polymorphisms related to oxidative stress and vitamin D levels, features of the metabolic syndrome, and RSBD-like parasomnias, may mediate the association between PTSD and neurodegenerative disorders, such as Alzheimer's and Parkinson's disease. It is possible to integrate these diverse findings into a biologically plausible framework. Though questions of causality and temporal sequence remain unsettled and certain methodological limitations need to be considered, these results are of importance from clinical, research, and public health perspectives. The current review can be considered complementary to existing reviews that emphasize the clinical and epidemiological links between PTSD and neurodegenerative disorders [46,113] and draws attention to the biological mechanisms and pathways that might link these conditions. Future research, ideally involving ethnically diverse populations, with a greater focus on civilians and an effort to minimize potential confounders, will hopefully clarify the true nature of the association between PTSD and these biological markers, as well as their value in predicting subsequent neurodegeneration and cognitive impairment. This would facilitate the development of interventions that target one or more of the biological pathways that these markers are associated with, hopefully leading to better pharmacological approaches to the prevention or early treatment of neurodegenerative disorders in those exposed to traumatic stress.

Supplementary Materials: The following supporting information can be downloaded at: https://www.mdpi.com/article/10.3390/biomedicines11051465/s1, Supplementary Table S1. Search strings and numerical results of citations retrieved from the PubMed database.

Funding: This research received no external funding.

Institutional Review Board Statement: Not applicable.

Informed Consent Statement: Not applicable.

Data Availability Statement: Not applicable.

Conflicts of Interest: The author declares no conflict of interest.

Abbreviations

Abbreviations used in the tables alone are explained in the footnotes to each table.

Aβ	Amyloid-beta protein
AD	Alzheimer's disease
ALOX12	Arachidonate 12-lipoxygenase
ALOX15	Arachidonate 15-lipoxygenase
BOLD	Blood oxygenation level-dependent
CRP	C-reactive protein
DTI	Diffusion tensor imaging
FDA	Food and Drug Administration (United States)
FKBP5	FK-506 binding protein 5
GC	Vitamin D-binding protein
HPA	Hypothalamic–pituitary–adrenal axis
IL-6	Interleukin-6
miR	microRNA
MRI	Magnetic resonance imaging
NIH	National Institutes of Health (United States)

PET	Positron emission tomography
PRISMA	Preferred Reporting Items for Systematic Reviews and Meta-Analyses
PTSD	Post-Traumatic Stress Disorder
REST	RE1-silencing transcription factor gene
RSBD	Rapid Eye Movement (REM) Sleep Behavior Disorder
SEPT-4	Septin-4
SNP	Single nucleotide polymorphism
SPECT	Single photon emission computerized tomography
TBI	Traumatic brain injury
TNF-α	Tumor necrosis factor alpha
WTC	World Trade Center

References

1. Kirkpatrick, H.A.; Heller, G.M. Post-traumatic stress disorder: Theory and treatment update. *Int. J. Psychiatry Med.* **2014**, *47*, 337–346. [CrossRef] [PubMed]
2. Greenberg, N.; Brooks, S.; Dunn, R. Latest developments in post-traumatic stress disorder: Diagnosis and treatment. *Br. Med. Bull.* **2015**, *114*, 147–155. [CrossRef]
3. Yehuda, R.; Hoge, C.W.; McFarlane, A.C.; Vermetten, E.; Lanius, R.A.; Nievergelt, C.A.; Hobfoll, S.E.; Koenen, K.C.; Neylan, T.C.; Hyman, S.E. Post-traumatic stress disorder. *Nat. Rev. Dis. Prim.* **2015**, *1*, 15057. [CrossRef] [PubMed]
4. Hoppen, T.H.; Priebe, S.; Vetter, I.; Morina, N. Global burden of post-traumatic stress disorder and major depression in countries affected by war between 1989 and 2019: A systematic review and meta-analysis. *BMJ Glob. Health* **2021**, *6*, e006303. [CrossRef] [PubMed]
5. Dewar, M.; Paradis, A.; Fortin, C.A. Identifying trajectories and predictors of response to psychotherapy for post-traumatic stress disorder in adults: A systematic review of the literature. *Can. J. Psychiatry* **2020**, *65*, 71–86. [CrossRef] [PubMed]
6. Williams, T.; Phillips, N.J.; Stein, D.J.; Ipser, J.C. Pharmacotherapy for post traumatic stress disorder. *Cochrane Database Syst. Rev.* **2022**, *3*, CD002795. [CrossRef] [PubMed]
7. Morina, N.; Wicherts, J.M.; Lobbrecht, J.; Priebe, S. Remission from post-traumatic stress disorder in adults: A systematic review and meta-analysis of long term outcome studies. *Clin. Psychol. Rev.* **2014**, *34*, 249–255. [CrossRef]
8. Benedict, T.M.; Keenan, P.G.; Nitz, A.J.; Moeller-Bertram, T. Post-traumatic stress disorder symptoms contribute to worse pain and health outcomes in veterans with PTSD compared to those without: A systematic review with meta-analysis. *Mil. Med.* **2020**, *185*, e1481–e1491. [CrossRef]
9. Al Jowf, G.I.; Ahmed, Z.T.; An, N.; Reijnders, R.A.; Ambrosino, E.; Rutten, B.P.F.; de Nijs, L.; Eijssen, L.M.T. A public health perspective of post-traumatic stress disorder. *Int. J. Environ. Res. Public Health* **2022**, *19*, 6474. [CrossRef]
10. Zammit, S.; Lewis, C.; Dawson, S.; Colley, H.; McCann, H.; Piekarski, A.; Rockliff, H.; Bisson, J. Undetected post-traumatic stress disorder in secondary-care mental health services: A systematic review. *Br. J. Psychiatry* **2018**, *212*, 11–18. [CrossRef]
11. Maria-Rios, C.E.; Morrow, J.D. Mechanisms of shared vulnerability to post-traumatic stress disorder and substance use disorders. *Front. Behav. Neurosci.* **2020**, *14*, 6. [CrossRef] [PubMed]
12. Britvic, D.; Anticevic, V.; Kaliterna, M.; Lusic, L.; Beg, A.; Brajevic-Gizdic, I.; Kudric, M.; Stupalo, Z.; Krolo, V.; Pivac, N. Comorbidities with posttraumatic stress disorder (PTSD) among combat veterans: 15 years postwar analysis. *Int. J. Clin. Health Psychol.* **2015**, *15*, 81–92. [CrossRef]
13. Pietrzak, R.H.; Goldstein, R.B.; Southwick, S.M.; Grant, B.F. Physical health conditions associated with posttraumatic stress disorder in U.S. older adults: Results from wave 2 of the National Epidemiologic Survey on Alcohol and Related Conditions. *J. Am. Geriatr. Soc.* **2012**, *60*, 296–303. [CrossRef] [PubMed]
14. Krysinska, K.; Lester, D. Post-traumatic stress disorder and suicide risk: A systematic review. *Arch. Suicide Res.* **2010**, *14*, 1–23. [CrossRef]
15. Hu, X.Y.; Wu, Y.L.; Cheng, C.H.; Liu, X.X.; Zhou, L. Association of Brain-Derived Neurotrophic Factor rs6265 G>A polymorphism and Post-traumatic Stress Disorder susceptibility: A systematic review and meta-analysis. *Brain Behav.* **2021**, *11*, e02118. [CrossRef] [PubMed]
16. Wang, Q.; Shelton, R.C.; Dwivedi, Y. Interaction between early-life stress and FKBP5 gene variants in major depressive disorder and post-traumatic stress disorder: A systematic review and meta-analysis. *J. Affect. Disord.* **2018**, *225*, 422–428. [CrossRef]
17. McLaughlin, K.A.; Koenen, K.A.; Bromet, E.J.; Karam, E.G.; Liu, H.; Petukhova, M.; Ruscio, A.M.; Sampson, N.A.; Stein, D.J.; Aguilar-Gaxiola, S.; et al. Childhood adversities and post-traumatic stress disorder: Evidence for stress sensitization in the World Mental Health Surveys. *Br. J. Psychiatry* **2017**, *211*, 280–288. [CrossRef]
18. McLaughlin, K.A.; Conron, K.J.; Koenen, K.C.; Gilman, S.E. Childhood adversity, adult stressful life events, and risk of past-year psychiatric disorder: A test of the stress sensitization hypothesis in a population-based sample of adults. *Psychol. Med.* **2010**, *40*, 1647–1658. [CrossRef]

19. Stefanovic, M.; Ehring, T.; Wittekind, C.E.; Kleim, B.; Rohde, J.; Kruger-Gottschalk, A.; Knaevelsrud, C.; Rau, H.; Schafer, I.; Schellong, J.; et al. Comparing PTSD symptom networks in type I vs. type II trauma survivors. *Eur. J. Psychotraumatol.* **2022**, *13*, 2114260. [CrossRef]
20. Hiscox, L.V.; Hiller, R.; Fraser, A.; Rabie, S.; Stewart, J.; Seedat, S.; Tomlinson, M.; Hallingan, S.L. Sex differences in post-traumatic stress disorder in a high adversity cohort of South African adolescents: An examination of depressive symptoms, age, and trauma type as explanatory factors. *Eur. J. Psychotraumatol.* **2021**, *12*, 1978669. [CrossRef]
21. Panagou, C.; MacBeth, A. Deconstructing pathways to resilience: A systematic review of associations between psychosocial mechanisms and transdiagnostic adult mental health outcomes in the context of adverse childhood experiences. *Clin. Psychol. Psychother.* **2022**, *29*, 1626–1654. [CrossRef]
22. Pankey, B.S.; Riedel, M.C.; Cowan, I.; Bartley, J.E.; Lobo, R.P.; Hill-Bowen, L.D.; Salo, T.; Musser, E.D.; Sutherland, M.T.; Laird, A.R. Extended functional connectivity of convergent structural alterations among individuals with PTSD: A neuroimaging meta-analysis. *Behav. Brain Funct.* **2022**, *18*, 9. [CrossRef]
23. Pan, X.; Wang, Z.; Wu, X.; Wen, S.W.; Liu, A. Salivary cortisol in post-traumatic stress disorder: A systematic review and meta-analysis. *BMC Psychiatry* **2018**, *18*, 324. [CrossRef] [PubMed]
24. Dell'Oste, V.; Fantasia, S.; Gravina, D.; Palego, L.; Betti, L.; Dell'Osso, L.; Giannaccini, G.; Carmassi, C. Metabolic and inflammatory response in post-traumatic stress disorder (PTSD): A systematic review on peripheral neuroimmune biomarkers. *Int. J. Environ. Res. Public Health* **2023**, *20*, 2937. [CrossRef]
25. Schiavone, S.; Jaquet, V.; Trabace, L.; Krause, K.H. Severe life stress and oxidative stress in the brain: From animal models to human pathology. *Antioxid. Redox Signal.* **2013**, *18*, 1475–1490. [CrossRef] [PubMed]
26. Krantz, D.S.; Shank, L.M.; Goodie, J.L. Post-traumatic stress disorder (PTSD) as a systemic disorder: Pathways to cardiovascular disease. *Health Psychol.* **2022**, *41*, 651–662. [CrossRef] [PubMed]
27. Polyak, H.; Galla, Z.; Nanasi, N.; Cseh, E.K.; Rajda, C.; Veres, G.; Spekker, E.; Szabo, A.; Klivenyi, P.; Tanaka, M.; et al. The tryptophan-kynurenine metabolic system is suppressed in cuprizone-induced model of demyelination simulating progressive multiple sclerosis. *Biomedicines* **2023**, *11*, 945. [CrossRef] [PubMed]
28. Tajti, J.; Szok, D.; Csati, A.; Szabo, A.; Tanaka, M.; Vecsei, L. Exploring novel therapeutic targets in the common pathogenic factors in migraine and neuropathic pain. *Int. J. Mol. Sci.* **2023**, *24*, 4114. [CrossRef] [PubMed]
29. Ippolito, G.; Bertaccini, R.; Tarasi, L.; Di Gregorio, F.; Trajkovic, J.; Battaglia, S.; Romei, V. The role of alpha oscillations among the main neuropsychiatric disorders in the adult and developing human brain: Evidence from the last 10 years of research. *Biomedicines* **2022**, *10*, 3189. [CrossRef]
30. Di Gregorio, F.; La Porta, F.; Petrone, V.; Battaglia, S.; Orlandi, S.; Ippolito, G.; Romei, V.; Piperno, R.; Lullini, G. Accuracy of EEG biomarkers in the detection of clinical outcome in disorders of consciousness after severe acquired brain injury: Preliminary results of a pilot study using a machine learning approach. *Biomedicines* **2022**, *10*, 1897. [CrossRef]
31. Harrison, B.J.; Fullana, M.A.; Via, E.; Soriano-Mas, C.; Vervliet, B.; Martinez-Zalacan, I.; Pujol, J.; Davey, C.G.; Kircher, T.; Straube, B.; et al. Human ventromedial prefrontal cortex and the positive affective processing of safety signals. *NeuroImage* **2017**, *152*, 12–18. [CrossRef] [PubMed]
32. Battaglia, S.; Cardellicchio, P.; Di Fazio, C.; Nazzi, C.; Fracasso, A.; Borgomaneri, S. Stopping in (e)motion: Reactive action inhibition when facing valence-independent emotional stimuli. *Front. Behav. Neurosci.* **2022**, *16*, 998714. [CrossRef] [PubMed]
33. Tanaka, M.; Szabo, A.; Vecsei, L. Integrating armchair, bench, and bedside research for behavioral neurology and neuropsychiatry: Editorial. *Biomedicines* **2022**, *10*, 2999. [CrossRef]
34. Battaglia, S.; Nazzi, C.; Thayer, J.F. Fear-induced bradycardia in mental disorders: Foundations, current advances, future perspectives. *Neurosci. Biobehav. Rev.* **2023**, *149*, 105163. [CrossRef] [PubMed]
35. Battaglia, S.; Di Fazio, C.; Vicario, C.M.; Avenanti, A. Neuropharmacological modulation of N-methyl-D-aspartate, noradrenaline and endocannabinoid receptors in fear extinction learning: Synaptic transmission and plasticity. *Int. J. Mol. Sci.* **2023**, *24*, 5926. [CrossRef]
36. Tanaka, M.; Torok, M.; Vecsei, L. Novel pharmaceutical approaches in dementia. In *Neuropsychopharmacotherapy*; Riederer, P., Laux, G., Nagatsu, T., Le, W., Riederer, C., Eds.; Springer: Cham, Switzerland, 2022. [CrossRef]
37. Rafferty, L.A.; Cawkill, P.E.; Stevelink, S.A.M.; Greenberg, K.; Greenberg, N. Dementia, post-traumatic stress disorder and major depressive disorder: A review of the mental health risk factors for dementia in the military veteran population. *Psychol. Med.* **2018**, *48*, 1400–1409. [CrossRef]
38. Gunak, M.M.; Billings, J.; Carratu, E.; Marchant, N.L.; Favarato, G.; Orgeta, V. Post-traumatic stress disorder as a risk factor for dementia: Systematic review and meta-analysis. *Br. J. Psychiatry* **2020**, *217*, 600–608. [CrossRef]
39. Bergman, B.P.; Mackay, D.F.; Pell, J.P. Dementia in Scottish military veterans: Early evidence from a retrospective cohort study. *Psychol. Med.* **2021**, *53*, 1015–1020. [CrossRef] [PubMed]
40. Song, H.; Sieurin, J.; Wirdefeldt, K.; Pedersen, N.L.; Almqvist, C.; Larsson, H.; Valdimarsdottir, U.A.; Fang, F. Association of stress-related disorders with subsequent neurodegenerative disorders. *JAMA Neurol.* **2020**, *77*, 700–709. [CrossRef]
41. Chan, Y.E.; Bai, Y.M.; Hsu, J.W.; Huang, K.L.; Su, T.P.; Li, C.T.; Lin, W.C.; Pan, T.L.; Chen, T.J.; Tsai, S.J.; et al. Post-traumatic stress disorder and risk of Parkinson disease: A nationwide longitudinal study. *Am. J. Geriatr. Psychiatry* **2017**, *25*, 917–923. [CrossRef]

42. White, D.L.; Kunik, M.E.; Yu, H.; Lin, H.L.; Richardson, P.A.; Moore, S.; Sarwar, A.I.; Marsh, L.; Jorge, R.E. Post-traumatic stress disorder is associated with further increased Parkinson's disease in veterans with traumatic brain injury. *Ann. Neurol.* **2020**, *88*, 33–41. [CrossRef] [PubMed]
43. Lohr, J.B.; Palmer, B.W.; Eidt, C.A.; Aailaboyina, S.; Mausbach, B.T.; Wolkowitz, O.M.; Thorp, S.R.; Jeste, D.V. Is post-traumatic stress disorder associated with premature senescence? A review of the literature. *Am. J. Geriatr. Psychiatry* **2015**, *23*, 709–725. [CrossRef] [PubMed]
44. Novellino, F.; Sacca, V.; Donato, A.; Zaffino, P.; Spadea, M.F.; Vismara, M.; Arcidiacono, B.; Malara, N.; Presta, I.; Donato, G. Innate immunity: A common denominator between neurodegenerative and neuropsychiatric diseases. *Int. J. Mol. Sci.* **2020**, *21*, 1115. [CrossRef] [PubMed]
45. Antonelli-Salgado, T.; Ramos-Lima, L.F.; Machado, C.S.; Cassidy, R.M.; Cardoso, T.A.; Kapczinski, F.; Passos, I.C. Neuroprogression in post-traumatic stress disorder: A systematic review. *Trends Psychiatry Psychother.* **2021**, *43*, 167–176. [CrossRef] [PubMed]
46. Desmarais, P.; Weidman, D.; Wassef, A.; Bruneau, M.A.; Friedland, J.; Bajsarowicz, P.; Thibodeau, M.P.; Herrmann, N.; Nguyen, Q.D. The interplay between post-traumatic stress disorder and dementia: A systematic review. *Am. J. Geriatr. Psychiatry* **2020**, *28*, 48–60. [CrossRef]
47. Elias, A.; Rowe, C.; Hopwood, M. Risk of dementia in posttraumatic stress disorder. *J. Geriatr. Psychiatry Neurol.* **2021**, *34*, 555–564. [CrossRef]
48. Tanaka, M.; Vecsei, L. Editorial of special issue 'Dissecting neurological and neuropsychiatric diseases: Neurodegeneration and neuroprotection'. *Int. J. Mol. Sci.* **2022**, *23*, 6991. [CrossRef]
49. Califf, R.M. Biomarker definitions and their applications. *Exp. Biol. Med.* **2018**, *243*, 213–221. [CrossRef]
50. Tricco, A.C.; Lillie, E.; Zarin, W.; O'Brien, K.K.; Colquhoun, H.; Levac, D.; Moher, D.; Peters, M.D.; Horsley, T.; Weeks, L.; et al. PRISMA extension for scoping reviews (PRISMA-ScR): Checklist and explanation. *Ann. Int. Med.* **2018**, *169*, 467–473. [CrossRef]
51. Chao, L.L.; Yaffe, K.; Samuelson, K.; Neylan, T.C. Hippocampal volume is inversely related to PTSD duration. *Psychiatry Res. Neuroimaging* **2014**, *222*, 119–123. [CrossRef]
52. Mueller, S.G.; Ng, P.; Neylan, T.; Mackin, S.; Wolkowitz, O.; Mellon, S.; Yan, X.; Flory, J.; Yehuda, R.; Marmar, C.R.; et al. Evidence for disrupted gray matter structural connectivity in posttraumatic stress disorder. *Psychiatry Res. Neuroimaging* **2015**, *234*, 194–201. [CrossRef]
53. Main, K.L.; Soman, S.; Pestilli, F.; Furst, A.; Noda, A.; Hernandez, B.; Kong, J.; Cheng, J.; Fairchild, J.K.; Taylor, J.; et al. DTI measures identify mild and moderate TBI cases among patients with complex health problems: A receiver operating characteristic analysis of U.S. veterans. *NeuroImage Clin.* **2017**, *16*, 1–16. [CrossRef]
54. Basavaraju, R.; France, J.; Maas, B.; Brickman, A.M.; Flory, J.D.; Szeszko, P.R.; Yehuda, R.; Rutherford, B.R.; Provenzano, F.A. Right hippocampal volume deficit in an older population with posttraumatic stress disorder. *J Psychiatr. Res.* **2021**, *17*, 368–375. [CrossRef]
55. Olivé, I.; Makris, N.; Densmore, M.; McKinnon, M.C.; Lanius, R.A. Altered basal forebrain BOLD signal variability at rest in posttraumatic stress disorder: A potential candidate vulnerability mechanism for neurodegeneration in PTSD. *Hum. Brain Mapp.* **2021**, *42*, 3561–3575. [CrossRef]
56. Brown, E.M.; Salat, D.H.; Milberg, W.P.; Fortier, C.B.; McGlinchey, R.E. Accelerated longitudinal cortical atrophy in OEF/OIF/OND veterans with severe PTSD and the impact of comorbid TBI. *Hum. Brain Mapp.* **2022**, *43*, 3694–3705. [CrossRef]
57. Kritikos, M.; Huang, C.; Clouston, S.A.P.; Pellecchia, A.C.; Mejia-Santiago, S.; Carr, M.A.; Hagan, T.; Kotov, R.; Gandy, S.; Sano, M.; et al. DTI connectometry analysis reveals white matter changes in cognitively impaired World Trade Center responders at midlife. *J. Alzheimers Dis.* **2022**, *89*, 1075–1089. [CrossRef]
58. Kuan, P.F.; Yang, X.; Clouston, S.; Ren, X.; Kotov, R.; Waszczuk, M.; Singh, P.K.; Glenn, S.T.; Gomez, E.C.; Wang, J.; et al. Cell type-specific gene expression patterns associated with posttraumatic stress disorder in World Trade Center responders. *Transl. Psychiatry* **2021**, *9*, 1. [CrossRef]
59. Sragovich, S.; Gershovits, M.; Lam, J.C.K.; Li, V.O.K.; Gozes, I. Putative somatic blood mutations in post-traumatic stress disorder-symptomatic soldiers: High impact of cytoskeletal and inflammatory proteins. *J. Alzheimers Dis.* **2021**, *79*, 1723–1734. [CrossRef]
60. Wolf, E.J.; Zhao, X.; Hawn, S.E.; Morrison, F.G.; Zhou, Z.; Fein-Schaffer, D.; Huber, B.; Miller, M.W.; Logue, M.W. Gene expression correlates of advanced epigenetic age and psychopathology in postmortem cortical tissue. *Neurobiol. Stress* **2021**, *15*, 100371. [CrossRef]
61. Clouston, S.A.P.; Deri, Y.; Diminich, E.; Kew, R.; Kotov, R.; Stewart, C.; Yang, X.; Gandy, S.; Sano, M.; Bromet, E.J.; et al. Posttraumatic stress disorder and total amyloid burden and amyloid-β 42/40 ratios in plasma: Results from a pilot study of World Trade Center responders. *Alzheimers Dement.* **2019**, *11*, 216–220. [CrossRef]
62. Cimino, N.; Kang, M.S.; Honig, L.S.; Rutherford, B.R. Blood-based biomarkers for Alzheimer's disease in older adults with posttraumatic stress disorder. *J. Alzheimers Dis. Rep.* **2022**, *6*, 49–56. [CrossRef] [PubMed]
63. Zhang, Y.; Rosen, R.; Reibman, J.; Shao, Y. Posttraumatic stress disorder mediates the association between traumatic World Trade Center dust cloud exposure and ongoing systemic inflammation in community members. *Int. J. Environ. Res. Public Health* **2022**, *19*, 8622. [CrossRef] [PubMed]

64. Elliott, J.E.; Opel, R.A.; Weymann, K.B.; Chau, A.Q.; Papesh, M.A.; Callahan, M.L.; Storzbach, D.; Lim, M.M. Sleep disturbances in traumatic brain injury: Association with sensory sensitivity. *J. Clin. Sleep Med.* 2018, *14*, 1177–1186. [CrossRef]
65. Elliott, J.E.; Opel, R.A.; Pleshakov, D.; Rachakonda, T.; Chau, A.Q.; Weymann, K.B.; Lim, M.M. Posttraumatic stress disorder increases the odds of REM sleep behavior disorder and other parasomnias in veterans with and without comorbid traumatic brain injury. *Sleep* 2020, *43*, zsz237. [CrossRef]
66. Feemster, J.C.; Steele, T.A.; Palermo, K.P.; Ralston, C.L.; Tao, Y.; Bauer, D.A.; Edgar, L.; Rivera, S.; Walters-Smith, M.; Gossard, T.R.; et al. Abnormal rapid eye movement sleep atonia control in chronic post-traumatic stress disorder. *Sleep* 2022, *45*, zsab259. [CrossRef]
67. Liu, Y.; Partinen, E.; Chan, N.Y.; Dauvilliers, Y.; Inoue, Y.; De Gennaro, L.; Piazzi, G.; Bolstad, C.J.; Nadorff, M.R.; Merikanto, I.; et al. Dream-enactment behaviours during the COVID-19 pandemic: An international COVID-19 sleep study. *J. Sleep Res.* 2023, *32*, e13613. [CrossRef] [PubMed]
68. Baker, D.G.; Ekhator, N.N.; Kasckow, J.W.; Hill, K.K.; Zoumakis, E.; Dashevsky, B.A.; Chrousos, G.P.; Geracioti, T.D. Plasma and cerebrospinal fluid interleukin-6 concentrations in posttraumatic stress disorder. *Neuroimmunomodulation* 2021, *9*, 209–217. [CrossRef]
69. Mohlenhoff, B.S.; Chao, L.L.; Buckley, S.T.; Weiner, M.W.; Neylan, T.C. Are hippocampal size difference in posttraumatic stress disorder mediated by sleep pathology? *Alzheimers Dement.* 2014, *10*, S146–S154. [CrossRef] [PubMed]
70. Miller, M.W.; Wolf, E.J.; Sadeh, N.; Logue, M.; Spielberg, J.M.; Hayes, J.P.; Sperbeck, E.; Schichman, S.A.; Stone, A.; Carter, W.C.; et al. A novel locus in the oxidative stress-related gene *ALOX12* moderates the association between PTSD and thickness of the prefrontal cortex. *Psychoneuroendocrinology* 2015, *62*, 359–365. [CrossRef]
71. O'Donovan, A.; Chao, L.L.; Paulson, J.; Samuelson, K.W.; Shigenaga, J.K.; Grunfeld, C.; Weiner, M.W.; Neylan, T.C. Altered inflammatory activity associated with reduced hippocampal volume and more severe posttraumatic stress symptoms in Gulf War veterans. *Psychoneuroendocrinology* 2015, *51*, 557–566. [CrossRef] [PubMed]
72. Wolf, E.J.; Sadeh, N.; Leritz, E.C.; Logue, M.W.; Stoop, T.; McGlinchey, R.; Milberg, W.; Miller, M.W. PTSD as a catalyst for the association between metabolic syndrome and reduced cortical thickness. *Biol. Psychiatry* 2016, *80*, 363–371. [CrossRef]
73. Hayes, J.P.; Logue, M.W.; Sadeh, N.; Spielberg, J.M.; Verfaelle, M.; Hayes, S.M.; Reagan, A.; Salat, D.H.; Wolf, E.J.; McGlinchey, R.E.; et al. Mild traumatic brain injury is associated with reduced cortical thickness in those at risk for Alzheimer's disease. *Brain* 2017, *140*, 813–825. [CrossRef]
74. Hayes, J.P.; Reagan, A.; Logue, M.W.; Hayes, S.M.; Sadeh, N.; Miller, D.R.; Verfaellie, M.; Wolf, E.J.; McGlinchey, R.E.; Milberg, W.P.; et al. BDNF genotype is associated with hippocampal volume in mild traumatic brain injury. *Genes Brain Behav.* 2018, *17*, 107–117. [CrossRef]
75. Kang, J.I.; Mueller, S.G.; Wu, G.W.Y.; Lin, J.; Ng, P.; Yehuda, R.; Flory, J.D.; Abu-Amara, D.; Reus, V.I.; Gautam, A.; et al. Effect of combat exposure and posttraumatic stress disorder on telomere length and amygdala volume. *Biol. Psychiatry Cogn. Neurosci. Neuroimaging* 2020, *5*, 678–687. [CrossRef] [PubMed]
76. Terock, J.; Hannemann, A.; Van der Auwera, S.; Janowitz, D.; Spitzer, C.; Bonk, S.; Volzke, H.; Grabe, H.J. Posttraumatic stress disorder is associated with reduced vitamin D levels and functional polymorphisms of the vitamin D-binding protein in a population-based sample. *Prog. Neuropsychopharmacol. Biol. Psychiatry* 2020, *96*, 109760. [CrossRef] [PubMed]
77. Guedes, V.A.; Lai, C.; Devoto, C.; Edwards, K.A.; Mithani, S.; Sass, D.; Vorn, R.; Qu, B.X.; Rusch, H.L.; Martin, C.A.; et al. Extracellular vesicle proteins and microRNAs are linked to chronic post-traumatic stress disorder symptoms in service members and veterans with mild traumatic brain injury. *Front. Pharmacol.* 2021, *12*, 745348. [CrossRef]
78. Weiner, M.W.; Harvey, D.; Landau, S.M.; Veitch, D.P.; Neylan, T.C.; Grafman, J.H.; Aisen, P.S.; Petersen, R.C.; Jack, C.R.; Tosun, D.; et al. Traumatic brain injury and post-traumatic stress disorder are not associated with Alzheimer's disease pathology measured with biomarkers. *Alzheimers Dement.* 2023, *19*, 884–895. [CrossRef] [PubMed]
79. Kritikos, M.; Diminich, E.D.; Meliker, J.; Mielke, M.; Bennett, D.A.; Finch, C.E.; Gandy, S.E.; Carr, M.A.; Yang, X.; Kotov, R.; et al. Plasma amyloid beta 40/42, phosphorylated tau 181, and neurofilament light are associated with cognitive impairment and neuropathological changes among World Trade Center responders: A prospective cohort study of exposures and cognitive aging at midlife. *Alzheimers Dement.* 2023, *15*, e12409. [CrossRef]
80. STRING: Functional Protein Association Networks. Available online: https://string-db.org/ (accessed on 28 March 2023).
81. Lugli, G.; Cohen, A.M.; Bennett, D.A.; Shah, R.C.; Fields, C.J.; Hernandez, A.G.; Smalheiser, N.R. Plasma exosomal miRNAs in persons with and without Alzheimer disease: Altered expression and prospects for biomarkers. *PLoS ONE* 2015, *10*, e0139233. [CrossRef]
82. Zhuang, K.; Chen, X.; Cassady, K.E.; Baker, S.L.; Jagust, W.J. Metacognition, cortical thickness, and tauopathy in aging. *Neurobiol. Aging* 2022, *118*, 44–54. [CrossRef]
83. Kim, S.; Park, S.; Chang, I.; Alzheimer's Disease Neuroimaging Initiative. Development of quantitative and continuous measure for severity degree of Alzheimer's disease evaluated from MRI images of 761 human brains. *BMC Bioinform.* 2022, *23*, 357. [CrossRef]
84. Sexton, C.E.; Kalu, U.G.; Fillippini, N.; Mackay, C.E.; Ebmeier, K.P. A meta-analysis of diffusion tensor imaging in mild cognitive impairment and Alzheimer's disease. *Neurobiol. Aging* 2011, *32*, e5–e2322. [CrossRef]
85. Qin, L.; Guo, Z.; McClure, M.A.; Mu, Q. White matter changes from mild cognitive impairment to Alzheimer's disease: A meta-analysis. *Acta Neurol. Belg.* 2021, *121*, 1435–1447. [CrossRef] [PubMed]

86. Herdick, M.; Dyrba, M.; Fritz, H.C.J.; Altenstein, S.; Ballarini, T.; Brosseron, F.; Buerger, K.; Cetindag, A.C.; Dechent, P.; Dobisch, L.; et al. Multimodal MRI analysis of basal forebrain structure and function across the Alzheimer's disease spectrum. *Neuroimage Clin.* **2020**, *28*, 102495. [CrossRef]
87. Atti, A.R.; Valente, S.; Iodice, A.; Caramella, I.; Ferrari, B.; Albert, U.; Mandelli, L.; De Ronchi, D. Metabolic syndrome, mild cognitive impairment, and dementia: A meta-analysis of longitudinal studies. *Am. J. Geriatr. Psychiatry* **2019**, *27*, 625–637. [CrossRef]
88. Zuin, M.; Roncon, L.; Passaro, A.; Cervellati, C.; Zuliani, G. Metabolic syndrome and the risk of late onset Alzheimer's disease: An updated review and meta-analysis. *Nutr. Metab. Cardiovasc. Dis.* **2021**, *31*, 2244–2252. [CrossRef]
89. Pillai, J.A.; Bena, J.; Bekris, L.; Kodur, N.; Kasumov, T.; Leverenz, J.B.; Kashyap, S.R.; Alzheimer's Disease Neuroimaging Initiative. Metabolic syndrome biomarkers relate to rate of cognitive decline in MCI and dementia stages of Alzheimer's disease. *Alzheimers Res. Ther.* **2023**, *15*, 54. [CrossRef]
90. Sommer, I.; Griebler, U.; Kien, C.; Auer, S.; Klerings, I.; Hammer, R.; Holzer, P.; Gartlehner, G. Vitamin D deficiency as a risk factor for dementia: A systematic review and meta-analysis. *BMC Geriatr.* **2017**, *17*, 16. [CrossRef] [PubMed]
91. Navale, S.S.; Mulugeta, A.; Zhou, A.; Llewellyn, D.J.; Hypponen, E. Vitamin D and brain health: An observational and Mendelian randomization study. *Am. J. Clin. Nutr.* **2022**, *116*, 531–540. [CrossRef]
92. Ghahremani, M.; Smith, E.E.; Chen, H.Y.; Creese, B.; Goodarzi, Z.; Ismail, Z. Vitamin D supplementation and incident dementia: Effects of sex, APOE, and baseline cognitive status. *Alzheimers Dement.* **2023**, *15*, e12404. [CrossRef] [PubMed]
93. Leng, F.; Hinz, R.; Gentleman, S.; Hampshire, A.; Dani, M.; Brooks, D.J.; Edison, P. Neuroinflammation is independently associated with brain network dysfunction in Alzheimer's disease. *Mol. Psychiatry* **2023**, *28*, 1303–1311. [CrossRef]
94. Chu, M.; Wen, L.; Jiang, D.; Liu, L.; Nan, H.; Yue, A.; Wang, Y.; Wang, Y.; Qu, M.; Wang, N.; et al. Peripheral inflammation in behavioural variant frontotemporal dementia: Associations with central degeneration and clinical measures. *J. Neuroinflammation* **2023**, *20*, 65. [CrossRef]
95. Chen, X.; Hu, Y.; Cao, Z.; Liu, Q.; Cheng, Y. Cerebrospinal fluid inflammatory cytokine aberrations in Alzheimer's disease, Parkinson's disease and amyotrophic lateral sclerosis: A systematic review and meta-analysis. *Front. Immunol.* **2018**, *9*, 2122. [CrossRef]
96. Renna, M.E.; O'Toole, M.S.; Spaeth, P.E.; Lekander, M.; Mennin, D.S. The association between anxiety, traumatic stress, and obsessive-compulsive disorders and chronic inflammation: A systematic review and meta-analysis. *Depress. Anxiety* **2018**, *35*, 1081–1094. [CrossRef] [PubMed]
97. Long, S.; Chen, Y.; Meng, Y.; Yang, Z.; Wei, M.; Li, T.; Ni, J.; Shi, J.; Tian, J. Peripheral high levels of CRP predict progression from normal cognition to dementia: A systematic review and meta-analysis. *J. Clin. Neurosci.* **2023**, *107*, 54–63. [CrossRef] [PubMed]
98. Custodero, C.; Ciavarella, A.; Panza, F.; Gnocchi, D.; Lenato, G.M.; Lee, J.; Mazzocca, A.; Sabba, C.; Solfrizzi, V. Role of inflammatory markers in the diagnosis of vascular contributions to cognitive impairment and dementia: A systematic review and meta-analysis. *Geroscience* **2022**, *44*, 1373–1392. [CrossRef]
99. Portilla-Fernandez, E.; Hwang, S.J.; Wilson, R.; Maddock, J.; Hill, D.W.; Teumer, A.; Mishra, P.P.; Brody, J.A.; Joehanes, R.; Litghart, S.; et al. Meta-analysis of epigenome-wide association studies of carotid intima-media thickness. *Eur. J. Epidemiol.* **2021**, *36*, 1143–1155. [CrossRef] [PubMed]
100. Ihara, M.; Tomimoto, H.; Kitayama, H.; Morioka, Y.; Akiguchi, I.; Shibasaki, H.; Noda, M.; Kinoshita, M. Association of the cytoskeletal GTP-binding protein Sept4/H5 with cytoplasmic inclusions found in Parkinson's disease and other synucleinopathies. *J. Biol. Chem.* **2003**, *278*, 24095–24102. [CrossRef] [PubMed]
101. Saba, R.; Goodman, C.D.; Huzarewich, R.L.; Robertson, C.; Booth, S.A. A miRNA signature of prion-induced neurodegeneration. *PLoS ONE* **2008**, *3*, e3652. [CrossRef]
102. Lemche, E. Early life stress and epigenetics in late-onset Alzheimer's Dementia: A systematic review. *Curr. Genomics* **2018**, *19*, 522–602. [CrossRef]
103. Galbiati, A.; Verga, L.; Giora, E.; Zucconi, M.; Ferini-Strambi, L. The risk of neurodegeneration in REM sleep behavior disorder: A systematic review and meta-analysis of longitudinal studies. *Sleep Med. Rev.* **2019**, *43*, 37–46. [CrossRef] [PubMed]
104. Germain, A. Sleep disturbances as the hallmark of PTSD: Where are we now? *Am. J. Psychiatry* **2013**, *170*, 172–182. [CrossRef] [PubMed]
105. Barone, D.A. Dream enactment behavior-a real nightmare: A review of post-traumatic stress disorder, REM sleep behavior disorder, and trauma-associated sleep disorder. *J. Clin. Sleep Med.* **2020**, *16*, 1943–1948. [CrossRef] [PubMed]
106. Mysliwiec, V.; Brock, M.S.; Creamer, J.L.; O'Reilly, B.M.; Germain, A.; Roth, B.J. Trauma induced sleep disorder: A parasomnia induced by trauma. *Sleep Med. Rev.* **2018**, *37*, 94–104. [CrossRef]
107. Eraly, S.A.; Nievergelt, C.A.; Maihofer, A.X.; Barkauskas, D.A.; Biswas, N.; Agorastos, A.; O'Connor, D.T.; Baker, D.G.; MRS Team. Assessment of plasma C-reactive protein as a biomarker of PTSD risk. *JAMA Psychiatry* **2014**, *71*, 423–431. [CrossRef]
108. Stein, D.J.; Karam, E.G.; Shahly, V.; Hill, E.D.; King, A.; Petukhova, M.; Atwoli, L.; Bromet, E.J.; Florescu, S.; Haro, J.M.; et al. Post-traumatic stress disorder associated with life-threatening motor vehicle collisions in the WHO World Mental Health Surveys. *BMC Psychiatry* **2016**, *16*, 257. [CrossRef]
109. Hawes, A.M.; Axinn, W.G.; Ghimire, D.J. Ethnicity and psychiatric disorders. *Ann. Psychiatry Ment. Health* **2016**, *4*, 1072.
110. Dworkin, E.R.; Schumacher, J.A. Preventing posttraumatic stress related to sexual assault through early intervention: A systematic review. *Trauma Violence Abus.* **2018**, *19*, 459–472. [CrossRef]

111. Peterson, K.; Veazie, S.; Bourne, D.; Anderson, J. Association between traumatic brain injury and dementia in veterans: A rapid systematic review. *J. Head Trauma Rehabil.* **2020**, *35*, 198–208. [CrossRef]
112. Islamoska, S.; Hansen, A.M.; Ishtiak-Ahmed, K.; Garde, A.H.; Andersen, P.K.; Garde, E.; Taudorf, L.; Waldemar, G.; Nabe-Nielsen, K. Stress diagnoses in midlife and risk of dementia: A register-based follow-up study. *Aging Ment. Health* **2021**, *25*, 1151–1160. [CrossRef]
113. van Dongen, D.H.E.; Havermans, D.; Deckers, K.; Olff, M.; Verhey, F.; Sobczak, S. A first insight into the clinical manifestation of posttraumatic stress disorder in dementia: A systematic literature review. *Psychogeriatrics* **2022**, *22*, 509–520. [CrossRef] [PubMed]

Disclaimer/Publisher's Note: The statements, opinions and data contained in all publications are solely those of the individual author(s) and contributor(s) and not of MDPI and/or the editor(s). MDPI and/or the editor(s) disclaim responsibility for any injury to people or property resulting from any ideas, methods, instructions or products referred to in the content.

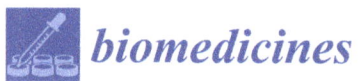

Article

Atorvastatin and Nitrofurantoin Repurposed in the Context of Breast Cancer and Neuroblastoma Cells

Catarina Moura [1,2,3], Ana Salomé Correia [1,2,3], Mariana Pereira [1,2,3], Eduarda Ribeiro [1,2,3], Joana Santos [1,2] and Nuno Vale [1,2,4,*]

1. OncoPharma Research Group, Center for Health Technology and Services Research (CINTESIS), Rua Doutor Plácido da Costa, 4200-450 Porto, Portugal
2. CINTESIS@RISE, Faculty of Medicine, University of Porto, Alameda Professor Hernâni Monteiro, 4200-319 Porto, Portugal
3. ICBAS-School of Medicine and Biomedical Sciences, University of Porto, Rua Jorge Viterbo Ferreira, 228, 4050-313 Porto, Portugal
4. Department of Community Medicine, Information and Health Decision Sciences (MEDCIDS), Faculty of Medicine, University of Porto, Rua Doutor Plácido da Costa, 4200-450 Porto, Portugal
* Correspondence: nunovale@med.up.pt; Tel.: +351-220426537

Abstract: Chemotherapy still plays a central role in the treatment of cancer. However, it is often accompanied by off-target effects that result in severe side-effects and development of drug resistance. The aim of this work was to study the efficacy of different repurposed drugs on the viability of MCF-7 and SH-SY5Y breast cancer and neuroblastoma cells, respectively. In addition, combinations of these repurposed drugs with a classical chemotherapeutic drug (doxorubicin) were also carried out. The cytotoxic effects of the repurposed drugs were evaluated individually and in combination in both cancer cell lines, assessed by MTT assays and morphological evaluation of the cells. The results demonstrated that atorvastatin reduced the viability of both cell lines. However, nitrofurantoin was able to induce cytotoxic effects in MCF-7 cells, but not in SH-SY5Y cells. The combinations of the repurposed drugs with doxorubicin induced a higher inhibition on cell viability than the repurposed drugs individually. The combination of the two repurposed drugs demonstrated that they potentiate each other. Synergism studies revealed that the combination of doxorubicin with the two repurposed drugs was more effective in SH-SY5Y cells, compared to MCF-7 cells. Taken together, our preliminary study highlights the potential use of atorvastatin and nitrofurantoin in the context of breast cancer and neuroblastoma.

Keywords: doxorubicin; drug combination; drug repurposing; MCF-7 cells; SH-SY5Y cells; atorvastatin; nitrofurantoin

Citation: Moura, C.; Correia, A.S.; Pereira, M.; Ribeiro, E.; Santos, J.; Vale, N. Atorvastatin and Nitrofurantoin Repurposed in the Context of Breast Cancer and Neuroblastoma Cells. *Biomedicines* 2023, 11, 903. https://doi.org/10.3390/biomedicines11030903

Academic Editor: Jun Lu

Received: 8 February 2023
Revised: 1 March 2023
Accepted: 13 March 2023
Published: 15 March 2023

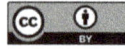

Copyright: © 2023 by the authors. Licensee MDPI, Basel, Switzerland. This article is an open access article distributed under the terms and conditions of the Creative Commons Attribution (CC BY) license (https://creativecommons.org/licenses/by/4.0/).

1. Introduction

Cancer is a disease that involves the abnormal and uncontrolled growth of cells. The fundamental approach of any cancer therapy is to suppress tumor growth, control metastases, and prevent relapse after elimination, thereby prolonging the patient's life. Conventionally used methods of cancer therapy include surgery, chemotherapy, and radiation therapy. Each method has its limitations and, therefore, is often not sufficient to produce satisfactory therapeutic results in patients, which leads to new studies being conducted to try to find new forms of treatments [1].

According to the World Health Organization (WHO), breast cancer is one of the main cancers affecting individuals worldwide, with 2.26 million new cases diagnosed in 2020 [2], which corresponds to the second cause of death from cancer in women [3]. It is assumed that one in eight women in the world will develop mammary gland cancer, and that only 5–10% of all cases of this cancer are caused by genetic diseases, while the remaining 90–95% of cases are linked to environmental and lifestyle factors [4].

Although treatment with single compounds can be beneficial, several recent studies have reported better results in combinations of two or more compounds compared to using a single compound. The combination of drugs has been used in several areas, one of them being cancer. When combining two or more drugs, the main goal is to achieve positive interaction effects that show superior evidence of the beneficial combination of two or more drugs compared to each drug individually, i.e., to achieve more with less [5]. The effects of the combination can be synergistic, antagonistic, or potentiating [6].

Several regimens that include two or more molecularly targeted agents have already been approved, and a number of combinations are in late-stage clinical development. The first combination of two HER2 (also known as ERBB2)-targeted drugs pertuzumab and trastuzumab, along with the chemotherapy agent docetaxel, was approved by the FDA in June 2012 for metastatic breast cancer. The second FDA-approved combination was the combination of a BRAF inhibitor and a MAPK/ERK kinase inhibitor (MEK), which was granted an accelerated approval by the FDA in January 2014 for the treatment of unconventional or metastatic BRAFV600E/K melanoma; both agents were developed by GlaxoSmithKline (GSK) and acquired by Novartis in March 2015. In October 2015, the FDA granted accelerated approval to the first combination immune checkpoint inhibitor, the programmed cell death protein 1 (PD1) inhibitor nivolumab and the cytotoxic T lymphocyte antigen 4 (CTLA4) inhibitor ipilimumab, for BRAFV600 unresectable or metastatic wildtype melanoma [7].

Drug repurposing refers to the application of a drug for another indication than was originally approved and has received increasing interest as an alternative strategy to the synthesis of new drugs. A major advantage of this use is that extensive data are often available, which reduces the need for additional studies to investigate the pharmacokinetic properties and toxicity of drugs. The repurposing of drugs for a new indication may, however, be accompanied by side-effects not previously found, which will require the validation of a new clinical trial [8].

The combination of a reference drug has the objective of already having a safe starting point, since the reference drug already has antitumor activity that is guaranteed in tumor cells. The combination with the repurposed drug, which already has an acceptable toxicological profile, aims to improve the activity of the reference drug and simultaneously reduce its therapeutic dose [9].

In this work, we aimed to focus on drug repurposing and drug combination studies, using atorvastatin (a statin), nitrofurantoin, and doxorubicin (DOX). We aimed to develop a combination model in which both repurposed drugs have synergistic effects when combined with a clinically used chemotherapeutic drug. We decided to choose atorvastatin since it has shown promising results in prostate cancer; moreover, in one study, it inhibited prostate cancer cell growth in a concentration-dependent manner [10]. Nitrofurantoin was chosen because it is a synthetic antibiotic which has been shown to have potential toxic effects attributable to the nitro group (NO_2) attached to the furan ring. The nitro group gives this molecule a toxicophore function, which acts as an electron acceptor, thereby inhibiting enzymes involved in pyruvate metabolism, an essential pathway of cellular metabolism. Nitrofurantoin has also been shown to be cytotoxic against cancer cells, inhibiting proliferation of human leukemia, colon, cervix, and prostate cancer cell lines [11].

There are few references to the interaction between the drugs nitrofurantoin together with atorvastatin, but a possible indication is that it may increase the risk of nerve damage. We intended to understand the effect of these drugs on cancer cells alone and then combined with a potent reference drug doxorubicin, as well as a combination of the three. No work of this kind has ever been performed, and new evidence was found to better understand the combination of nitrofurantoin with atorvastatin.

Statins belong to a group of drugs that work by decreasing blood cholesterol levels through specific inhibition of the enzyme 3-hydroxy-3-methylglutaryl coenzyme A (HMG-CoA) reductase. In addition to these effects on lipid metabolism, statins induce immunomodulatory, anti-inflammatory, and antioxidant activity. During the last few years, antineoplastic effects of statins have also been reported [12]. Atorvastatin (Figure 1A) is one of the most frequently prescribed statins for the prevention of cardiovascular and cerebrovascular diseases. This drug also shows antiproliferative effects on different cancer cells, including breast cancer cells. Thus, atorvastatin has gained increasing interest as a potential therapeutic agent for use as an anticancer treatment. Although the exact mechanism of its antiproliferative effects is currently unknown, atorvastatin both modifies the cell cycle and induces growth suppression or apoptosis of malignant cells. Furthermore, the lipophilic nature of atorvastatin allows it to easily cross the cell membrane and induce these effects [12]. In one study, atorvastatin was shown to have proapoptotic and antimetastatic effects on prostate cancer cells. Parikh et al. hypothesized that atorvastatin may induce autophagy-associated cell death in PC3 cells. However, the biological mechanisms underlying the anticancer effects of atorvastatin have yet to be elucidated [10].

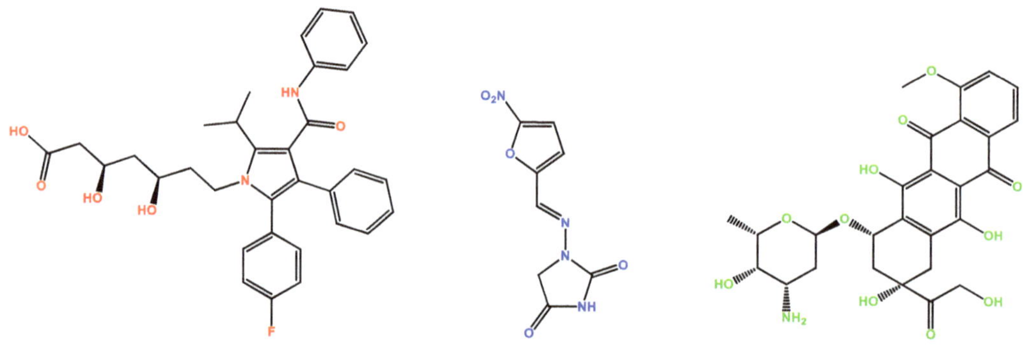

Figure 1. Chemical structure of the drugs applied in this project: (**A**) atorvastatin, (**B**) nitrofurantoin, and (**C**) doxorubicin.

Nitrofurantoin (Figure 1B), an antibiotic drug [13], is a synthetic nitrofuran derivative of hydantoin used for the prevention and treatment of urinary tract infections. The mode of action of this drug involves the reduction of the nitro group by bacterial flavoenzymes producing reactive intermediates and the formation of hydroxyl radicals. These radicals can interact with DNA, resulting in inhibition of nucleic acid synthesis and breaks of single- and double-stranded DNA. Nitrofurantoin has been shown to be cytotoxic against cancer cells, inhibiting proliferation of human leukemia, colon, cervical, and prostate cancer cell lines [11].

Doxorubicin (DOX) (Figure 1C) is an anthracycline antibiotic, isolated from the species *Streptomyces peucetius*, and it is used effectively in several types of cancer [14]. In the cancer cell, DOX intercalates into the DNA and disrupts topoisomerase-II mediated DNA repair. This also generates free radicals that damage cell membranes, DNA, and proteins [1]. Unfortunately, despite being highly effective, doxorubicin is also not selective for cancer cells, meaning its use is significantly limited due to its toxicity [14]. Although DOX is a popular anticancer drug, its clinical results are still unsatisfactory due to the dominant effect of drug resistance mechanisms. In this way, if a higher dosage is prescribed to increase its effectiveness, it may have adverse side-effects on normal tissue cells, primarily affecting the heart and kidneys [1].

As mentioned earlier, doxorubicin is a widely used drug in the treatment of various cancers. Thus, we decided to choose two different cancer cell lines for this work, MCF-7 and SH-SY5Y. MCF-7 cells and SH-SY5Y cells are, respectively, human breast cancer and neuroblastoma cells. Both cell lines are epithelial and were collected from metastatic tumors, having high proliferative capabilities [15,16]. These cell lines represent commonly used human cell lines in research, particularly for the study of breast cancer and neurological diseases, such as Parkinson's disease [17]. Indeed, the MCF-7 cell line is the most studied human breast cancer cell line in the world [18]. In fact, drug repurposing studies are frequently performed in these two cell lines [19,20].

Thus, the main goal of this work was to evaluate the efficacy of atorvastatin and nitrofurantoin on the viability of MCF-7 and SH-SY5Y cells (Scheme 1). We also aimed to analyze the combination of doxorubicin (a reference drug already used in the treatment of breast cancer) with the mentioned repurposed drugs and evaluate whether together these drugs had a greater inhibition in the breast cancer line MCF-7 or in human neuroblastoma SH-SY5Y, and consequently compare the drug combination with the drugs individually.

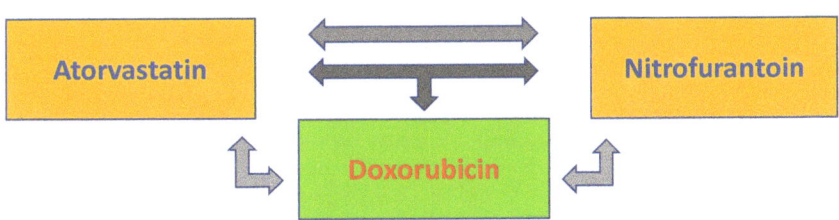

Scheme 1. Drug combination model used in this project.

2. Materials and Methods

2.1. Drug Solutions

For the treatment of the cells with the drugs under study, DOX (Cayman Chemical Company cat. 15007, Cayman Europe, Tallinn, Estonia), ATOR (Sigma-Aldrich cat. PHR1422-1G, Sintra, Portugal), and NITRO (Cayman Chemical Company cat. 23510, Cayman Europe, Tallinn, Estonia), were dissolved in dimethyl sulfoxide (DMSO). A stock solution of each compound was prepared at a concentration of 100 mM for ATOR, at a concentration of 10 mM for DOX, and at a concentration of 200 mM for NITRO. In addition to these stock concentrations, a new stock solution for 200 mM ATOR was then needed. All these stock solutions were kept in the refrigerator at approximately 4 °C. The concentrations used in each assay for DOX were 0.01, 0.1, 1, 5, and 10 µM; those for ATOR and NITRO were 0.1, 1, 10, 25, 50, and 100 µM.

2.2. Cell Culture

The experimental work was performed with MCF-7 and SH-SY5Y (ATCC, American Type Culture Collection, Manassas, VA, USA) cell lines. The cells were incubated at 37 °C in a humidified atmosphere with 95% air and 5% CO_2. Cells were cultured Dulbecco's modified Eagle medium (DMEM), supplemented with 10% fetal bovine serum (FBS) and 1% penicillin/streptomycin mixture (1000 U/mL; 10 mg/mL). For maintenance, cells were cultured in a monolayer and sub-cultured by trypsinization in the same medium when a confluence of ~80% was reached. Cells were maintained in logarithmic growth phase at all timepoints.

2.3. MTT Reduction Assay

Cells were plated in 96-well plates at a seeding density of 5.0×10^4 cells/mL, kept in a 37 °C incubator for 24 h before exposure to the drug. After this time, the cell culture media were replaced with 200 µL of media containing drugs with different treatments and different concentrations for 48 h. The cells were kept at 37 °C for the mentioned time. Then, the cell medium was removed, and 100 µL of MTT solution (0.5 mg/mL in PBS) was added to each well. Subsequently, the cells were incubated at 37 °C for 2 h, protected from light. At the end of this time, MTT was removed, and 100 µL of DMSO was added to each well. The last step consisted of absorbance readings at 570 nm in an automated microplate reader

(Sinergy HT, BioTek Instruments, Winooski, VT, USA) to evaluate the effects with the drugs alone and in combination on the cell viability of MCF-7 and SH-SY5Y cells.

2.4. Evaluation of the Effect of Drugs

Half of the maximum inhibitory concentration (IC_{50}) value was first determined for each drug alone in MCF-7 and SH-SY5Y cells. The concentrations of the drugs used ranged from 0.1 to 100 μM for single drug treatment. The combination studies were performed by combining DOX (Drug 1) with the repurposed drugs (Drug 2), combining DOX with two repurposed drugs, and combining the two repurposed drugs with each other. Only the drugs that showed the most promising pharmacological profile, such as ATOR and NITRO, were tested in combination with DOX and presented in this paper. The concentrations of both Drug 1 and Drug 2 were variable.

2.5. Cell Morphology Visualization

After the treatment with the drugs, the morphological characteristics of MCF-7 and SH-SY5Y cells were captured using a Leica DMI 6000B microscope coupled to a Leica DFC350 FX camera (Leica Microsystems, Wetzlar, Germany). The plate containing the cells was placed on the microscope, and the images of the cells were analyzed on the computer using Leica Las X imaging software (v3.7.4) (Leica Microsystems, Wetzlar, Germany).

2.6. Data Analysis

GraphPad Prism 8 (GraphPad Software Inc., San Diego, CA, USA) was used to create bar graphs of cell viability and to produce concentration–response curves by nonlinear regression analysis. The viability of cells treated with each drug was normalized to the viability of control cells and cell viability fractions were plotted versus drug concentrations on a logarithmic scale.

2.7. Statistical Analysis

Statistical analysis was performed in all experiments. The results are expressed as the arithmetic mean ± standard error of the mean (SEM) for n experiments performed, explicit in the legends of the graphs. Differences between the treated cells and the corresponding untreated control were tested using one-way ANOVA.

2.8. Synergism Studies

Using the CompuSyn software (version 1.0; ComboSyn, Paramus, NJ, USA) and through the Chou–Talalay equation, the combination index (CI) and the fractional effect (Fa) of the combinations were assessed, using a non-fixed ratio. In this context, a CI inferior to 1 indicates synergism between the drugs, while values equal to 1 indicate additivity, and CI values superior to 1 indicate antagonism. The Fa ranges between 0 and 1, representing cellular death, with 0 being no cell death and 1 being total cell death.

3. Results and Discussion

3.1. Effect of the Repurposed Drugs on MCF-7 and SH-SY5Y Cell Viability

To evaluate the effects of atorvastatin (ATOR) on the viability of MCF-7 and SH-SY5Y cells, the cells were treated with this drug in a concentration range between 0.1 and 100 μM for 48 h. The percentage cell viability was evaluated by MTT assay (Figure 2).

Our results demonstrate that ATOR had a significant inhibitory effect for the highest concentrations of 25, 50, and 100 μM (Figures 2 and 3E–G,L–N) for both cells tested; for SH-SY5Y cells, the effect was much more accentuated, which evidences that ATOR had greater cytotoxic effects in these cells, compared to MCF-7 cells. Being neuronal cells, SH-SY5Y cells may be more sensitive to the effects of this drug, explaining these differences between cell lines. Indeed, in a study, statins demonstrated to induce apoptosis in SH-SY5Y cells by reducing the levels of dolichol, required for the biosynthesis of biologically important N-linked glycoproteins [21].

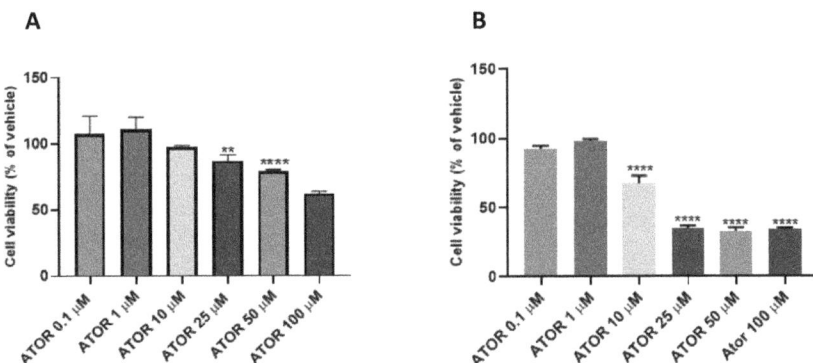

Figure 2. Effect of ATOR on the viability of MCF-7 (**A**) and SH-SY5Y (**B**) cells. The cells were cultured in the presence of increasing concentrations of ATOR. After 48 h, MTT assay was performed to measure cell viability. Values are expressed as percentages and represent the means ± SEM. Each experiment was performed three times independently (n = 3). One-way ANOVA was used as statistical test. Statistically significant ** $p < 0.01$, and **** $p < 0.0001$ vs. vehicle.

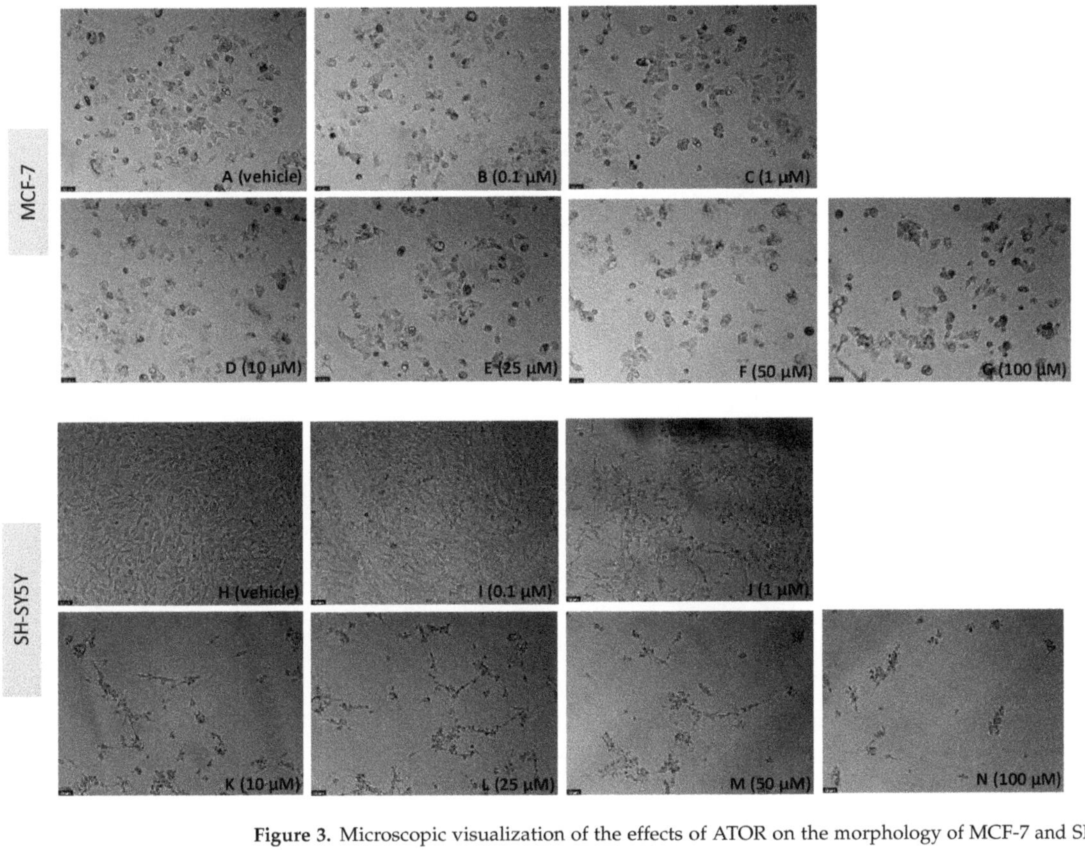

Figure 3. Microscopic visualization of the effects of ATOR on the morphology of MCF-7 and SH-SY5Y cells over 48 h. Cells were treated with (**A,H**) 0.1% DMSO (vehicle) or (**B,I**) 0.1 μM, (**C,J**) 1 μM, (**D,K**) 10 μM, (**E,L**) 25 μM, (**F,M**) 50 μM, or (**G,N**) 100 μM ATOR. Scale bar: 50 μm; 100× total magnification.

For SH-SY5Y cells, viability values of about 35%, 33%, and 34% were obtained for the 25, 50, and 100 µM concentrations, respectively, while, for MCF-7 cells, the cell viability values obtained were 87%, 79%, and 62%, respectively, for the 25, 50, and 100 µM concentrations of ATOR. These cell viability values were also confirmed by cell morphology (Figure 3), whereby, at these concentrations, the cells were rounded and smaller in shape compared to the control (Figure 3A), which shows that these cells are unviable and that, consequently, ATOR had a concentration-dependent inhibitory effect on MCF-7 and SH-SY5Y cells, with this anticancer effect being highest for SH-SY5Y cells. Therefore, it was possible to obtain an IC50 for ATOR for both cell lines tested; with MCF-7, the IC50 obtained was 37.95 µM, whereas, for SH-SY5Y, an IC50 of 10.10 µM was obtained, as evidenced in Table 1. These findings demonstrated that ATOR is a repurposed drug intended for the reduction in blood cholesterol, but it evidenced anticancer effects in MCF-7 and SH-SY5Y cells. Indeed, studies indicate that the growth/survival of some types of cancer depend on the mevalonate pathway, being vulnerable to statin therapy because these drugs inhibit HMG-CoA reductase, an important enzyme of the mevalonate pathway. In fact, statins have been shown to induce tumor-specific apoptosis, being also associated with reduced cancer risk [22].

Table 1. IC50 (half of the maximum inhibitory concentration) values for repurposed drugs atorvastatin and nitrofurantoin against MCF-7 and SY-SY5Y cells.

Drug	IC50 (MCF-7, µM)	IC50 (SH-SY5Y, µM)
Atorvastatin	37.98	10.10
Nitrofurantoin	5.70	>100

The effects of nitrofurantoin (NITR) were evaluated on the viability of MCF-7 and SH-SY5Y cells; for this purpose, cells were treated with NITR in a concentration range between 0.1 and 100 µM for 48 h. The percentage cell viability was assessed by MTT assay (Figure 4).

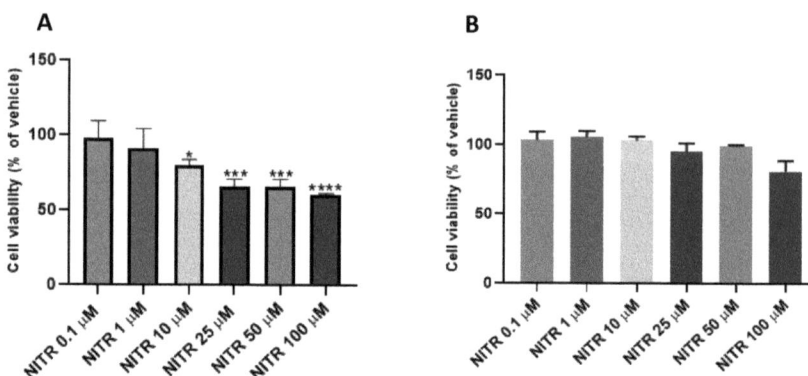

Figure 4. Effects of NITR on cell viability of MCF-7 (**A**) and SH-SY5Y (**B**) cells. The cells were cultured in the presence of increasing concentrations of NITR. After 48 h, MTT assay was performed to evaluate cell viability. Values are expressed as percentages and represent means ± SEM. Each experiment was performed three times independently (n = 3). One-way ANOVA was used as statistical test. Statistically significant * $p < 0.05$, *** $p < 0.001$, and **** $p < 0.0001$ vs. vehicle.

The morphology of MCF-7 and SH-SY5Y cells treated with different concentrations of NITR for 48 h is evidenced in Figure 5.

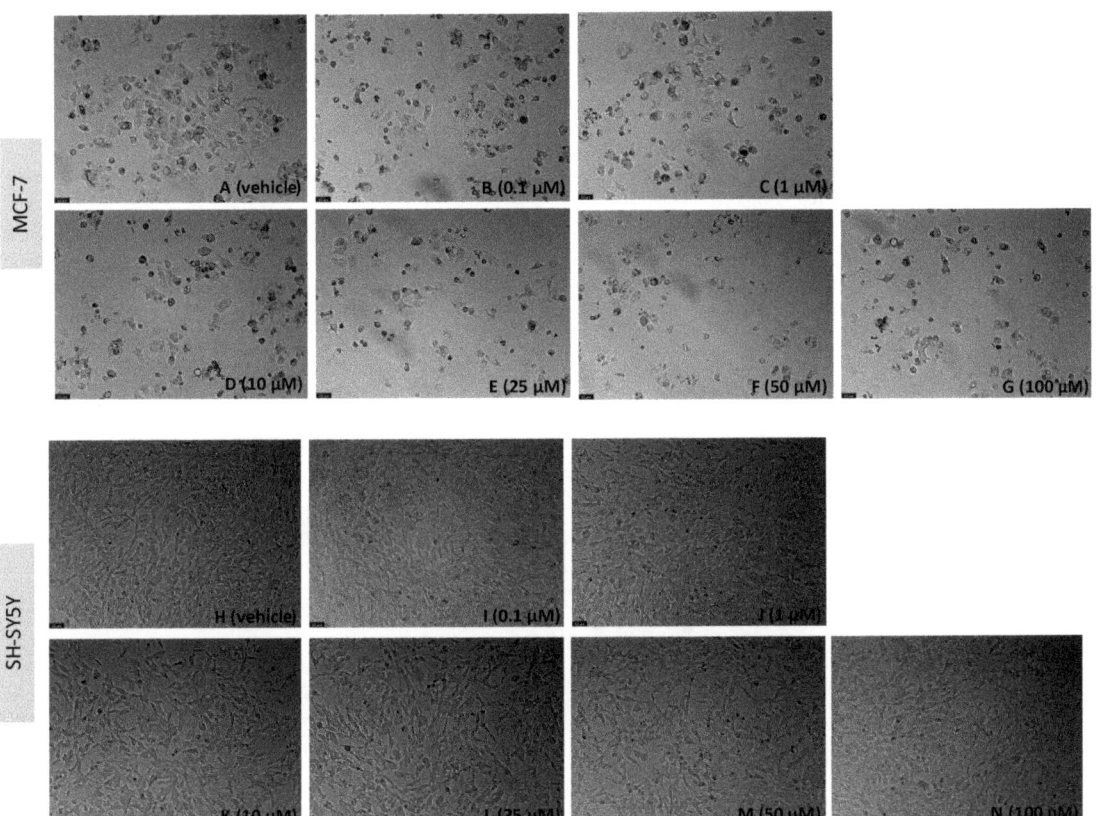

Figure 5. Microscopic visualization of the effects of NITR on the morphology of MCF-7 and SH-SY5Y cells over 48 h. Cells were treated with (**A,H**) 0.1% DMSO (vehicle) or (**B,I**) 0.1 μM, (**C,J**) 1 μM, (**D,K**) 10 μM, (**E,L**) 25 μM, (**F,M**) 50 μM, or (**G,N**) 100 μM NITR. Scale bar: 50 μm; 100× total magnification.

Our results demonstrate that NITR was effective in reducing the cell viability of MCF-7 cells (Figure 4A) for almost all concentrations (10, 25, 50, and 100 μM), for which viability percentages of 80%, 66%, 66%, and 61%, respectively, were obtained. In Figure 5, this effect can also be observed, revealing that the morphology of MCF-7 cells for the previously mentioned concentrations of the NITR was different from the morphology of the control cells (Figure 5A); that is, in the images, it can be observed that there are fewer cells compared to the control and that the cells have a rounded and smaller shape, a characteristic of cells that are unviable. For the SH-SY5Y cell line, a very effective inhibitory effect was not observed, since there was no noticeable decrease in cell viability for any of the concentrations tested. The only concentration that showed a decrease in cell viability was 100 μM, but it only reached a percentage viability of about 81%, and the remaining concentrations tested were close to 100% cell viability. Thus, for MCF-7 cells, it was possible to obtain an IC50 of 5.7 μM (Table 1), a very low and very good value, since this drug is a repurposed drug used for the prevention and treatment of urinary tract infections, now demonstrating anticancer effects for these cells. For the SH-SY5Y cell line, it was not possible to obtain an IC50, since the results showed that NITR in these cells did not have an inhibitory effect on cell viability. Indeed, this pronounced effect on MCF-7 cells may be explained by the evidence that nitrofurantoin interacts with the human BCRP (breast cancer resistance protein) (https://pubmed.ncbi.nlm.nih.gov/15709111/, accessed on

1 September 2022). However, there are few studies about the effect of this drug in both breast cancer and neuroblastoma, making it interesting to explore the differential effects of this drug in this cell cultures. Nevertheless, some studies demonstrated cytotoxic activity of this drug. For example, in HL-60 leukemia cells, this drug upregulated BAX and downregulated BCL-xL expression, inducing apoptosis [11].

3.2. Effect of Different Combinations of DOX and Repurposed Drugs on the Cell Viability of MCF-7 and SH-SY5Y Cells

To evaluate the different combinations of DOX with ATOR on the viability of MCF-7 and SH-SY5Y cells, cells were treated with 0.17 μM DOX (IC50 obtained for doxorubicin by the research group) [23] and with ATOR in a concentration range between 0.1 and 100 μM for 48 h. The percentage cell viability was assessed by MTT assay (Figure 6).

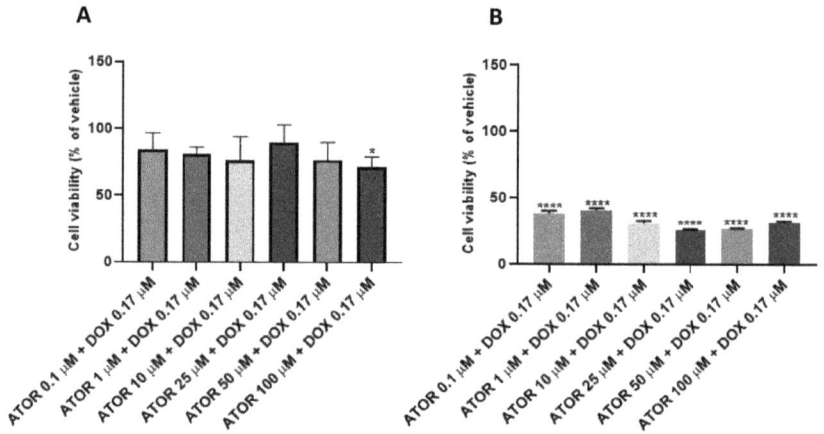

Figure 6. Effects of combining DOX with ATOR on cell viability of MCF-7 (**A**) and SH-SY5Y (**B**) cells. Cells were cultured in the presence of a single concentration of DOX (0.17 μM) and with increasing concentrations of ATOR. After 48 h, the MTT assay was performed to measure cell viability. Values are expressed as percentages and represent means ± SEM. Each experiment was performed three times independently (n = 3). One-way ANOVA was used as statistical test. Statistically significant * $p < 0.05$, and **** $p < 0.0001$ vs. vehicle.

Through the results obtained for the combination of DOX with ATOR for the SH-SY5Y cell line (Figures 6B and 7), it is possible to observe that this combination was very beneficial for both DOX and ATOR, since, for almost all the results obtained (except ATOR 100 μM + DOX 0.17 μM), the cell viability decreased greatly compared to ATOR individually, and the cell viability for all combinations always remained below 50%. A possible explanation for these achievements may be that DOX may increase the sensitivity of cells to the effect of other drugs, potentiating their apoptotic effects. Indeed, chemosensitization is a strategy to overcome chemoresistance, based on the use of one drug to potentiate the activity of another [24].

The combination for this cell line that obtained the best results was 0.17 μM DOX with 25 μM ATOR, which achieved a cell viability of about 26%, i.e., a cell death rate of about 74%. Contrary to SH-SY5Y cells, MCF-7 cell viability did not stay below 50% for any of the tested combinations, but this combination still managed to be very beneficial for ATOR, since, for almost all combinations, it was possible to decrease cell viability and consequently increase cell death, except for the concentration of 0.17 μM DOX with 25 μM ATOR, where this decrease was not visible and, therefore, cell viability remained the same for the combination and for ATOR alone. Thus, we can see that these two drugs together showed quite marked cytotoxic effects in SH-SY5Y cells and little effect in MCF-7 cells compared to the drugs tested individually; consequently, each drug was able to potentiate the other to have better effects, increasing cell death in the cells tested.

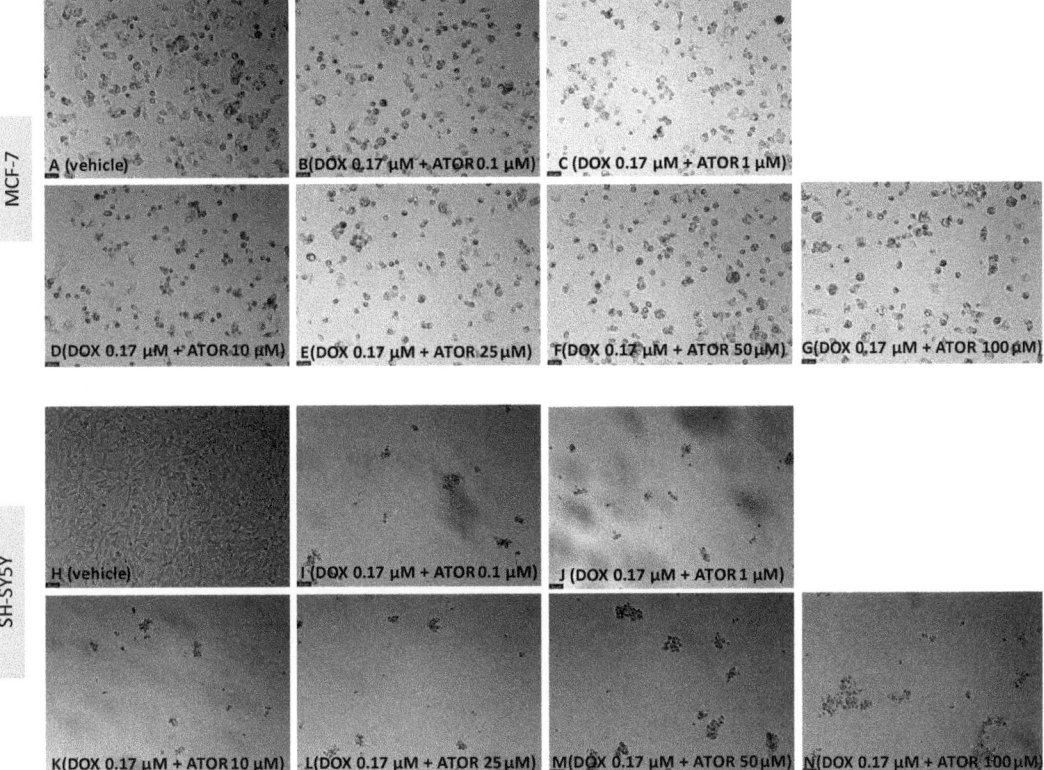

Figure 7. Microscopic visualization of the effects of combining DOX with ATOR on the morphology of MCF-7 and SH-SY5Y cells for 48 h. Cells were treated with (**A,H**) 0.1% DMSO (control), (**B,I**) 0.17 μM DOX + 0.1 μM ATOR, (**C,J**) 0.17 μM DOX + 1 μM ATOR, (**D,K**) 0, 17 μM DOX + 10 μM ATOR, (**E,L**) 0.17 μM DOX + 25 μM ATOR, (**F,M**) 0.17 μM DOX + 50 μM ATOR, or (**G,N**) 0.17 μM DOX + 100 μM ATOR. Scale bar: 50 μm; 100× total magnification.

The effects of different combinations of DOX with NITR were evaluated on the viability of MCF-7 cells; for this purpose, MCF-7 cells were treated with 0.17 μM DOX and with NITR in a range of concentrations between 0.1 and 100 μM for 48 h. The percentage cell viability was assessed by MTT assay (Figure 8).

Figure 9 shows the microscopic visualization of the MCF-7 breast cancer cell line and the SH-SY5Y cell line treated with the different combinations of DOX with NITR over a period of 48 h.

Through the results obtained for the combination of DOX with NITR (Figures 8 and 9), we can observe that this combination of these two drugs was very effective for SH-SY5Y cells, since, for all tested combinations, a very low cell viability was reached (always below 40%) when compared to the individual drugs. For NITR, no decrease in cell viability was evident, which demonstrates that these two drugs together potentiated each other. For the MCF-7 cell line, slight decreases in cell viability were also observed, which shows that this combination was also beneficial for these cells; however, the increases in cell death observed were not as sharp as for the SH-SY5Y cells.

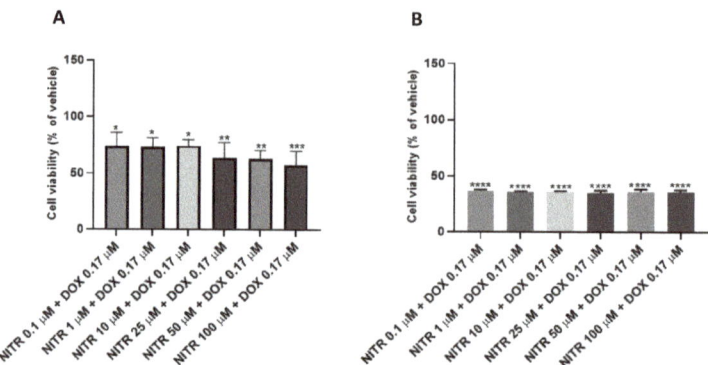

Figure 8. Effects of combining DOX with NITR on cell viability of MCF-7 (**A**) and SH-SY5Y (**B**) cells. The cells were cultured in the presence of a single concentration of DOX (0.17 µM) and with increasing concentrations of NITR. After 48 h, MTT assay was performed to measure cell viability. Values are expressed as percentages and represent means ± SEM. Each experiment was performed three times independently (n = 3). One-way ANOVA was used as statistical test. Statistically significant * $p < 0.05$, ** $p < 0.01$, *** $p < 0.001$, and **** $p < 0.0001$ vs. vehicle.

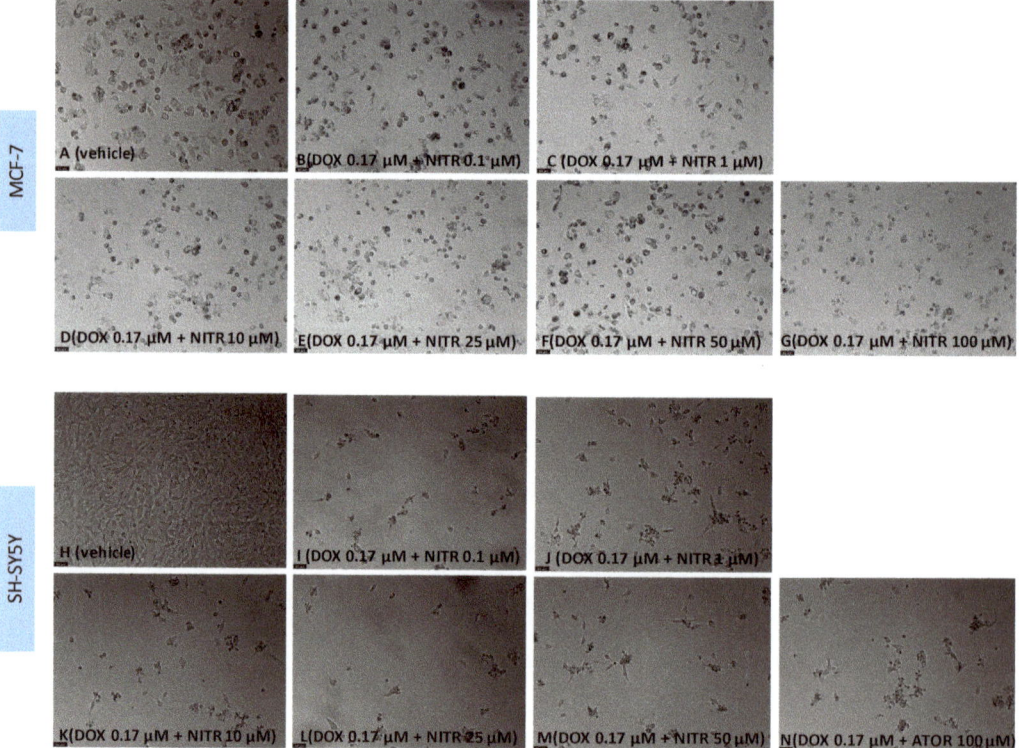

Figure 9. Microscopic visualization of the effects of combining DOX with NITR on the morphology of MCF-7 cells for 48 h. Cells were treated with (**A,H**) 0.1% DMSO (control), (**B,I**) 0.17 µM DOX + 0.1 µM NITR, (**C,J**) 0.17 µM DOX + 1 µM NITR, (**D,K**) 0.17 µM DOX + 10 µM NITR, (**E,L**) 0.17 µM DOX + 25 µM NITR, (**F,M**) 0.17 µM DOX + 50 µM NITR, or (**G,N**) 0.17 µM DOX + 100 µM NITR. Scale bar: 50 µm; 100× total magnification.

To evaluate the different combinations of ATOR with NITR on the viability of MCF-7 and SH-SY5Y cells, cells were treated with ATOR and NITR at concentrations between 0.1 and 100 µM for 48 h. The percentage of cell viability was assessed by MTT assay (Figure 10).

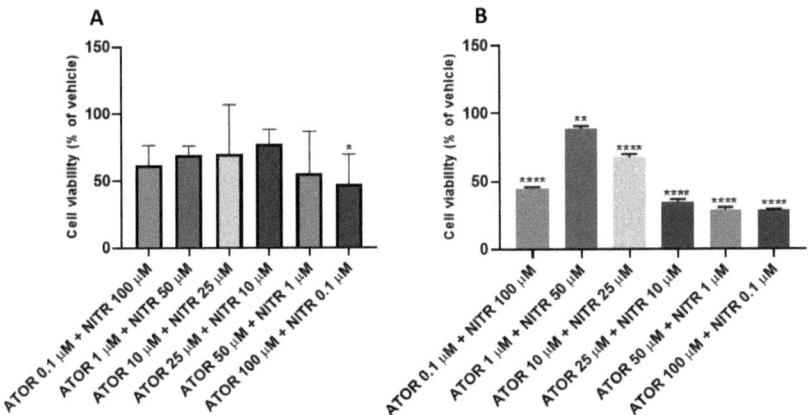

Figure 10. Effects of the combination of ATOR and NITR on cell viability of MCF-7 (**A**) and SH-SY5Y (**B**) cells. The cells were cultured in the presence of concentrations between 0.1 and 100 µM of ATOR and NITR. After 48 h, MTT assay was performed to measure cell viability. Values are expressed as percentages and represent means ± SEM. Each experiment was performed three times independently (n = 3). One-way ANOVA was used as statistical test. Statistically significant * $p < 0.05$, ** $p < 0.01$, and **** $p < 0.0001$ vs. vehicle.

Figure 11 shows the microscopic visualization of the MCF-7 breast cancer cell line and the SH-SY5Y cell line treated with the different combinations of ATOR with NITR over a period of 48 h.

Through the results obtained for the combination of ATOR with NITR (Figures 10 and 11), it is visible that this combination was beneficial, since, for all combinations, there was a decrease in cell viability compared to the drugs separately. Observing Figure 10, it is possible to verify that, the combination of 0.1 µM ATOR with 100 µM NITR yielded the best effect. When compared with the individual results of these drugs (Figures 2 and 4), we can affirm that, for this combination, there was a very sharp increase in cell death, since the cell viability of the drugs individually was around 108% for the concentration of 0.1 ATOR and 61% for the concentration of 100 NITR, whereas, when combined, these two drugs for these concentrations managed to achieve a cell death of about 38% for MCF-7 cells. For SH-SY5Y cells, the cell death of the individual drugs was around 7% for the concentration of 0.1 ATOR and 19% for the concentration of 100 NITR; when combined, these two drugs for this concentration achieved a cell death of about 55% for SH-SY5Y cells. Thus, we can state that both drugs potentiate each other; furthermore, for MCF-7 cells, NITR potentiates ATOR more than vice versa, whereas, for SH-SY5Y cells, it is ATOR that potentiates NITR. These results may be sustained by the effects of these drugs individually, demonstrated above.

The effects of different combinations of DOX with ATOR and with NITR were evaluated on the viability of MCF-7 and SH-SY5Y cells; for this purpose, cells were treated with 0.17 µM DOX and with concentrations between 0.1 and 100 µM ATOR and NITR for 48 h. The percentage cell viability was assessed by MTT (Figure 12).

Figure 13 shows the microscopic visualization of the MCF-7 breast cancer cell line and the SH-SY5Y cell line treated with the different combinations of DOX with ATOR and with NITR over a period of 48 h.

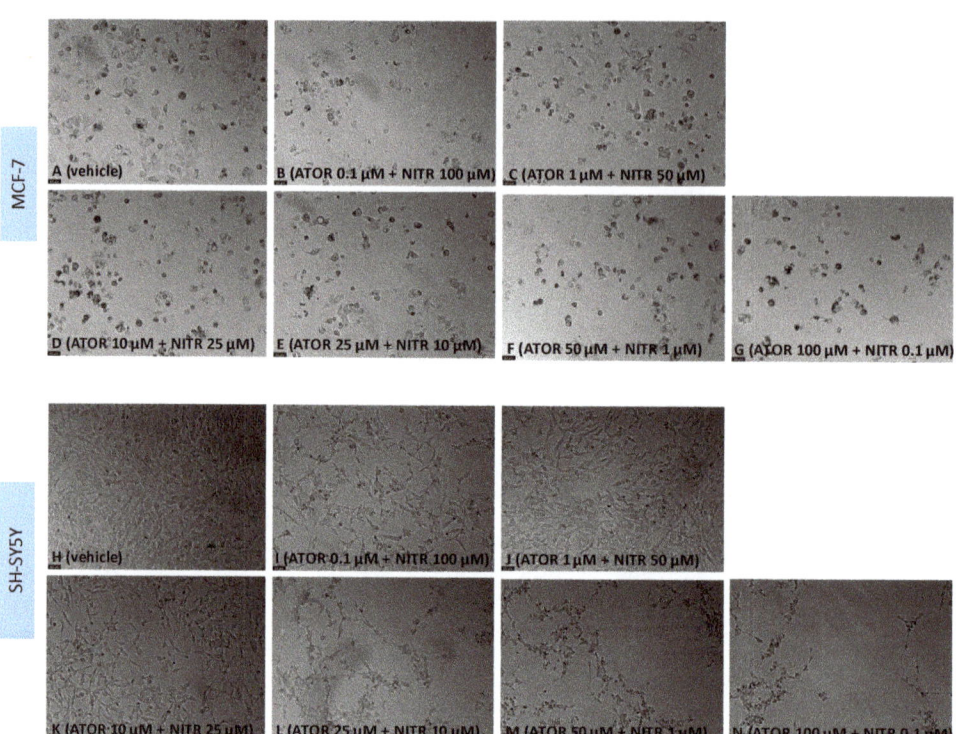

Figure 11. Microscopic visualization of the effects of combining ATOR with NITR on the morphology of MCF-7 cells for 48 h. Cells were treated with (**A,H**) 0.1% DMSO (control), (**B,I**) 0.1 μM ATOR + 100 μM NITR, (**C,J**) 1 μM ATOR + 50 μM NITR, (**D,K**) 10 μM ATOR + 25 μM NITR, (**E,L**) 25 μM ATOR + 10 μM NITR, (**F,M**) 50 μM ATOR + 1 μM NITR, or (**G,N**) 100 μM ATOR + 0.1 μM NITR. Scale bar: 50 μm; 100× total magnification.

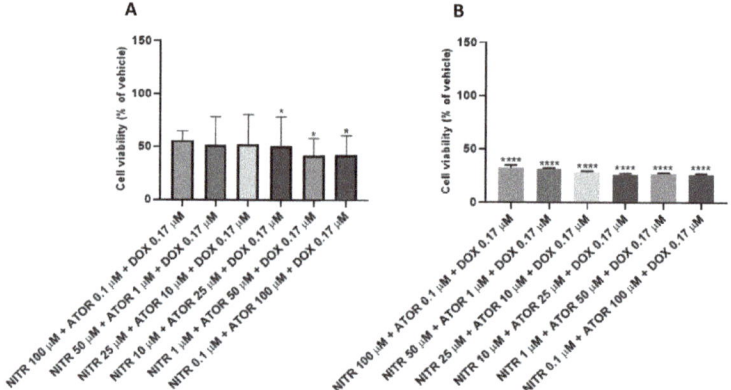

Figure 12. Effects of combining DOX with ATOR and with NITR on cell viability of MCF-7 (**A**) and SH-SY5Y (**B**) cells. The cells were cultured in the presence of concentrations between 0.1 and 100 μM of ATOR and NITR. After 48 h, MTT assay was performed to measure cell viability. Values are expressed as percentages and represent means ± SEM. Each experiment was performed three times independently (n = 3). One-way ANOVA was used as statistical test. Statistically significant * $p < 0.05$, and **** $p < 0.0001$ vs. vehicle.

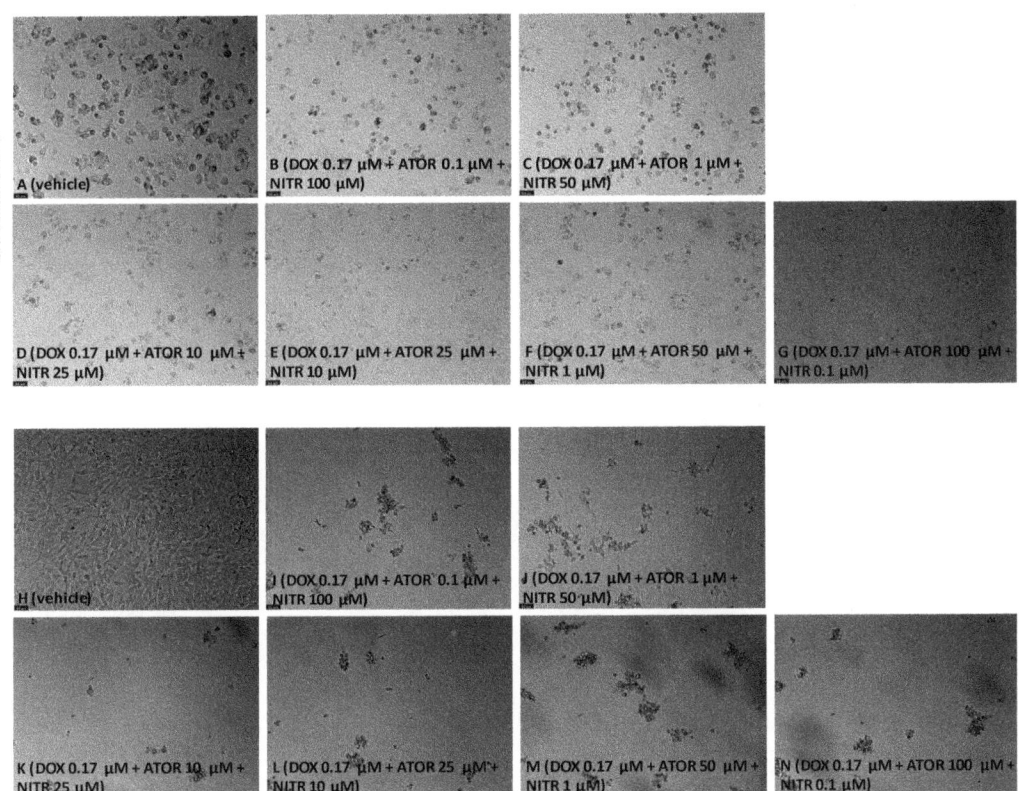

Figure 13. Microscopic visualization of the effects of combining DOX with ATOR and with NITR on the morphology of MCF-7 and SH-SY5Y cells for 48 h. Cells were treated with (**A,H**) 0.1% DMSO (control), (**B,I**) 0.17 µM DOX + 0.1 µM ATOR + 100 µM NITR, (**C,J**) 0.17 µM DOX + 1 µM ATOR + 50 µM NITR, (**D,K**) 0, 17 µM DOX + 10 µM ATOR + 25 µM NITR, (**E,L**) 0.17 µM DOX + 25 µM ATOR + 10 µM NITR, (**F,M**) 0.17 µM DOX + 50 µM ATOR + 1 µM NITR, or (**G,N**) 0.17 µM DOX + 100 µM ATOR + 0.1 µM NITR. Scale bar: 50 µm; 100× total magnification.

Through the results obtained for the combination of DOX with ATOR and NITR (Figures 12 and 13), we can observe that, for the three tested combinations, all managed to achieve lower cell viability compared to the cell viability of all drugs separately for both cell lines tested. From Figure 12, we can see that the combination that achieved the highest cell death for MCF-7 cells was 0.17 µM DOX with 50 µM ATOR and with 1 µM NITR, which reached a cell viability of about 42%; for SH-SY5Y cells, 0.17 µM DOX with 100 µM ATOR and with 0.1 µM NITR reached a cell viability of about 26%. Thus, we can observe that the combination of DOX with ATOR and NITR was able to further potentiate these drugs to achieve higher cell death, and we can conclude that the combination of DOX with ATOR and with NITR was quite good in reducing the viability of MCF-7 and SH-SY5Y cells; consequently, all drugs potentiated each other.

3.3. Synergistic Combinations of DOX and Repurposed Drugs

To investigate the effects of the combinations of DOX with the repurposed drugs, atorvastatin and nitrofurantoin, and of the repurposed drugs with each other, the combi-nation index (CI) was calculated according to the Chou–Talalay method using CompuSyn software. The Chou–Talalay method is based on the median effect equation, derived from the principle of the law of mass action. This unified theory encompasses the Michaelis–Menten, Hill, Henderson–Hasselbalch, and Scatchard equations in biochemistry and biophysics and provides a quantitative definition for additive effect (CI = 1), synergism (CI < 1), and antagonism (CI > 1) in drug combinations [25]. The fractional effect is a value between 0 and 1, where 0 means that the drug did not affect cell viability, and 1 means that the drug had a full effect in decreasing cell viability [19,26]. The combination of DOX with atorvastatin in MCF-7 cells did not show synergism for any of the combinations tested (Table 2), showing that these two drugs had an antagonistic action in these cells, with a CI greater than 1 for all pairs of combinations. For SH-SY5Y cells, this combination was very promising, since the combination of 0.17 µM DOX with 100 µM ATOR was the only one that did not show synergism, while all other synergistic pairs showed synergism in this cell line and an Fa value of 0.74 (Table 2).

Table 2. Fractional effect (Fa) and combination index (CI) values ATOR and DOX combinations for 48 h in MCF-7 and SH-SY5Y cells. CI < 1 synergism, CI = 1 additivity, and CI > 1 antagonism. Fa values range from 0 (no cellular death) to 1 (complete cellular death).

Dose DOX (µM)	Dose ATOR (µM)	MCF-7		SH-SY5Y	
		Effect (Fa)	CI	Effect (Fa)	CI
0.17	0.1	0.15985	3.16E20	0.61633	0.38916
	1.0	0.19309	2.64E31	0.59243	0.45248
	10.0	0.23632	3.52E43	0.68567	0.38837
	25.0	0.10102	10.5377	0.73556	0.40282
	50.0	0.2349	8.02E43	0.73363	0.60022
	100.0	0.28865	1.88E56	0.68255	1.41110

For the combination of DOX with NITRO, for MCF-7 cells, this was the most promising combination for this cell line, with three synergistic pairs and an Fa value reaching 0.54 (Table 3); for SH-SY5Y cells, this combination was one of the most promising with all pairs of combinations being synergistic, i.e., with CI < 1 and with almost all Fa values reaching 0.65 (Table 3).

Table 3. Fractional effect (Fa) and CI (combination index) values of NITRO and DOXO combinations for 48 h in MCF-7 and SH-SY5Y cells. CI < 1 synergism, CI = 1 additivity, and CI > 1 antagonism. Fa values range from 0 (no cellular death) to 1 (complete cellular death).

Dose DOXO (µM)	Dose NITRO (µM)	MCF-7		SH-SY5Y	
		Effect (Fa)	CI	Effect (Fa)	CI
0.17	0.1	0.26221	1.67662	0.63341	0.35821
	1.0	0.26396	1.65830	0.64722	0.33785
	10.0	0.25571	1.81996	0.64172	0.36880
	25.0	0.53983	0.28529	0.65123	0.38937
	50.0	0.37222	0.79532	0.64143	0.46750
	100.0	0.42196	0.58248	0.64410	0.58474

For the combination of ATOR with NITRO, in MCF-7 cells, this combination did not result in any synergism, with CI > 1 for all concentration pairs (Table 4); for SH-SY5Y cells, this combination resulted in four synergistic pairs, with an Fa value of 0.71 (Table 4).

Lastly, for the combination of DOX with ATOR and with NITRO, in MCF-7 cells, this combination did not show synergism in any of the combinations tested (Table 5); in SH-SY5Y cells, this combination was one of the most promising, with all synergistic pairs showing synergism, i.e., CI < 1 for all combinations tested (Table 5). These results, thus, demonstrated that NITRO and ATOR may be promising combinations.

Table 4. Fractional effect (Fa) and CI (combination index) values of ATOR and NITRO combinations for 48 h in MCF-7 and SH-SY5Y cells. CI < 1 synergism, CI = 1 additivity, and CI > 1 antagonism. Fa values range from 0 (no cellular death) to 1 (complete cellular death).

Dose ATOR (µM)	Dose NITRO (µM)	MCF-7		SH-SY5Y	
		Effect (Fa)	CI	Effect (Fa)	CI
0.1	100.0	0.38063	1.71E71	0.55072	0.29008
1.0	50.0	0.30337	2.14E57	0.11475	1.24825
10.0	25.0	0.29898	2.68E57	0.32571	1.25105
25.0	10.0	0.22573	2.32E41	0.65215	0.37312
50.0	1.0	0.44593	4.03E85	0.71205	0.45641
100.0	0.1	0.52423	3.16E99	0.7135	0.8988

Table 5. Fractional effect (Fa) and CI (combination index) values of ATOR, NITRO, and DOX combinations for 48 h in MCF-7 and SH-SY5Y cells. CI < 1 synergism, CI = 1 additivity, and CI > 1 antagonism. Fa values range from 0 (no cellular death) to 1 (complete cellular death).

Dose ATOR (µM)	Dose NITRO (µM)	Dose DOX (µM)	MCF-7		SH-SY5Y	
			Effect (Fa)	CI	Effect (Fa)	CI
0.1	100.0		0.44234	1.89E82	0.67706	0.52120
1.0	50.0		0.48526	5.62E90	0.68137	0.40941
10.0	25.0	0.17	0.47763	2.68E90	0.71715	0.37664
25.0	10.0		0.49533	7.79E93	0.73526	0.42406
50.0	1.0		0.58165	1.8E109	0.73081	0.61436
100.0	0.1		0.57114	5.0E107	0.73571	0.96965

Figures 14 and 15 show the Fa–CI plots of the combinations in the MCF-7 and SH-SY5Y cell lines, respectively.

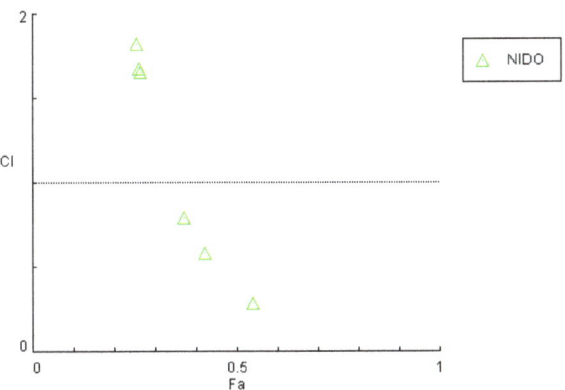

Figure 14. Fa–CI plot of combinations in MCF-7 cell line. Only the NIT + DOX combination (green) had CI values in this graph range of CI (0–2).

The dose reduction index (DRI) was also calculated; this index refers to the percentage of dose reduction for each drug within the combination that can be reduced to generate a specific effect as a result of the synergy. A DRI > 1 indicates a favorable dose reduction, while a DRI < 1 represents an unfavorable dose reduction, and a DRI = 1 shows no corresponding dose reduction. It is also necessary to mention that DRI is associated with CI, but it is only the CI values that effectively verify the synergism or antagonism of drug combinations. It should then be considered that, once the dose of a drug is reduced, the toxicity of this drug will eventually decrease [27].

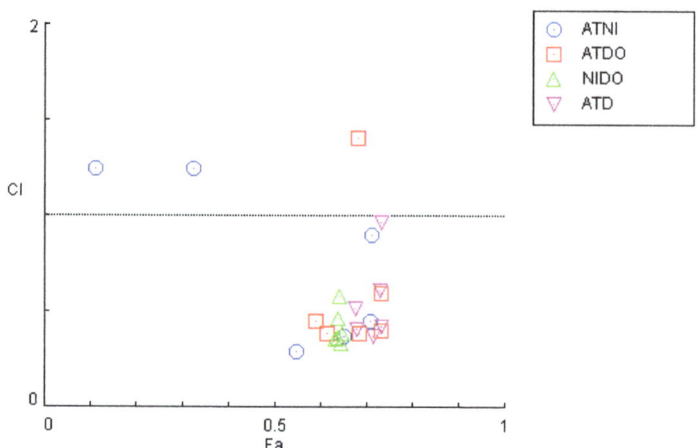

Figure 15. Fa–CI plot of combinations in SH-SY5Y cell line. Combinations: ATOR + NIT (blue), ATOR + DOX (red), NIT + DOX (green), and ATOR + NIT + DOX (pink).

Figures 16 and 17 show the Fa–DRI plots of the combinations in the MCF-7 and SH-SY5Y cell lines, respectively.

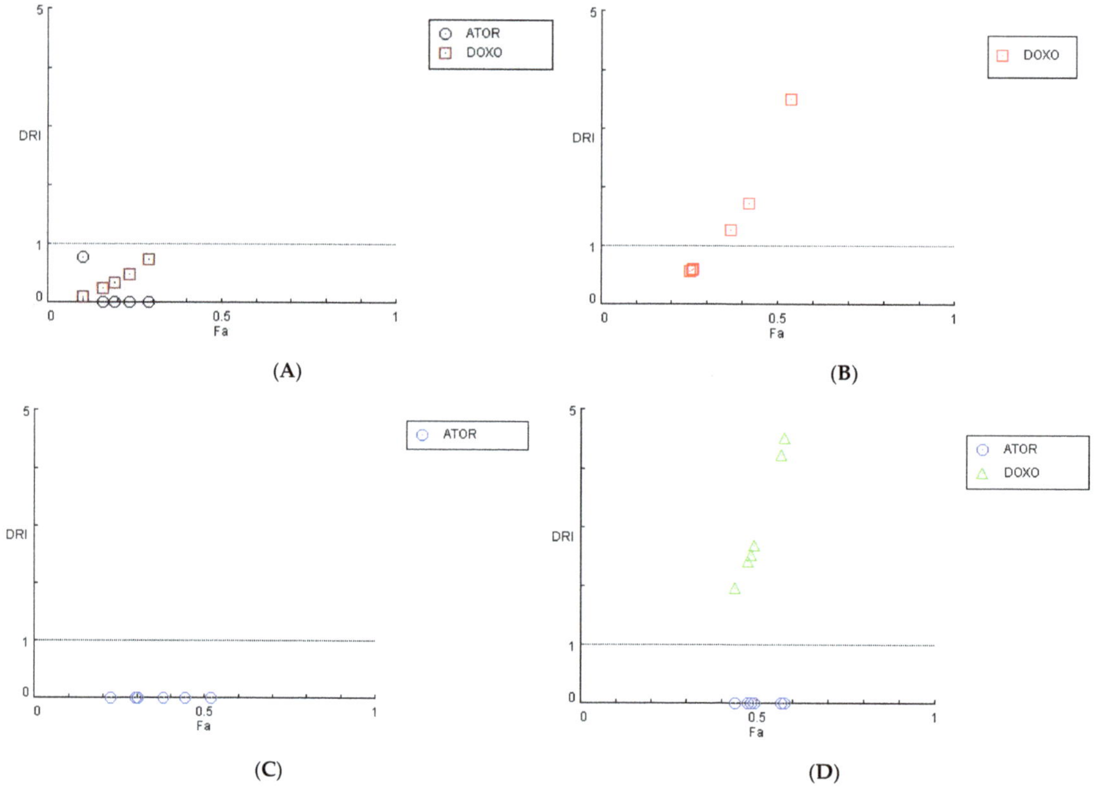

Figure 16. Fa–DRI plot of combinations in MCF-7 cell line. Combinations: ATOR + DOX (**A**), NIT + DOX (**B**), ATOR + NIT (**C**), and ATOR + NIT + DOX (**D**).

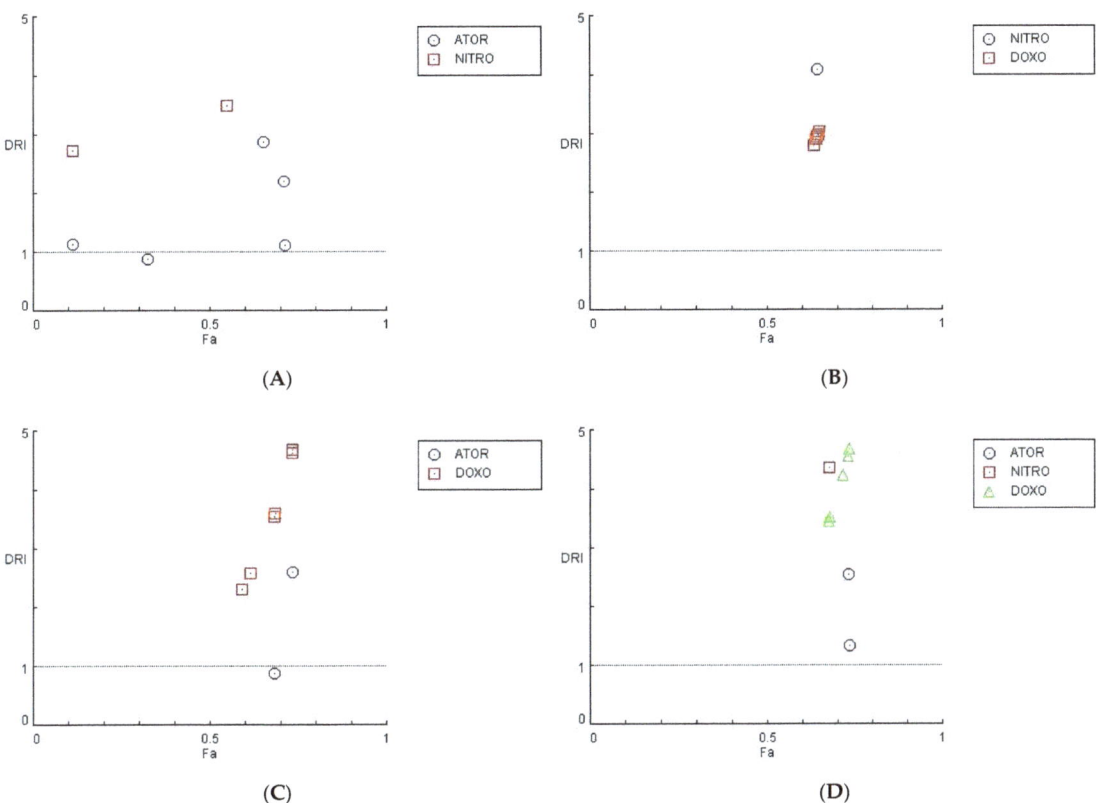

Figure 17. Fa–DRI plot of combinations in SH-SY5Y cell line. Combinations: ATOR + DOX (**A**), NIT + DOX (**B**), ATOR + NIT (**C**), and ATOR + NIT + DOX (**D**).

For MCF-7 cells, the combinations of DOX with ATOR and ATOR with NIT showed a DRI < 1 (Figure 16A,C), which indicates that there should be no dose reduction, i.e., these combinations show an unfavorable dose reduction. In contrast, the combinations of DOX with NIT and of DOX with ATOR and NIT (Figure 16B,D) had a DRI > 1, which shows that these combinations can benefit from favorable dose reduction.

For SH-SY5Y cells, for all combinations tested, a DRI > 1 was evidenced (Figure 17), which highlights that all these combinations in this cell line can benefit from a favorable dose reduction.

Through this synergy analysis, we demonstrated that the two repurposed drugs tested in this study can synergistically decrease cell viability when combined with DOX for SH-SY5Y cells. Our results revealed more synergistic pairs for SH-SY5Y compared to MCF-7 cells, with almost all the combinations tested resulting in synergistic pairs for the lowest concentrations. For MCF-7 cells, the results evidenced that almost all the tested combinations did not result in synergistic pairs; hence, ATOR and NITRO cannot synergistically decrease the cell viability of MCF-7 cells when combined with DOX.

Although the exact mechanism of its antiproliferative effects is currently unknown, atorvastatin both modifies the cell cycle and induces suppression of growth or apoptosis of malignant cells. Furthermore, the lipophilic nature of atorvastatin allows it to easily cross the cell membrane and induce these effects. Indeed, a previous study reported that ATOR treatment at concentrations of up to 80 µM caused a decrease in the viability of MCF-7 cells after 24 h and 48 h [12]. These results are in concordance with our results in which cell viability decreases were also observed for MCF-7 cells. The other repurposed drug, NTRO, is a synthetic antibiotic that has potential toxic effects attributable to the nitro group (NO_2) attached to the furan ring. The nitro group gives this molecule a toxicophoric function, which acts as an electron acceptor, thus inhibiting enzymes involved in pyruvate metabolism, an essential pathway of cellular metabolism [11].

As explained above, SH-SY5Y cells are neuronal cells. These kinds of cells are known to be more sensitive to cytotoxic effects than breast cells. Indeed, this study is innovative because there are few reports about these drugs in these types of cells. Future studies focused on the molecular mechanisms underlying the differences between these cells regarding the obtained responses in this study are very important. Nevertheless, this study revealed the potential of drug combination and repurposing in the context of cancer treatment.

4. Conclusions

We concluded that ATOR had inhibitory effects on the viability of both tumor cell lines tested, MCF-7 and SH-SY5Y, and that NITRO showed inhibitory effects on the growth and viability of MCF-7 cells, while, in SH-SY5Y cells, this repurposed drug did not show any cytotoxic effects. Regarding the combination of DOX, the reference drug used in breast cancer, with the repurposed drugs, it is possible to conclude that, for all tested combinations, there was a reduction in cell viability and, consequently, an increase in cell death. Thus, DOX was able to potentiate ATOR and NITRO in both cells tested. Concerning the combination of ATOR with NITRO, it is possible to see that both drugs were able to potentiate each other, but that NITRO showed a greater potentiation on ATOR for MCF-7 cells; on the other hand, for human neuroblastoma cells (SH-SY5Y), the opposite occurred, i.e., ATOR showed a higher potentiation on NITRO, since it had no inhibitory effect on these cells when isolated and, when combined with ATOR, showed quite high cytotoxic effects. Through synergism, it was possible to conclude that the combinations of DOX with the repurposed drugs were more advantageous in SH-SY5Y cells than in MCF-7 cells, since, for all tested combinations, synergism was always evidenced for almost all studied combination pairs. This new drug combination model opens the door to a new pharmacological interaction between different reused drugs combined with each other or combined again but with a reference drug in oncology.

Author Contributions: Conceptualization, N.V.; methodology, C.M., A.S.C., M.P., E.R. and J.S.; formal analysis, C.M., A.S.C., M.P., E.R., J.S. and N.V.; investigation, C.M. and N.V.; writing—original draft preparation, C.M.; writing—review and editing, N.V.; supervision, N.V.; project administration, N.V.; funding acquisition, N.V. All authors have read and agreed to the published version of the manuscript.

Funding: This work was financed by FEDER—Fundo Europeu de Desenvolvimento Regional through the COMPETE 2020—Operational Program for Competitiveness and Internationalization (POCI), Portugal 2020, and by Portuguese funds through FCT—Fundação para a Ciência e a Tecnologia, in the framework of the projects in CINTESIS, R&D Unit (reference UIDB/4255/2020) and within the scope of the project RISE—LA/P/0053/2020. N.V. also acknowledges the support from FCT and FEDER (European Union), award number IF/00092/2014/CP1255/CT0004 and CHAIR in Onco-Innovation at FMUP.

Institutional Review Board Statement: Not applicable.

Informed Consent Statement: Not applicable.

Data Availability Statement: Not applicable.

Acknowledgments: A.S.C. thanks FCT for the PhD Grant (SFRH/BD/146093/2019). M.P. acknowledges FCT for funding her PhD grant (2021.07450.BD). N.V. acknowledges support from FCT and FEDER (European Union), award number IF/00092/2014/CP1255/CT0004 and CHAIR in Onco-Innovation from FMUP.

Conflicts of Interest: The authors declare no conflict of interest.

References

1. Lakkakula, J.R.; Gujarathi, P.; Pansare, P.; Tripathi, S. A comprehensive review on alginate-based delivery systems for the delivery of chemotherapeutic agent: Doxorubicin. *Carbohydr. Polym.* **2021**, *259*, 117696. [CrossRef] [PubMed]
2. Wu, T.; Arevalo, C.; Hsu, F.-C.; Hong, S.; Parada, H.; Yang, M.; Pierce, J.P. Independent and Joint Associations of Pessimism, Total Calorie Intake and Acid-Producing Diets with Insomnia Symptoms among Breast Cancer Survivors. *J. Clin. Med.* **2022**, *11*, 2828. [CrossRef] [PubMed]
3. Wild, C.P.; Weiderpass, E.; Stewart, B.W. (Eds.) *World Cancer Report: Cancer Research for Cancer Prevention*; International Agency for Research on Cancer: Lyon, France, 2020. Available online: http://publications.iarc.fr/586 (accessed on 12 January 2023).
4. Kolak, A.; Kamińska, M.; Sygit, K.; Budny, A.; Surdyka, D.; Kukiełka-Budny, B.; Burdan, F. Primary and secondary prevention of breast cancer. *Ann. Agric. Environ. Med. AAEM* **2017**, *24*, 549–553. [CrossRef]
5. Duarte, D.; Vale, N. Evaluation of synergism in drug combinations and reference models for future orientations in oncology. *Curr. Res. Pharmacol. Drug Discov.* **2022**, *3*, 100110. [CrossRef] [PubMed]
6. Batra, H.; Pawar, S.; Bahl, D. Curcumin in combination with anti-cancer drugs: A nanomedicine review. *Pharmacol. Res.* **2019**, *139*, 91–105. [CrossRef]
7. Webster, R.M. Combination therapies in oncology. *Nat. Rev. Drug Discov.* **2016**, *15*, 81–82. [CrossRef]
8. Sleire, L.; Førde, H.E.; Netland, I.A.; Leiss, L.; Skeie, B.S.; Enger, P.Ø. Drug repurposing in cancer. *Pharmacol. Res.* **2017**, *124*, 74–91. [CrossRef]
9. Duarte, D.; Vale, N. New Trends for Antimalarial Drugs: Synergism between Antineoplastics and Antimalarials on Breast Cancer Cells. *Biomolecules* **2020**, *10*, 1623. [CrossRef]
10. He, Z.; Yuan, J.; Qi, P.; Zhang, L.; Wang, Z. Atorvastatin induces autophagic cell death in prostate cancer cells in vitro. *Mol. Med. Rep.* **2015**, *11*, 4403–4408. [CrossRef]
11. Andrade, J.K.F.; Souza, M.I.F.; Gomes Filho, M.A.; Silva, D.M.F.; Barros, A.L.S.; Rodrigues, M.D.; Silva, P.B.N.; Nascimento, S.C.; Aguiar, J.S.; Brondani, D.J.; et al. N-pentyl-nitrofurantoin induces apoptosis in HL-60 leukemia cell line by upregulating BAX and downregulating BCL-xL gene expression. *Pharmacol. Rep.* **2016**, *68*, 1046–1053. [CrossRef]
12. Alarcon Martinez, T.; Zeybek, N.D.; Müftüoğlu, S. Evaluation of the Cytotoxic and Autophagic Effects of Atorvastatin on MCF-7 Breast Cancer Cells. *Balk. Med. J.* **2018**, *35*, 256–262. [CrossRef] [PubMed]
13. Squadrito, F.J.; Del Portal, D. *Nitrofurantoin*; StatPearls Publishing: St. Petersburg, FL, USA, 2019. Available online: https://www.ncbi.nlm.nih.gov/books/NBK470526/ (accessed on 15 January 2023).
14. Meredith, A.-M.; Dass, C.R. Increasing role of the cancer chemotherapeutic doxorubicin in cellular metabolism. *J. Pharm. Pharmacol.* **2016**, *68*, 729–741. [CrossRef] [PubMed]
15. ATCC. MCF7—HTB-22. Available online: https://www.atcc.org/products/htb-22 (accessed on 9 September 2022).
16. ATCC. SH-SY5Y—CRL-2266. Available online: https://www.atcc.org/products/crl-2266 (accessed on 9 September 2022).
17. Singh, J. Applications of cell lines as bioreactors and in vitro models. *Artic. Int. J. Appl. Biol. Pharm. Technol.* **2012**, *2*, 178–198.
18. Lee, A.V.; Oesterreich, S.; Davidson, N.E. MCF-7 Cells—Changing the Course of Breast Cancer Research and Care for 45 Years. *JNCI J. Natl. Cancer Inst.* **2015**, *107*, 73. [CrossRef] [PubMed]
19. Duarte, D.; Cardoso, A.; Vale, N. Synergistic Growth Inhibition of HT-29 Colon and MCF-7 Breast Cancer Cells with Simultaneous and Sequential Combinations of Antineoplastics and CNS Drugs. *Int. J. Mol. Sci.* **2021**, *22*, 7408. [CrossRef]
20. Zhou, J.; Li, Q.; Wu, W.; Zhang, X.; Zuo, Z.; Lu, Y.; Zhao, H.; Wang, Z. Discovery of Novel Drug Candidates for Alzheimer's Disease by Molecular Network Modeling. *Front. Aging Neurosci.* **2022**, *14*, 233. [CrossRef]
21. Atil, B.; Sieczkowski, E.; Hohenegger, M. Statins reduce endogenous dolichol levels in the neuroblastoma cell line SH-SY5Y. *BMC Pharmacol. Toxicol.* **2012**, *13*, A51. [CrossRef]
22. Longo, J.; van Leeuwen, J.E.; Elbaz, M.; Branchard, E.; Penn, L.Z. Statins as Anticancer Agents in the Era of Precision Medicine. *Clin. Cancer Res.* **2020**, *26*, 5791–5800. [CrossRef]
23. Duarte, D.; Rêma, A.; Amorim, I.; Vale, N. Drug Combinations: A New Strategy to Extend Drug Repurposing and Epithelial-Mesenchymal Transition in Breast and Colon Cancer Cells. *Biomolecules* **2022**, *12*, 190. [CrossRef]
24. Gupta, S.C.; Kannappan, R.; Reuter, S.; Kim, J.H.; Aggarwal, B.B. Chemosensitization of tumors by resveratrol. *Ann. N. Y. Acad. Sci.* **2011**, *1215*, 150–160. [CrossRef]
25. Nunes, M.; Duarte, D.; Vale, N.; Ricardo, S. Pitavastatin and Ivermectin Enhance the Efficacy of Paclitaxel in Chemoresistant High-Grade Serous Carcinoma. *Cancers* **2022**, *14*, 4357. [CrossRef] [PubMed]
26. Pereira, M.; Vale, N. Repurposing Alone and in Combination of the Antiviral Saquinavir with 5-Fluorouracil in Prostate and Lung Cancer Cells. *Int. J. Mol. Sci.* **2022**, *23*, 12240. [CrossRef] [PubMed]
27. Sharma, A.; Mehta, V.; Parashar, A.; Malairaman, U. Combinational effect of Paclitaxel and Clotrimazole on human breast cancer: Proof for synergistic interaction. *Synergy* **2017**, *5*, 13–20. [CrossRef]

Disclaimer/Publisher's Note: The statements, opinions and data contained in all publications are solely those of the individual author(s) and contributor(s) and not of MDPI and/or the editor(s). MDPI and/or the editor(s) disclaim responsibility for any injury to people or property resulting from any ideas, methods, instructions or products referred to in the content.

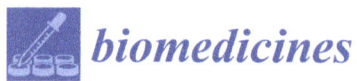

Review

The Beneficial Role of Apigenin against Cognitive and Neurobehavioural Dysfunction: A Systematic Review of Preclinical Investigations

Tosin A. Olasehinde [1,*] and Oyinlola O. Olaokun [2]

1 Nutrition and Toxicology Division, Food Technology Department, Federal Institute of Industrial Research Oshodi, Lagos 100261, Nigeria
2 Department of Biology and Environmental Science, School of Science and Technology, Sefako Makgatho Health Science University, Pretoria 0204, South Africa; oyinolaokun@yahoo.com
* Correspondence: tosinolasehinde26@yahoo.com

Abstract: Apigenin is a flavone widely present in different fruits and vegetables and has been suggested to possess neuroprotective effects against some neurological disorders. In this study, we systematically reviewed preclinical studies that investigated the effects of apigenin on learning and memory, locomotion activity, anxiety-like behaviour, depressive-like behaviour and sensorimotor and motor coordination in rats and mice with impaired memory and behaviour. We searched SCOPUS, Web of Science, PubMed and Google Scholar for relevant articles. A total of 34 studies were included in this review. The included studies revealed that apigenin enhanced learning and memory and locomotion activity, exhibited anxiolytic effects, attenuated depressive-like behaviour and improved sensorimotor and motor coordination in animals with cognitive impairment and neurobehavioural deficit. Some of the molecular and biochemical mechanisms of apigenin include activation of the ERK/CREB/BDNF signalling pathway; modulation of neurotransmitter levels and monoaminergic, cholinergic, dopaminergic and serotonergic systems; inhibition of pro-inflammatory cytokine production; and attenuation of oxidative neuronal damage. These results revealed the necessity for further research using established doses and short or long durations to ascertain effective and safe doses of apigenin. These results also point to the need for a clinical experiment to ascertain the therapeutic effect of apigenin.

Keywords: cognitive dysfunction; neurobehavioural function; neurodegenerative diseases; neuroinflammation; anxiety; depression; learning and memory; sensorimotor function; locomotion

Citation: Olasehinde, T.A.; Olaokun, O.O. The Beneficial Role of Apigenin against Cognitive and Neurobehavioural Dysfunction: A Systematic Review of Preclinical Investigations. *Biomedicines* **2024**, *12*, 178. https://doi.org/10.3390/biomedicines12010178

Academic Editors: Simone Battaglia and Masaru Tanaka

Received: 4 December 2023
Revised: 22 December 2023
Accepted: 4 January 2024
Published: 13 January 2024

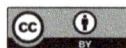

Copyright: © 2024 by the authors. Licensee MDPI, Basel, Switzerland. This article is an open access article distributed under the terms and conditions of the Creative Commons Attribution (CC BY) license (https://creativecommons.org/licenses/by/4.0/).

1. Introduction

Neurological disorders are diseases that affect the nervous system, ranging from common migraine to severe brain, spine and nerve diseases [1]. Some common neurological diseases include dementia, stroke, Parkinson's disease, lateral amyotrophic sclerosis epilepsy and multiple-system atrophy. Neurological diseases have been identified as the leading cause of mortality and disability among adults. These diseases have become a major health burden, especially among aged individuals, as they affect millions of people across the world and the cost of treatment is high [2]. The high incidence rate of neurological diseases has been linked to an increase in the age of the population, as this disease is mostly common in adults [3,4]. Apart from other pathological characteristics, some neurological disorders, especially neurodegenerative diseases, are accompanied by cognitive and neurobehavioural changes which affect quality of life [5,6]. Neuronal degeneration leads to cognitive decline and neurobehavioural impairment and has been identified in patients with AD, PD, epilepsy, stroke and MS [7]. Cognitive decline is usually characterized by impaired working memory, learning abilities, executive function and attention memory, while neurobehavioural dysfunction is commonly accompanied by anxiety, depression and loss of motor function and coordination, which are attributed to the loss and death of specific neurons such as cholinergic, dopaminergic and motor neurons in the central nervous system [8]. Several therapeutic strategies have been developed to treat the symptoms and mitigate the progression of these impairments to improve quality of life.

In the last few years, the impact of flavonoids on neurological function has been studied extensively. This class of polyphenols has shown potent neuroprotective effects against some neurodegenerative diseases in different experimental models. Apigenin is a flavone-kind of flavonoid present in fruits, teas and vegetables. It is a potent antioxidant and has been shown to exhibit anti-inflammatory, antitumorigenic and antimicrobial activities [9]. Its ability to cross the blood–brain barrier is important as it contributes to its pharmacological activity against neurological disorders [10]. Kim et al. [10] reported that apigenin exhibited a neuroprotective effect against peripheral nerve degeneration. Some studies have also established that apigenin confers antidepressant activity, which is mediated by its effect on α-adrenergic, dopaminergic and serotonergic receptors [11–14]. Apigenin improved serotonin, dopamine and epinephrine levels, which were altered in depressive animals [15,16]. Apigenin further regulates the cAMP-CREB-BDNF signalling pathway and N-methyl-D-aspartate (NMDA) receptors, which play important roles in neuronal survival, synaptic plasticity, cognitive function and mood behaviour [15]. Some experimental evidence and expert reviews have shown the pharmacological activities of apigenin, especially against some neurological diseases [17,18]. However, no systematic review has assessed the effect of apigenin on cognitive dysfunction and neurobehavioural deficit in preclinical models. This study aims to systematically review preclinical investigations that explored the cognitive-enhancing effects of apigenin and identify research gaps for further studies where needed. In this study, we explored different paradigms, including learning and memory, sensorimotor function and motor coordination, locomotion activity, anxiety-like behaviour and depressive-like behaviour, to assess the effect of apigenin on cognitive impairment and neurobehavioural deficit. We also highlighted some possible biochemical and molecular mechanisms of its therapeutic actions.

2. Materials and Methods

A search was conducted in four different databases (SCOPUS, Google Scholar, PubMed and Web of Science) to identify relevant studies that reported the effect of apigenin on cognitive and neurobehavioural function in preclinical experiments without limitations to regions/location or language using the Preferred Reporting Items for Systematic Reviews and Meta-Analyses (PRISMA) guidelines. The following search terms were used: "Apigenin AND (memor* OR cogniti* OR *behav* OR neuroinflammati* OR neurodegenerat* OR Alzheim* OR Parkinso*)". Interventional studies must list the authority that provided approval and the corresponding ethical approval code.

2.1. Study Selection

The selection of studies for inclusion in this review was based on the following criteria: (1) that they are preclinical studies or animal studies that used mice or rats; (2) studies that used any dosage of apigenin administered for any duration versus a control group treated with stress or any chemical capable of inducing memory deficit or neurobehavioural dysfunction; and (3) that they measured outcomes that focused on memory and learning (Morris Water Maze, Barnes maze, Y-maze, T-maze, novel object recognition, passive avoidance test, inhibitory avoidance), anxiety-like behaviour (elevated plus maze, dark–light model of anxiety), depressive-like behaviour (forced swimming test, sucrose preference test, splash test, tail suspension test, sucrose splash test), sensorimotor and motor coordination (rotarod activity, grip strength, catalepsy, SG mount, sensorimotor test) and locomotion activity (open field test, locomotion activity). Articles that reported plant extracts containing apigenin were not included. Also, articles involving the use of other models such as *Drosophila melanogaster*, *Caenorhabditis elegans* and cell cultures were excluded from this study. Review articles, theses and conference papers that reported the role of apigenin on cognitive function were also excluded. Studies that reported the use of apigenin in mixtures with other compounds or bioactive constituents were also excluded. Studies that focused on the effect of apigenin on biochemical markers associated with cognitive and neurobehavioural function not indicating relevant behavioural paradigms were also excluded. Two investigators thoroughly reviewed the titles and abstracts of the articles for eligibility for inclusion in the study. Disagreement in the evaluation of eligibility for inclusion was planned to be resolved based on consensus. However, no case of disagreement emerged during the evaluation for eligibility for inclusion.

2.2. Data Extraction

One of the authors extracted data from the included studies while the other author checked and confirmed the extracted data. The following information was extracted from the included studies: (1) subjects; (2) dosage and route of administration; (3) duration of experiment; (4) study description; and (5) type of outcome measured. To examine the effect of apigenin using different cognitive and neurobehavioural paradigms, we categorized the measured outcome identified in the included studies into the following: learning and memory; anxiety-like behaviour, depressive-like behaviour; sensorimotor and motor coordination; and locomotion activity.

3. Results
3.1. Study Characteristics

As shown in Figure 1, 461 studies were identified from PubMed, Scopus, Web of Science and Google Scholar. However, 32 studies were included in the systematic review after screening with the eligibility criteria. These studies specifically address the effect of apigenin on cognitive function and behavioural outcomes in preclinical models. The hypothesis was associated with the effect of apigenin on cognitive and behavioural impairment compared to the disease group. All the included studies were performed either in mice or rats, some induced with rotenone, streptozotocin, corticosterone, chronic or mild stress, high-fat diet or fructose, lipopolysaccharide, scopolamine, methotrexate, pentylenetetrazole and acetonitrile (Table 1). The lowest dose of apigenin in the included studies was 2 mg/kg, while 351 mg/kg was the highest. Most studies used 10, 20, 40, 50 and 100 mg/kg. Also, different administration routes were used, including intragastric, intraperitoneal and oral routes, as shown in Table 1. Most of the studies used male subjects, except two studies that reported female animals. All the studies included mice or rats (Sprague Dawley or Wistar strains). The duration of the experiments in the included studies ranged from 4 days to 22 months. Twenty-two (22) cognitive and behavioural outcomes were identified in all the included studies. These include the Morris Water Maze, Barnes test, open field test, forced swimming test, splash test, rotarod test, catalepsy, elevated plus maze, Y-maze, T-maze, novel object recognition test, sucrose preference test, tail suspension test, grip strength test, passive avoidance test, locomotor activity test, inhibitory avoidance test, shuttle avoidance test, dark–light model of anxiety, pentobarbital sleeping and sensorimotor test (Table 1).

3.2. Learning and Memory

In the learning and memory paradigm, eight different cognitive tests were identified in the included studies (Table 2). Of the 32 included studies, only 24 reported the effect of apigenin on learning and memory. Out of these 24 studies, 12 were on the Morris Water Maze, 1 on the Barnes test, 3 studies were on the Y-maze, 2 studies on the T-maze, 2 studies reported novel recognition tests, 3 studies reported passive avoidance tests, while 1 study reported the inhibitory avoidance test. All the studies showed that apigenin improved learning and memory, except for two studies.

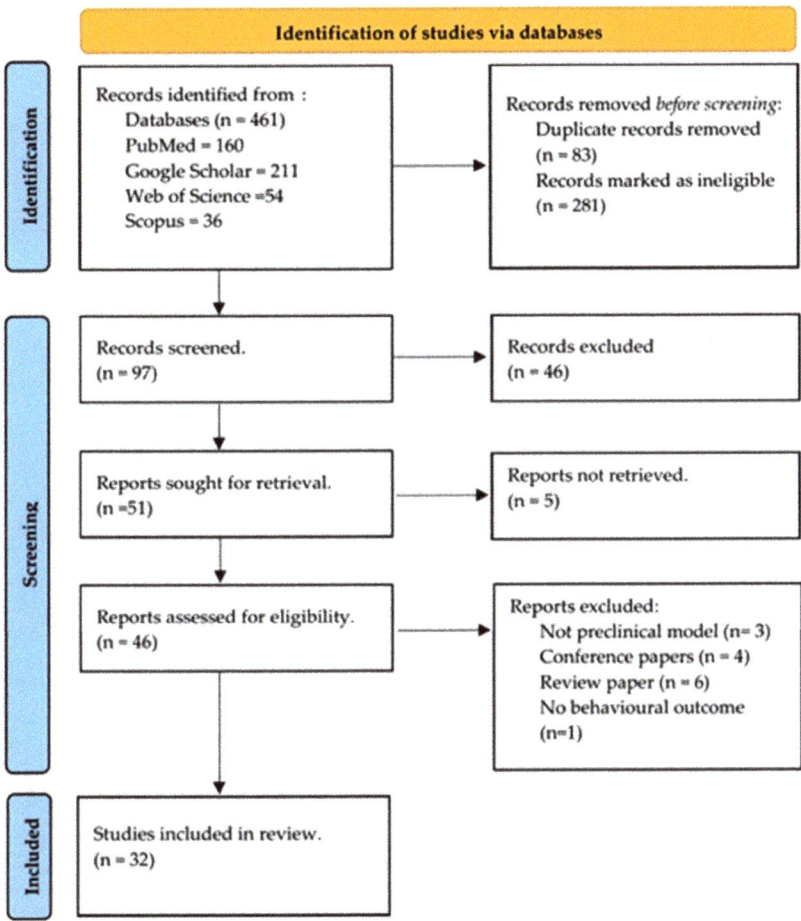

Figure 1. Flow diagram of article selection (based on Page et al. [19]).

Table 1. Description of included studies.

Authors	Subjects	Dosage and Route of Administration	Duration of Experiment	Study Description	Cognitive and Behavioural Parameters Studies
Chen et al. [20]	100 male Sprague Dawley rats	50 and 100 mg/kg/intraperitoneal	7 days	Isoflurane-induced cognitive dysfunction and neuroinflammation	Morris Water Maze
Chesworth et al. [21]	Male and female (C57BL/6) and GFAP-IL6 heterozygous mice	110 mg/kg/oral	22 months	Mouse model of chronic neuroinflammation	Barnes maze
Bijani et al. [22]	Male mice of NMRI	10, 20 and 40 mg/kg intraperitoneal	4 days	Streptozotocin-induced depressive-like behaviour	Open field test Forced swimming test Splash test
Anusha and Sumathi [23]	Male Wistar rats	10 and 20 mg/kg intraperitoneal	14 days	Rotenone-induced model of Parkinson's disease	Rotarod activity Catalepsy Rearing behaviour
Anusha et al. [24]	Male Sprague Dawley rats	10 and 20 mg/kg intraperitoneal		Rotenone-induced model of Parkinson's disease	Rotarod test
Amin et al. [25]	Sprague Dawley rats	50 mg/kg oral	21 days	Diabetes-induced depression and anxiety	Elevated plus maze Forced swimming test
Ahmedy et al. [26]	Male Swiss Albino mice	40 mg/kg oral	7 days	Lipopolysaccharide-induced cognitive impairment in mice	Morris Water Maze Y Maze
Hashemi et al. [27]	Male Wistar rats	50 mg/kg	5 days	Kainite temporal lobe epilepsy model	Morris Water Maze Y Maze
Jameie et al. [28]	Female Wistar rats	2 mg intraperitoneal	5 weeks	Longterm ovariectomy-induced cognitive decline	Morris Water Maze
Kim et al. [29]	Male ICR mice	10 and 20 mg/kg oral	14 days	Scopolamine-induced cognitive dysfunction	T-maze Morris Water Maze Novel object recognition test
Mao et al. [30]	Male Wistar rats	10, 20 and 40 mg/kg intraperitoneal	7 weeks	Diabetes-induced cognitive deficit	Morris water maze
Nikbakht et al. [31]	Wistar rats	50 mg/kg oral	28 days	Aβ25-35-induced neurotoxicity	Y-Maze
Li et al. [32]	Male Sprague Dawley rats	20 mg/kg intragastric	3 weeks	Chronic mild stress-induced depressive behaviour	Sucrose preference test Open field test

Table 1. Cont.

Authors	Subjects	Dosage and Route of Administration	Duration of Experiment	Study Description	Cognitive and Behavioural Parameters Studies
Li et al. [33]	Male ICR mice	25 and 50 mg/kg intraperitoneal	7 days	Lipopolysaccharide-induced depressive behaviour	Tail suspension test Sucrose preference test Open field test
Liu et al. [34]	Male Kunming mice	10 and 20 mg/kg oral	8 days	Amyloid-25-35-induced toxicity in mice	Morris Water Maze
Olayinka et al. [11]	Male Mice	12.5 and 25 mg/kg intraperitoneal	14 days	Chronic stress-induced depressive-like behaviour in mice	Sucrose splash test Elevated plus maze Forced swim test Tail suspension test
Patel and Singh [35]	Male Wistar rats	25 and 50 mg P.O.	14 days	LPS-induced parkinsonism	Open field test Rotarod Grip strength test
Patil et al. [36]	Swiss Mice	5, 10 and 20 mg/kg intraperitoneal	7 dats	LPS-induced cognitive impairment	Passive avoidance test Elevated plus maze Locomotor activity Rotarod
Popovic et al. [10]	Male Wistar rats	20 mg/kg intraperitoneal	56 days	Scopolamine-induced memory impairment	Passive avoidance test
Salgueiro et al. [37]	Male Wistar rats	10 mg/kg intraperitoneal		Normal rats	Inhibitory avoidance Open field test Shuttle avoidance
Sharma et al. [38]	Swiss Albino male mice	10 and 20 mg/kg P.O.	20 days	Pentylenetetrazole-kindling-associated cognitive and behavioural impairment	T-maze Elevated plus maze Tail suspension test Forced swimming test
Taha et al. [39]	Male Sprague Dawley rats	20 mg/kg P.O.	30 days	Methotrexate-induced cognitive dysfunction	Novel object recognition Morris Water Maze
Tu et al. [40]	Male Sprague Dawley rats	20 and 40 mg/kg intraperitoneal	28 days	Post-stroke cognitive deficit in rats	Morris Water Maze

Table 1. Cont.

Authors	Subjects	Dosage and Route of Administration	Duration of Experiment	Study Description	Cognitive and Behavioural Parameters Studies
Weng et al. [41]	Male ICR mice	20 and 40 mg/kg oral	21 days	Corticosterone-induced depression-like behaviour	Sucrose preference test Forced swimming test
Yadav et al. [42]	Wistar rats	40 and 80 mg/kg P.O.		Methylmercury-induced behavioural impairment	Morris Water Maze Grip strength test Open field test Forced swim test
Yarim et al. [43]	Male C57BL/6 mice	50 mg/kg intraperitoneal	10 days	1-methyl-4-phenyl-1,2,3,6-tetrahydropyridine (MPTP)-induced Parkinson's disease	Sensorimotor test - Challenging beam traversal procedure - Spontaneous activity in the cylinder procedure - Pole test
Yi et al. [16]	Male ICR mice and Wistar rats	10 and 20 mg/kg gastric gavage 7 and 14 mg/kg oral	2 weeks 4 weeks	Chronic mild stress-induced depressive-like behaviour	Forced swimming test Sucrose preference test
Zanoli et al. [44]	Male Sprague Dawley rats	25 mg/kg and 50 mg/kg intraperitoneal	<1 h	Behavioural characterization of apigenin	Open field test Dark-light model of anxiety Pentobarbital sleeping time
Zhang et al. [15]	C57BL/6 male mice	10, 20 and 40 mg/kg/P.O.	3 weeks	Corticosterone-induced depressive-like behaviour	Sucrose preference test Tail suspension test Open field test
Zhao [45]	Male Sprague Dawley rats	117, 234, 351 mg/kg intragastric	28 days	Acetonitrile-induced neuroinflammation in rats	Open field Test
Zhao et al. [46]	APP/PS1 double-transgenic mice and wild-type littermates	40 mg/kg oral gavage	12 weeks	AβPPswe Alzheimer's disease mouse model	Morris Water Maze
Zhao et al. [47]	Mice	10, 20 and 40 mg/kg		Senescence-accelerated mouse prone 8 (SAMP8) mouse model	Morris Water Maze

Table 2. Effect of apigenin on learning and memory.

Study	Behavioural Paradigm	Results
Chen et al. [20]	Morris Water Maze	- Reduced escape latency - Improved learning and memory
Chesworth et al. [21]	Barnes maze	- High primary latency in mice (apigenin did not have any effect on primary latency) - Apigenin did not affect path length - Apigenin had no effect on error acquired during acquisition - Apigenin did not improve spatial memory in GFAP-IL6 transgenic mice
Ahmedy et al. [26]	Morris Water Maze Y-maze	- Apigenin improved time spent in the quadrant - Improved spontaneous alternation performance - Improved ability to retrieve spatial memory and form short term memories
Hashemi et al. [27]	Morris Water Maze Y-maze	- Reduced first entry to the target quadrant - Increased number of crossing into the platform region - Increased time spent in target region - Increased percentage of alternative behaviour - Restored reference memory impairment - Restored working memory deficit induced by KA
Jameie et al. [28]	Morris Water Maze	- Increased elapsed time in the target quadrant
Kim et al. [29]	Morris Water Maze Tmaze Novel object recognition	- Reduced latency to reach hidden platform - Increased time spent in the target quadrant - Increased exploration of new and old routes - Increased exploration for novel objects - Improved spatial cognitive ability - Improved scopolamine-induced recognition deficit
Mao et al. [30]	Morris Water Maze	- Reduced escape latency - Significantly reduced mean path length - Increased time spent in target quadrant
Liu et al. [34]	Morris Water Maze	- Significantly reduced escape latency - Significantly increased staying time to cross the first quadrant - Significantly increased time to cross the platform. - Improved learning and memory capabilities
Patil et al. [36]	Passive avoidance test	- Increased step-through latency
Popovic et al. [10]	Passive avoidance test	- Apigenin delayed forgetting of passive avoidance response
Salgueiro et al. [37]	Inhibitory avoidance Passive avoidance performance	- Apigenin slightly induced increase in number of crossings - No significant effect on performance of test session rearing responses - Apigenin did not show significant effect on passive avoidance performance
Sharma et al. [38]	T-maze	- Increased percentage of spontaneous alternation (T-maze)
Taha et al. [39]	Novel object recognition Morris Water Maze	- Apigenin increased discrimination index - Significantly increased preference index - Improved learning ability by reducing escape latency time
Tu et al. [40]	Morris Water Maze	- Attenuated memory acquisition deficit
Yadav et al. [42]	Morris Water Maze	- Restored long-term memory deficit via reduction in escape latency and increase in time spent in target quadrant

Table 2. *Cont.*

Study	Behavioural Paradigm	Results
Zhao et al. [46]	Morris Water Maze	- Exhibited significant effect on escape latency and recovered spatial learning deficit - In the probe trail, apigenin increased time spent in the target quadrant - Increased number of crossings, thereby improving spatial memory capability
Zhao et al. [47]	Morris Water Maze	- Reduced escape latency - Increased time spent in target quadrant and number of crossings of the platform
Nikbakht et al. [31]	Y-maze	- Improved spatial working memory

From the Morris Water Maze tests, eight studies showed that apigenin reduced escape latency [20,30], improved the time spent in the target quadrant [26–28,30], reduced first entry to the target quadrant and increased the number of crossings into the platform region [27]. Only one study reported the effect of apigenin on spatial memory using the Barnes test. The study showed that apigenin did not affect primary latency or error acquired during acquisition and did not improve spatial memory. Three studies also revealed that apigenin improved spatial working memory in animals using the Y-maze test. In these studies, apigenin restored impaired reference memory and working memory deficit by increasing the percentage of alternating behaviour in the test animals [26,27,31]. Two studies also reported that apigenin improved cognitive function using the T-maze test. In these two studies, apigenin increased the exploration of new routes and objects [29] and the percentage of spontaneous alternation [29]. Two studies that reported novel recognition tests showed that apigenin improved scopolamine-induced recognition deficit and methotrexate-induced recognition impairment.

The results from the passive avoidance test reported in two studies showed that apigenin improved retention deficit by increasing step-through latency [36] and delayed forgetting of passive avoidance response [10], while one study showed no effect on passive avoidance performance [37]. One study also revealed that apigenin did not significantly affect inhibitory avoidance activity.

3.3. Locomotor Activity

Two neurobehavioural paradigms were identified in the included studies, locomotor test and open field, as presented in Table 3. A total of 10 studies reported the effect of apigenin on locomotion using open field tests and locomotion tests. In the open field test, apigenin improved locomotor activity [32,35,37,42,44]. However, apigenin did not significantly affect locomotor activity in three studies, as shown by the effect on crossing [22,36], grooming and rearing [33].

3.4. Depressive-like Behaviour

Our findings revealed that seven studies reported the effect of apigenin on depression-like behaviour using the forced swimming test, as shown in Table 4. All the studies showed that apigenin improved immobility time in the forced swimming test. Six studies reported the use of a sucrose preference test to assess the effect of apigenin on depression-like behaviour in the intervention studies, Table 4. The results from these studies revealed that apigenin improved sucrose preference and consumption, and grooming time, and alleviated anhedonic-like behaviour in depressive mice. The tail suspension test was reported in four studies, which revealed that apigenin reduced the duration of immobility time. The splash test was also reported in one study (Table 4). The splash test revealed that apigenin improved grooming activity and locomotion in streptozotocin-induced depressive-like behaviour in a mouse model via an improvement in grooming activity.

Table 3. Effect of apigenin on locomotor behaviour.

Study	Behavioural Paradigm	Results
Bijani et al. [22]	Open field test	- Apigenin showed no effect on the alteration in locomotion
Li et al. [32]	Open field test	- Improved locomotor activity
Li et al. [33]	Open field test	- Apigenin did not show significant effect on crossing, grooming or rearing
Patel and Singh [35]	Open field test	- Increased locomotor activity
Patil et al. [36]	Locomotor activity	- Apigenin did not show any effect on locomotor activity.
Salgueiro et al. [37]	Open field test	- No significant effect on performance of test session rearing responses
Yadav et al. [42]	Open field test	- Improved locomotion and rearing activity
Zanoli et al. [44]	Open field test	- Reduced number of crossings and rearings - Reduced locomotor behaviour
Zhang et al. [15]	Open field test	- Reduced immobility time - Increased total moving distance and reduced immobility time
Zhao et al. [45]	Open field test	- Reduced total distance of motion via reduction in autonomic activity

3.5. Anxiety-like Behaviour Test

Of the five studies that reported the effect of apigenin on anxiety-like behaviour, four studies each reported the impact of the intervention using the elevated plus maze paradigm (Table 5). The four studies showed that apigenin attenuated anxiety-like behaviour by reducing the anxiety index and increasing the time spent in open arms and the number of entries into open arms. One study used the dark–light model of anxiety to examine the effect of apigenin on anxiety-like behaviour (Table 5). The results showed that apigenin did not exhibit an antianxiolytic effect as it did not alter the latency to the first crossing, and not did it show an effect on the time spent in the light compartment.

3.6. Sensorimotor Behaviour and Coordination Activity

Four studies reported the impact of apigenin on motor behaviour and performance using the rotarod test (Table 6). All the studies revealed that apigenin improved rotarod performance and enhanced muscle coordination by delaying the fall time. Two studies reported the use of the grip strength test to assess the effect of apigenin on motor coordination and muscular performance. The results showed that apigenin ameliorated the reduction in grip strength performance and improved motor coordination [23,35]. Only one study examined the effect of apigenin on motor coordination using the catalepsy test. The result from this study showed that apigenin reversed the change in cataleptic behaviour and postural instability in streptozotocin-induced depression-like behaviour in rats. Other sensorimotor function and behavioural paradigms that revealed the effect of apigenin on muscular coordination include the pole test, spontaneous activity in the cylinder and the challenging beam transversal procedure (Table 6). These tests were reported in a study by Yarim et al. [43], and the results revealed that apigenin reduced total steps but did not show any effect on step errors or error per step. Furthermore, apigenin reduced pole test scores, increased hindlimb and forelimb test scores and improved rearing and grooming in a Parkinson's mouse model.

Table 4. Effect of apigenin on depressive-like behaviour.

Study	Behavioural Paradigm	Results
Bijani et al. [22]	Forced swimming test Splash test	- Apigenin improved immobility time in FST - Apigenin improved grooming activity in splash test
Amin et al. [25]	Forced swimming test	- Improved mobility time in forced swimming test
Li et al. [32]	Sucrose preference test	- Improved sucrose consumption and prevented elicited anhedonia and antidepressant-like symptoms
Li et al. [33]	Tail suspension test Sucrose preference test	- Reduced immobility duration - Increased percentage sucrose consumption
Olayinka et al. [11]	Sucrose splash test Forced swim test Tail suspension test	- Significantly increased duration of grooming - Alleviated anhedonic-like behaviour in depressive mice via increase in grooming time - Reduced the duration of immobility
Sharma et al. [38]	Tail suspension test Forced swimming test	- Significant reduction in the duration of immobility time
Weng et al. [41]	Sucrose preference test Forced swimming test	- Apigenin improved sucrose preference in mice - Reduced immobility time in mice
Yadav et al. [42]	Forced swim test	- Markedly reduced immobility time
Yi et al. [16]	Forced swimming test Sucrose preference test	- Apigenin at 10 and 20 mg/kg reduced immobility time - Attenuated CMS-induced deficit in sucrose intake by increasing levels of sucrose consumption
Zhang et al. [15]	Sucrose preference test Tail suspension test	- Significantly reversed reduction in sucrose consumption in rats - Reduced immobility time

Table 5. Effect of apigenin on anxiety-like behaviours.

Study	Behavioural Paradigm	Results
Amin et al. [25]	Elevated plus maze	- Increased time spent in open arms, and also increased number entries into open arms
Olayinka et al. [11]	Elevated plus maze	- Increased frequency of open arm entry - Increased duration of mice in the open arm
Patil et al. [36]	Elevated plus maze	- Decreased transfer latency (EPM)
Sharma et al. [38]	Elevated plus maze	- Markedly reduced anxiety index
Zanoli et al. [44]	Dark–light model of anxiety	- Did not alter latency to the first crossing nor time spent in the light compartment.

Table 6. Effect of apigenin on sensorimotor function and motor coordination.

Study	Behavioural Paradigm	Results
Anusha and Sumathi [23]	Rotarod activity Grip strength Catalepsy	- Apigenin improved muscle grip strength but did not produce a significant effect on grip strength performance - Reversed change in cataleptic behaviour - Reversed postural instability
Anusha et al. [24]	Rotarod	- Apigenin improved muscle coordination by delaying fall time Improved grip strength performance
Patel and Singh [35]	Rotarod Grip strength test SG mount	- Ameliorated reduction in rotarod activity - Ameliorated reduction in grip strength performance (motor coordination) - Significantly attenuated increased climbing and get off time
Patil et al. [36]	Rotarod	- Apigenin improved rotarod performance in aged mice at higher doses (20 mg); lower doses did not show any effect
Yadav et al. [42]	Grip strength test	- Improved grip strength force
Yarim et al. [43]	Sensorimotor test - Challenging beam traversal procedure - Spontaneous activity in the cylinder procedure - Pole test	- Apigenin reduced total steps - Did not show any effect on step errors or errors per step - Reduced forelimb steps - Increased forelimb and hindlimb steps - Increased rearing number and grooming time

4. Discussion

To the best of our knowledge, this is the first systematic review on the effect of apigenin on cognitive and neurobehavioural outcomes in preclinical studies. Our findings revealed that apigenin exhibited cognitive-enhancing effects and improved neurobehavioural function in stress-induced animals. The studies included in this systematic review showed that apigenin improved cognitive function and neurobehaviour in impaired or stressed animals. In this study, we identified the effects of apigenin on different cognitive and neurobehavioural paradigms: learning and memory, locomotor activity, anxiety-like behaviour, depression-like behaviour and sensorimotor function.

The memory and learning paradigm revealed that apigenin exhibited nootropic effects. A significant improvement in memory and learning abilities was observed in impaired rats. Apigenin improved spatial and long-term memory, short-term and spatial working memory, recognition memory and learning abilities. However, one study reported that apigenin did not improve cognitive function in a chronic neuroinflammatory mouse model induced with glial fibrillary acidic protein-interleukin-6 (GFAP-IL-6), as revealed by the Barnes maze test [21]. The authors suggested that though other studies established that apigenin improved memory function in different models, in the context of their study, which involved chronic neuroinflammation, no improvement in cognitive function was observed.

Moreover, the study only employed the Barnes maze and did not explore other learning and memory paradigms. The molecular mechanisms of apigenin's effect on learning and memory have been linked to synaptic transduction of the ERK/CREB/BDNF signalling pathway in the cortical cholinergic system. cAMP response element binding protein (CREB)-mediated transcription genes are essential for learning and memory. CREB also mediates the activity of glucagon-like peptide-1 (GLP-1), which in turn activates the CREB-regulated BDNF promoter [48]. Impaired ERK/CREB/BDNF signalling pathway and an inhibition of CaMK-II/PKC/PKA-ERK-CREB signalling lead to cognitive deficit and disruption of long-term potentiation in the hippocampus [49]. Furthermore, depletion of CREB and withdrawal of BDNF lead to a drastic reduction in synaptic markers in the hippocampus, which may impair long-term potentiation [50,51]. Hence, the learning and memory-enhancing effect of apigenin could be linked to its influence on CREB-BDNF signalling. Apigenin improved BDNF levels and enhanced ERK1/2 and CREB expression [21,51]. Apigenin also improved GLP-1 expression [51]. The memory-enhancing effects of apigenin were also attributed to the attenuation of oxidative stress, inhibition of apoptosis, antiamyloidegonic effects and activation of BDNF.TrkB signalling pathways [29]. Treatment with apigenin reduced Bax/Bcl-2 ratio, caspase-3 and PARP expression, hence inhibiting neuronal apoptosis and degeneration. The influence of apigenin on these signalling pathways explains the observed memory-enhancing effects.

Apigenin improved locomotion behaviour in stressed animals, as shown through three major neurobehavioural paradigms. The open field test was commonly used in all the identified studies. Two studies that reported open field tests showed that apigenin had no effect on locomotion in rats with behavioural deficits. Moreover, one of the studies revealed that apigenin did not affect locomotion. In contrast, seven other studies involving open field tests, including one that used the locomotion test, showed that apigenin improved locomotion.

Our findings also showed that apigenin markedly reduced depressive-like behaviour in preclinical studies, as shown by the results of the forced swimming test, sucrose preference test and tail suspension test from 10 included studies. Depressive-like behaviour is associated with low monoamine levels due to high monoamine oxidase activity [17,25,52]. The improvement in immobility time exhibited by apigenin in animals with depressive-like behaviour could be due to increased monoamine and serotonin levels. Hence, the mechanism of action of apigenin could be linked to the modulation of monoaminergic systems [25]. Apigenin is a potent inhibitor of monoamine oxidase [11,17]. Results from the included studies revealed apigenin as an effective natural antidepressant comparable to synthetic compounds. Some findings also attributed the antidepressant effect of apigenin to the modulation of some neurochemicals and proteins in the brain. Yi, Li, Li, Pan, Xu and Kong [16] suggested that the antidepressive effect of apigenin could be associated with multiple biochemical mechanisms, including modulation of brain monoamine, serotonin and dopamine levels; normalization of HPA axis alterations; and downregulation of the cAMP pathway. The antidepressive effect of apigenin has also been linked with its interaction with the serotonergic pathway, increasing serotonin levels and BDNF expression. Other studies also showed that apigenin exhibited antidepressive effects via increased phosphorylation of CREB and elevated levels of BDNF [38,41]. After oral treatment with apigenin, changes in the levels of serotonin and high BDNF expression were observed, and these are suggested to activate the PKA-CREB signalling pathways. Experimental investigations have also shown a link between the pathophysiology of depression and neuroinflammation. The production of pro-inflammatory cytokines contributes to the development of depression, and antidepressants have been identified as a potent inhibitor of the production of neuroinflammatory biomarkers such as cytokines. The antidepressant effect of apigenin is partly due to its anti-neuroinflammatory effects [32,33]. Apigenin inhibited cytokine production, iNos and COX-2 expression, and NF-kB activation in lipopolysaccharide depressive-like mice. Apigenin also inhibited NLRP3 inflammasome activation through the upregulation of PPAR-γ [33].

The results from the included studies showed that apigenin could be an effective alternative approach for the treatment of anxiety. There are indications that anxiety is linked to alterations in the monoaminergic system [53]. The extensive period spent in the open arms in the elevated plus maze test could be due to increased monoamine levels in the brain [54]. Amin, Ibrahim, Rizwan-ul-Hasan, Khaliq, Gabr, Muhammad,

Khan, Sidhom, Tikmani, Shawky, Ahmad and Abidi [25] reported that apigenin reduced anxiety-like symptoms in rodents, and this was attributed to the modulation of brain monoamine levels and interactions with serotonin receptors. Furthermore, inflammatory processes are triggered by anxiety, which is caused by high levels of pro-inflammatory cytokines such as IL-6, IL-1β and TNF-α. This is due to the impact of these cytokines on neurotransmitters related to the anxiety response. Apigenin also inhibited proinflammatory cytokine production, which could be associated with its anxiolytic effect [11,36]. The role of oxidative stress and inflammatory-related transcription factors in the development of anxiety-like disorders has also been established [55,56]. Sharma, Sharma and Singh [38] also reported that apigenin exhibited anxiolytic effects via modulation of CREB phosphorylation and elevated BDNF levels.

The results from the sensorimotor tests presented in the included studies revealed that apigenin improved motor coordination and prevented loss of muscle control. In Parkinson's disease and amyotrophic lateral sclerosis models, apigenin improved grip strength and rotarod activity, hence improving sensorimotor function [35,42,43]. Impaired motor coordination and balance in Parkinson's disease is linked to alterations in some neurotransmitters such as dopamine, glutamate and γ-amino butyric acid (GABA) [35,57,58]. Oxidative stress and neuroinflammatory processes also contribute to motor neuron degeneration, which is important for motor coordination and sensorimotor function [35,42,43]. The identified studies showed that apigenin improved sensorimotor function and motor coordination by improving antioxidant defence and the inhibition of neuroinflammation, hence attenuating dopaminergic degeneration and, ultimately, motor neuron degeneration (Figure 2).

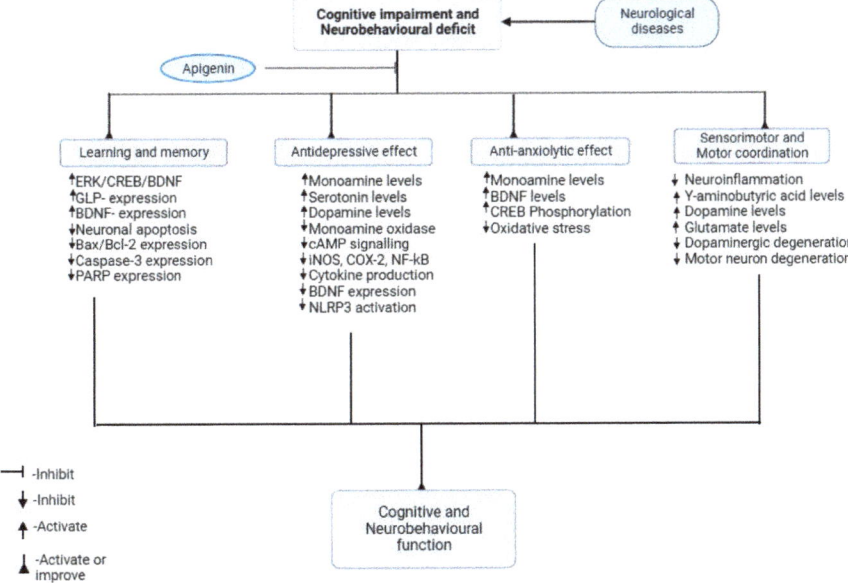

Figure 2. Biochemical and molecular mechanisms of apigenin against cognitive and neurobehavioural deficit.

5. Conclusions

Apigenin is a less toxic flavone widely present in many fruits and vegetables. This systematic review of preclinical trials adds to existing individual studies suggesting that apigenin can improve cognitive and neurobehavioural function. Apigenin improved learning and memory, locomotion activity, sensorimotor and motor coordination and depressive-like and anxiety-like behaviour. The learning and memory-enhancing effects of apigenin could be attributed to the modulation of BDNF levels and expression of ERL1/1 and CREB. Apigenin improved ERK/CREB/BDNF signalling which, in turn, contributed to long-term potentiation and memory function. Apigenin also attenuated hippocampal cholinergic deficit and improved acetylcholine levels, which are important for cholinergic neurotransmission and required for memory function. In addition, the antidepressive and antianxiolytic effects of apigenin are related to the inhibition of inflammatory markers (TNF-α, IL-6, IL-1β, iNOS and COX-2) and NF-kB activation; the modulation of monoamine, dopamine and serotonin levels; the normalization of HPA axis alterations; and downregulation of the cAMP pathway. Apigenin also improved sensorimotor function and motor coordination via attenuation of motor and dopaminergic degeneration; modulation of dopamine, glutamate and γ-amino butyric acid (GABA); and inhibition of ROS production and neuroinflammation.

These results show very good potential for exploring apigenin in clinical studies. Further studies can employ clinical experiments in different populations using short- and long-term trials to examine the effect of apigenin on cognitive and neurobehavioural disorders. Furthermore, different delivery systems can also be examined to establish therapeutic efficacy and minimize challenges associated with absorption, distribution and metabolism. Also, different doses of apigenin can be further explored to ascertain the safety levels around its use in treatment and its consumption through food substances.

Author Contributions: Conceptualization T.A.O.; methodology, T.A.O. and O.O.O.; validation, T.A.O. and O.O.O.; formal analysis, T.A.O. and O.O.O.; investigation, T.A.O. and O.O.O.; resources, T.A.O. and O.O.O.; data curation, T.A.O. and O.O.O.; writing—original draft preparation, T.A.O.; writing—review and editing, T.A.O. and O.O.O. All authors have read and agreed to the published version of the manuscript.

Funding: This research received no external funding.

Institutional Review Board Statement: Not applicable.

Informed Consent Statement: Not applicable.

Data Availability Statement: Not applicable.

Conflicts of Interest: The authors declare no conflict of interest.

References

1. Dumurgier, J.; Tzourio, C. Epidemiology of neurological diseases in older adults. *Rev. Neurol.* **2020**, *176*, 642–648. [CrossRef] [PubMed]
2. Van Schependom, J.; D'Haeseleer, M. Advances in Neurodegenerative Diseases. *J. Clin. Med.* **2023**, *12*, 1709. [CrossRef]
3. Morris, J.C. Neurodegenerative disorders of aging: The down side of rising longevity. *Mo. Med.* **2013**, *110*, 393–394. [PubMed]
4. Gómez-Gómez, M.E.; Zapico, S.C. Frailty, Cognitive Decline, Neurodegenerative Diseases and Nutrition Interventions. *Int. J. Mol. Sci.* **2019**, *20*, 2842. [CrossRef] [PubMed]
5. Levenson, R.W.; Sturm, V.E.; Haase, C.M. Emotional and behavioral symptoms in neurodegenerative disease: A model for studying the neural bases of psychopathology. *Annu. Rev. Clin. Psychol.* **2014**, *10*, 581–606. [CrossRef] [PubMed]
6. Ayeni, E.A.; Aldossary, A.M.; Ayejoto, D.A.; Gbadegesin, L.A.; Alshehri, A.A.; Alfassam, H.A.; Afewerky, H.K.; Almughem, F.A.; Bello, S.M.; Tawfik, E.A. Neurodegenerative Diseases: Implications of Environmental and Climatic Influences on Neurotransmitters and Neuronal Hormones Activities. *Int. J. Environ. Res. Public Health* **2022**, *19*, 12495. [CrossRef] [PubMed]
7. Migliaccio, R.; Tanguy, D.; Bouzigues, A.; Sezer, I.; Dubois, B.; Le Ber, I.; Batrancourt, B.; Godefroy, V.; Levy, R. Cognitive and behavioural inhibition deficits in neurodegenerative dementias. *Cortex* **2020**, *131*, 265–283. [CrossRef]
8. Calina, D.; Buga, A.M.; Mitroi, M.; Buha, A.; Caruntu, C.; Scheau, C.; Bouyahya, A.; El Omari, N.; El Menyiy, N.; Docea, A.O. The Treatment of Cognitive, Behavioural and Motor Impairments from Brain Injury and Neurodegenerative Diseases through Cannabinoid System Modulation-Evidence from In Vivo Studies. *J. Clin. Med.* **2020**, *9*, 2395. [CrossRef]
9. Cirmi, S.; Ferlazzo, N.; Lombardo, G.E.; Ventura-Spagnolo, E.; Gangemi, S.; Calapai, G.; Navarra, M. Neurodegenerative Diseases: Might *Citrus* Flavonoids Play a Protective Role? *Molecules* **2016**, *21*, 1312. [CrossRef]
10. Popović, M.; Caballero-Bleda, M.; Benavente-García, O.; Castillo, J. The flavonoid apigenin delays forgetting of passive avoidance conditioning in rats. *J. Psychopharmacol.* **2014**, *28*, 498–501. [CrossRef]
11. Olayinka, J.N.; Akawa, O.B.; Ogbu, E.K.; Eduviere, A.T.; Ozolua, R.I.; Soliman, M. Apigenin attenuates depressive-like behavior via modulating monoamine oxidase A enzyme activity in chronically stressed mice. *Curr. Res. Pharmacol. Drug Discov.* **2023**, *5*, 100161. [CrossRef] [PubMed]

12. Al-Yamani, M.J.; Mohammed Basheeruddin Asdaq, S.; Alamri, A.S.; Alsanie, W.F.; Alhomrani, M.; Alsalman, A.J.; Al Mohaini, M.; Al Hawaj, M.A.; Alanazi, A.A.; Alanzi, K.D.; et al. The role of serotonergic and catecholaminergic systems for possible antidepressant activity of apigenin. *Saudi J. Biol. Sci.* **2022**, *29*, 11–17. [CrossRef] [PubMed]
13. Zhang, X.; Bu, H.; Jiang, Y.; Sun, G.; Jiang, R.; Huang, X.; Duan, H.; Huang, Z.; Wu, Q. The antidepressant effects of apigenin are associated with the promotion of autophagy via the mTOR/AMPK/ULK1 pathway. *Mol. Med. Rep.* **2019**, *20*, 2867–2874. [CrossRef] [PubMed]
14. Alghamdi, A.; Almuqbil, M.; Alrofaidi, M.A.; Burzangi, A.S.; Alshamrani, A.A.; Alzahrani, A.R.; Kamal, M.; Imran, M.; Alshehri, S.; Mannasaheb, B.A.; et al. Potential Antioxidant Activity of Apigenin in the Obviating Stress-Mediated Depressive Symptoms of Experimental Mice. *Molecules* **2022**, *27*, 9055. [CrossRef] [PubMed]
15. Zhang, L.; Lu, R.R.; Xu, R.H.; Wang, H.H.; Feng, W.S.; Zheng, X.K. Naringenin and apigenin ameliorates corticosterone-induced depressive behaviors. *Heliyon* **2023**, *9*, e15618. [CrossRef] [PubMed]
16. Yi, L.T.; Li, H.M.; Li, Y.C.; Pan, Y.; Xu, Q.; Kong, L.D. Antidepressant-like behavioral and neurochemical effects of the citrus-associated chemical apigenin. *Life Sci.* **2008**, *82*, 741–751. [CrossRef] [PubMed]
17. Nabavi, S.F.; Khan, H.; D'Onofrio, G.; Šamec, D.; Shirooie, S.; Dehpour, A.R.; Argüelles, S.; Habtemariam, S.; Sobarzo-Sanchez, E. Apigenin as neuroprotective agent: Of mice and men. *Pharmacol. Res.* **2018**, *128*, 359–365. [CrossRef]
18. Gaur, K.; Siddique, Y.H. Effect of apigenin on neurodegenerative diseases. In *CNS & Neurological Disorders-Drug Targets*; Bentham Science Publishers: Hilversum, The Netherlands, 2023.
19. Page, M.J.; McKenzie, J.E.; Bossuyt, P.M.; Boutron, I.; Hoffmann, T.C.; Mulrow, C.D.; Shamseer, L.; Tetzlaff, J.M.; Akl, E.A.; Brennan, S.E.; et al. The PRISMA 2020 statement: An updated guideline for reporting systematic reviews. *Syst. Rev.* **2021**, *10*, 89. [CrossRef]
20. Chen, L.; Xie, W.; Xie, W.; Zhuang, W.; Jiang, C.; Liu, N. Apigenin attenuates isoflurane-induced cognitive dysfunction via epigenetic regulation and neuroinflammation in aged rats. *Arch. Gerontol. Geriatr.* **2017**, *73*, 29–36. [CrossRef]
21. Chesworth, R.; Gamage, R.; Ullah, F.; Sonego, S.; Millington, C.; Fernandez, A.; Liang, H.; Karl, T.; Münch, G.; Niedermayer, G. Spatial memory and microglia activation in a mouse model of chronic neuroinflammation and the anti-inflammatory effects of apigenin. *Front. Neurosci.* **2021**, *15*, 699329. [CrossRef]
22. Bijani, S.; Dizaji, R.; Sharafi, A.; Hosseini, M.J. Neuroprotective Effect of Apigenin on Depressive-Like Behavior: Mechanistic Approach. *Neurochem. Res.* **2022**, *47*, 644–655. [CrossRef]
23. Anusha, C.; Sumathi, T. Protective role of apigenin against rotenone induced model of parkinson's disease: Behavioral study. *Int. J. Toxicol. Pharmacol. Res.* **2016**, *8*, 79–82.
24. Anusha, C.; Sumathi, T.; Joseph, L.D. Protective role of apigenin on rotenone induced rat model of Parkinson's disease: Suppression of neuroinflammation and oxidative stress mediated apoptosis. *Chem.-Biol. Interact.* **2017**, *269*, 67–79. [CrossRef] [PubMed]
25. Amin, F.; Ibrahim, M.A.A.; Rizwan-ul-Hasan, S.; Khaliq, S.; Gabr, G.A.; Muhammad; Khan, A.; Sidhom, P.A.; Tikmani, P.; Shawky, A.M.; et al. Interactions of Apigenin and Safranal with the 5HT1A and 5HT2A Receptors and Behavioral Effects in Depression and Anxiety: A Molecular Docking, Lipid-Mediated Molecular Dynamics, and In Vivo Analysis. *Molecules* **2022**, *27*, 8658. [CrossRef]
26. Ahmedy, O.A.; Abdelghany, T.M.; El-Shamarka, M.E.A.; Khattab, M.A.; El-Tanbouly, D.M. Apigenin attenuates LPS-induced neurotoxicity and cognitive impairment in mice via promoting mitochondrial fusion/mitophagy: Role of SIRT3/PINK1/Parkin pathway. *Psychopharmacology* **2022**, *239*, 3903–3917. [CrossRef] [PubMed]
27. Hashemi, P.; Fahanik Babaei, J.; Vazifekhah, S.; Nikbakht, F. Evaluation of the neuroprotective, anticonvulsant, and cognition-improvement effects of apigenin in temporal lobe epilepsy: Involvement of the mitochondrial apoptotic pathway. *Iran. J. Basic Med. Sci.* **2019**, *22*, 752–758.
28. Jameie, S.B.; Pirasteh, A.; Naseri, A.; Jameie, M.S.; Farhadi, M.; Babaee, J.F.; Elyasi, L. β-Amyloid Formation, Memory, and Learning Decline Following Long-term Ovariectomy and Its Inhibition by Systemic Administration of Apigenin and β-Estradiol. *Basic Clin. Neurosci.* **2021**, *12*, 383–394.
29. Kim, Y.; Kim, J.; He, M.; Lee, A.; Cho, E. Apigenin Ameliorates Scopolamine-Induced Cognitive Dysfunction and Neuronal Damage in Mice. *Molecules* **2021**, *26*, 5192. [CrossRef]
30. Mao, X.Y.; Yu, J.; Liu, Z.Q.; Zhou, H.H. Apigenin attenuates diabetes-associated cognitive decline in rats via suppressing oxidative stress and nitric oxide synthase pathway. *Int. J. Clin. Exp. Med.* **2015**, *8*, 15506–15513.
31. Nikbakht, F.; Khadem, Y.; Haghani, S.; Hoseininia, H.; Moein Sadat, A.; Heshemi, P.; Jamali, N. Protective Role of Apigenin Against Aβ 25-35 Toxicity Via Inhibition of Mitochondrial Cytochrome c Release. *Basic Clin. Neurosci.* **2019**, *10*, 557–566.
32. Li, R.; Wang, X.; Qin, T.; Qu, R.; Ma, S. Apigenin ameliorates chronic mild stress-induced depressive behavior by inhibiting interleukin-1β production and NLRP3 inflammasome activation in the rat brain. *Behav. Brain Res.* **2016**, *296*, 318–325. [CrossRef]
33. Li, R.; Zhao, D.; Qu, R.; Fu, Q.; Ma, S. The effects of apigenin on lipopolysaccharide-induced depressive-like behavior in mice. *Neurosci. Lett.* **2015**, *594*, 17–22. [CrossRef] [PubMed]
34. Liu, R.; Zhang, T.; Yang, H.; Lan, X.; Ying, J.; Du, G. The flavonoid apigenin protects brain neurovascular coupling against amyloid-$β_{25-35}$-induced toxicity in mice. *J. Alzheimers Dis.* **2011**, *24*, 85–100. [CrossRef] [PubMed]
35. Patel, M.; Singh, S. Apigenin Attenuates Functional and Structural Alterations via Targeting NF-kB/Nrf2 Signaling Pathway in LPS-Induced Parkinsonism in Experimental Rats: Apigenin Attenuates LPS-Induced Parkinsonism in Experimental Rats. *Neurotox. Res.* **2022**, *40*, 941–960. [CrossRef] [PubMed]

36. Patil, C.S.; Singh, V.P.; Satyanarayan, P.S.; Jain, N.K.; Singh, A.; Kulkarni, S.K. Protective effect of flavonoids against aging- and lipopolysaccharide-induced cognitive impairment in mice. *Pharmacology* **2003**, *69*, 59–67. [CrossRef] [PubMed]
37. Salgueiro, J.B.; Ardenghi, P.; Dias, M.; Ferreira, M.B.; Izquierdo, I.; Medina, J.H. Anxiolytic natural and synthetic flavonoid ligands of the central benzodiazepine receptor have no effect on memory tasks in rats. *Pharmacol. Biochem. Behav.* **1997**, *58*, 887–891. [CrossRef] [PubMed]
38. Sharma, P.; Sharma, S.; Singh, D. Apigenin reverses behavioural impairments and cognitive decline in kindled mice via CREB-BDNF upregulation in the hippocampus. *Nutr. Neurosci.* **2020**, *23*, 118–127. [CrossRef]
39. Taha, M.; Eldemerdash, O.M.; Elshaffei, I.M.; Yousef, E.M.; Soliman, A.S.; Senousy, M.A. Apigenin Attenuates Hippocampal Microglial Activation and Restores Cognitive Function in Methotrexate-Treated Rats: Targeting the miR-15a/ROCK-1/ERK1/2 Pathway. *Mol. Neurobiol.* **2023**, *60*, 3770–3787. [CrossRef]
40. Tu, F.; Pang, Q.; Huang, T.; Zhao, Y.; Liu, M.; Chen, X. Apigenin ameliorates post-stroke cognitive deficits in rats through histone acetylation- mediated neurochemical alterations. *Med. Sci. Monit.* **2017**, *23*, 4004–4013. [CrossRef]
41. Weng, L.; Guo, X.; Li, Y.; Yang, X.; Han, Y. Apigenin reverses depression-like behavior induced by chronic corticosterone treatment in mice. *Eur. J. Pharmacol.* **2016**, *774*, 50–54. [CrossRef]
42. Yadav, R.K.; Mehan, S.; Sahu, R.; Kumar, S.; Khan, A.; Makeen, H.A.; Al Bratty, M. Protective effects of apigenin on methylmercury-induced behavioral/neurochemical abnormalities and neurotoxicity in rats. *Hum. Exp. Toxicol.* **2022**, *41*, 9603271221084276. [CrossRef]
43. Yarim, G.F.; Kazak, F.; Yarim, M.; Sozmen, M.; Genc, B.; Ertekin, A.; Gokceoglu, A. Apigenin alleviates neuroinflammation in a mouse model of Parkinson's disease. *Int. J. Neurosci.* **2022**. ahead of print. [CrossRef] [PubMed]
44. Zanoli, P.; Avallone, R.; Baraldi, M. Behavioral characterisation of the flavonoids apigenin and chrysin. *Fitoterapia* **2000**, *71*, S117–S123. [CrossRef] [PubMed]
45. Zhao, F.; Dang, Y.; Zhang, R.; Jing, G.; Liang, W.; Xie, L.; Li, Z. Apigenin attenuates acrylonitrile-induced neuro-inflammation in rats: Involved of inactivation of the TLR4/NF-κB signaling pathway. *Int. Immunopharmacol.* **2019**, *75*, 105697. [CrossRef] [PubMed]
46. Zhao, L.; Wang, J.-L.; Liu, R.; Li, X.-X.; Li, J.-F.; Zhang, L. Neuroprotective, anti-amyloidogenic and neurotrophic effects of apigenin in an Alzheimer's disease mouse model. *Molecules* **2013**, *18*, 9949–9965. [CrossRef]
47. Zhao, Y.; Li, F.; Zeng, Y. Effects of apigenin on learning and memory and synaptic plicity in SAMP8 mice. *Chin. J. Gerontol.* **2015**, *35*, 4113–4116.
48. Bourtchuladze, R.; Frenguelli, B.; Blendy, J.; Cioffi, D.; Schutz, G.; Silva, A.J. Deficient long-term memory in mice with a targeted mutation of the cAMP-responsive element-binding protein. *Cell* **1994**, *79*, 59–68. [CrossRef]
49. Lyu, Y.; Ren, X.K.; Zhang, H.F.; Tian, F.J.; Mu, J.B.; Zheng, J.P. Sub-chronic administration of benzo[a]pyrene disrupts hippocampal long-term potentiation via inhibiting CaMK II/PKC/PKA-ERK-CREB signaling in rats. *Environ. Toxicol.* **2020**, *35*, 961–970. [CrossRef]
50. Velmurugan, K.; Balamurugan, A.N.; Loganathan, G.; Ahmad, A.; Hering, B.J.; Pugazhenthi, S. Antiapoptotic actions of exendin-4 against hypoxia and cytokines are augmented by CREB. *Endocrinology* **2012**, *153*, 1116–1128. [CrossRef]
51. Kalivarathan, J.; Chandrasekaran, S.P.; Kalaivanan, K.; Ramachandran, V.; Carani Venkatraman, A. Apigenin attenuates hippocampal oxidative events, inflammation and pathological alterations in rats fed high fat, fructose diet. *Biomed. Pharmacother.* **2017**, *89*, 323–331. [CrossRef]
52. Miura, H.; Naoi, M.; Nakahara, D.; Ohta, T.; Nagatsu, T. Changes in monoamine levels in mouse brain elicited by forced-swimming stress, and the protective effect of a new monoamine oxidase inhibitor, RS-8359. *J. Neural Transm.* **1993**, *95*, 175–187. [CrossRef] [PubMed]
53. Liu, Y.; Zhao, J.; Guo, W. Emotional Roles of Mono-Aminergic Neurotransmitters in Major Depressive Disorder and Anxiety Disorders. *Front. Psychol.* **2018**, *9*, 2201. [CrossRef] [PubMed]
54. Cryan, J.F.; Page, M.E.; Lucki, I. Differential behavioral effects of the antidepressants reboxetine, fluoxetine, and moclobemide in a modified forced swim test following chronic treatment. *Psychopharmacology* **2005**, *182*, 335–344. [CrossRef] [PubMed]
55. Salim, S.; Chugh, G.; Asghar, M. Inflammation in anxiety. In *Advances in Protein Chemistry and Structural Biology*; Donev, R., Ed.; Elsevier: Amsterdam, The Netherlands, 2012; Volume 88, pp. 1–25.
56. Quesseveur, G.; David, D.J.; Gaillard, M.C.; Pla, P.; Wu, M.V.; Nguyen, H.T.; Nicolas, V.; Auregan, G.; David, I.; Dranovsky, A.; et al. BDNF overexpression in mouse hippocampal astrocytes promotes local neurogenesis and elicits anxiolytic-like activities. *Transl. Psychiatry* **2013**, *3*, e253. [CrossRef]
57. Moore, A.H.; Bigbee, M.J.; Boynton, G.E.; Wakeham, C.M.; Rosenheim, H.M.; Staral, C.J.; Morrissey, J.L.; Hund, A.K. Non-Steroidal Anti-Inflammatory Drugs in Alzheimer's Disease and Parkinson's Disease: Reconsidering the Role of Neuroinflammation. *Pharmaceuticals* **2010**, *3*, 1812–1841. [CrossRef]
58. Gardoni, F.; Bellone, C. Modulation of the glutamatergic transmission by Dopamine: A focus on Parkinson, Huntington and Addiction diseases. *Front. Cell. Neurosci.* **2015**, *9*, 25. [CrossRef]

Disclaimer/Publisher's Note: The statements, opinions and data contained in all publications are solely those of the individual author(s) and contributor(s) and not of MDPI and/or the editor(s). MDPI and/or the editor(s) disclaim responsibility for any injury to people or property resulting from any ideas, methods, instructions or products referred to in the content.

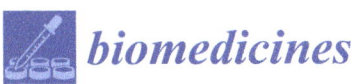

Systematic Review

Mercury and Autism Spectrum Disorder: Exploring the Link through Comprehensive Review and Meta-Analysis

Aleksandar Stojsavljević [1,*], Novak Lakićević [2] and Slađan Pavlović [3]

[1] Innovative Centre, Faculty of Chemistry, University of Belgrade, Studentski Trg 12–16, 11000 Belgrade, Serbia
[2] Clinical Centre of Montenegro, Clinic for Neurosurgery, Ljubljanska bb, 81000 Podgorica, Montenegro; novak.lakicevic@kccg.me
[3] Institute for Biological Research "Siniša Stanković"—National Institute of the Republic of Serbia, University of Belgrade, Bulevar Despota Stefana 142, 11060 Belgrade, Serbia; sladjan@ibiss.bg.ac.rs
* Correspondence: aleksandars@chem.bg.ac.rs

Abstract: Mercury (Hg) is a non-essential trace metal with unique neurochemical properties and harmful effects on the central nervous system. In this study, we present a comprehensive review and meta-analysis of peer-reviewed research encompassing five crucial clinical matrices: hair, whole blood, plasma, red blood cells (RBCs), and urine. We assess the disparities in Hg levels between gender- and age-matched neurotypical children (controls) and children diagnosed with autism spectrum disorder (ASD) (cases). After applying rigorous selection criteria, we incorporated a total of 60 case-control studies into our meta-analysis. These studies comprised 25 investigations of Hg levels in hair (controls/cases: 1134/1361), 15 in whole blood (controls/cases: 1019/1345), 6 in plasma (controls/cases: 224/263), 5 in RBCs (controls/cases: 215/293), and 9 in urine (controls/cases: 399/623). This meta-analysis did not include the data of ASD children who received chelation therapy. Our meta-analysis revealed no statistically significant differences in Hg levels in hair and urine between ASD cases and controls. In whole blood, plasma, and RBCs, Hg levels were significantly higher in ASD cases compared to their neurotypical counterparts. This indicates that ASD children could exhibit reduced detoxification capacity for Hg and impaired mechanisms for Hg excretion from their bodies. This underscores the detrimental role of Hg in ASD and underscores the critical importance of monitoring Hg levels in ASD children, particularly in early childhood. These findings emphasize the pressing need for global initiatives aimed at minimizing Hg exposure, thus highlighting the critical intersection of human–environment interaction and neurodevelopment health.

Keywords: mercury (Hg); autism spectrum disorder (ASD); clinical matrices; comprehensive meta-analysis

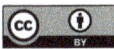

1. Introduction

Autism spectrum disorder (ASD) is a disturbance associated with brain development that causes problems in social interaction and communication, along with restricted and/or repetitive behaviors or interests [1,2]. Terminologically, in 2022, the World Health Organization (WHO) published the latest International Classification of Disease and Related Problems-11th Revision (ICD-11), and the official name of autism is ASD [3]. Additionally, according to the European Autism Information System (EAIS), the official name/observation ASD should be used [4].

The incidence of ASD has risen to such an extent that it has become known as the "ASD epidemic" in scientific literature [5]. According to the latest WHO report, one in every 100 children receives a diagnosis of ASD [6]. In the United States (US), one out of every 36 children carries a confirmed ASD diagnosis [7]. Notably, ASD is considerably more prevalent in boys, with a nearly fourfold higher incidence compared to girls [8,9]. Symptoms of ASD typically manifest within the first year of life, becoming most conspicuous between 18 and 24 months [10,11]. Currently, no prenatal biomarker for ASD exists, and regrettably, ASD remains without a cure. However, with appropriate treatments, it is a condition that can be effectively managed [12–14].

It is widely accepted that the etiology of ASD is multifactorial, with various contributing factors [15,16]. In addition to genetic, epigenetic, and certain environmental factors, there is a growing suspicion that non-essential trace metals, particularly those with neurotoxic properties, could play a crucial role in the etiology of ASD. It is known that Hg is not the only toxic metal associated with ASD. Other metals related to ASD are aluminum (Al), antimony (Sb), arsenic (As), beryllium (Be), cadmium (Cd), chromium (Cr), lead (Pb), and nickel (Ni) [17,18]. Non-essential trace elements have no known function in the human body and can be toxic even in low levels. Non-essential trace elements include heavy metals and metalloids such as aluminum Al, As, Cd, Hg, Pb, Sb, tin (Sn), uranium (U), and vanadium (V). Their toxicity is related to their ability to damage vital organs such as the brain, kidney, liver, and others. Long-term exposure to non-essential elements can lead to physical (e.g., chronic pain, changes in blood pressure, changes in blood composition, etc.) and psychological (e.g., anxiety, passivity, etc.) disorders, neurodegenerative diseases, and cancer [19]. Exposure to trace metals commences in utero, as the placental barrier often proves insufficient in preventing their transport to the developing fetus [20]. Furthermore, during the initial year of life, the immature blood–brain barrier leaves infants vulnerable to the effects of non-essential trace metals [21,22]. As a result, trace metals can disrupt critical biochemical processes essential for sustaining life [23]. However, the etiology of ASD is still unclear. Environmental factors that could prenatally influence the onset of ASD include immune abnormalities, zinc deficiency, abnormal melatonin synthesis, maternal diabetes, stress, toxins, and parental age. Postnatal environmental factors include stress, immune abnormalities, and toxic metal. There is extensive evidence of the connection between many prenatal environmental factors and increased development of ASD [24].

The hazardous, non-essential/toxic trace metal Hg has garnered notable attention due to its potent neurotoxic properties and specific neurobiochemistry within the human body. According to its role in the body, Hg is classified as a non-essential toxic element, while it is considered a heavy metal according to its physical and chemical properties [25]. The WHO classifies Hg as one of the 10 priority environmental pollutants [26]. Industrial development has led to a nearly threefold increase in Hg emissions into the environment, with atmospheric Hg levels rising by nearly 1.5% annually [27].

Hg exists in various forms, including elemental (Hg^0), inorganic (Hg^{2+}), and organic (alkyl Hg) forms [28]. While elemental Hg can be ingested orally with minimal adverse effects, it becomes toxic when chemically converted into the Hg^{2+} species [26,29]. Further bioconversion into alkyl Hg results in a highly toxic compound with a strong affinity for lipid-rich organs, specifically the brain [30]. Organic forms of Hg (such as methylmercury, MeHg and ethylmercury, EtHg) are notably more toxic than inorganic forms [31,32].

Even at relatively low levels, Hg can be deleterious, primarily to young children [33,34]. Hg easily crosses both the placental and blood–brain barriers, accumulating in the central nervous system, particularly in the cerebral cortex and cerebellum. MeHg and EtHg are fat-soluble and have a high affinity for thiol groups, allowing them to easily penetrate the placental and the blood–brain barrier [35]. Within cells, Hg binds to mitochondria, the endoplasmic reticulum, and the Golgi apparatus, disrupting their essential biochemical functions [36]. The buildup of Hg in brain structures results in neuroinflammation, oxidative stress, and elevated levels of autoantibodies against brain proteins and other components [37,38]. Chronic childhood Hg poisoning, known as acrodynia or "pink disease", resulting from exposure to Hg chloride-containing tooth powder, underscores the vulnerability of children to Hg compared to adults [39,40]. Moreover, offspring of acrodynia survivors face a higher risk of developing ASD, with an earlier incidence rate of one in 22 compared to the general child population's one in 160 [39].

During pregnancy, the main sources of Hg exposure stem from maternal consumption of seafood and the number of dental Hg amalgam fillings [41,42]. Seafood consumption poses a common and potentially hazardous route, primarily due to the ingestion of MeHg through contaminated fish, shellfish, and sea mammals [43]. According to the Food and Drug Administration (FDA), pregnant women, women of childbearing age, and young children are advised to avoid shark, swordfish, mackerel, and tilefish, due to their higher Hg concentrations [44]. In contrast, Hg exposure from dental fillings remains relatively constant over time, with dental Hg amalgam fillings largely being replaced by composite fillings [31]. Airborne Hg exposure, primarily resulting from industrial waste, such as coal burning and mining activities, cannot be ruled out [45,46].

Children have been exposed to Hg later in life through thimerosal, a compound containing EtHg used in some vaccines, and anti-Rho(D) immune globulins for Rh-negative mothers during pregnancy [47,48]. Thimerosal, with approximately 50% of its weight consisting of Hg, has been used as a preservative in numerous vaccines since the 1930s to prevent microbial growth [2,49]. Due to substantial public concern and controversy, the FDA proposed the removal of thimerosal from vaccines between 1999 and 2001 [5]. The CDC, following several multi-year studies, declared that "exposure to thimerosal during pregnancy and in young children was not associated with an increased risk of ASD" [7]. It is worth noting that the incidence of ASD continued to rise even after the removal or reduction of thimerosal from many vaccines in the USA, Europe, and certain Asian countries [7]. Consequently, due to controversy, thimerosal was removed from anti-Rho(D) immune globulins [48]. Presently, the scientific community places substantial focus on the environmental Hg exposure of pregnant women, nursing mothers, and young children, suggesting that environmental triggers could play a more important role in the Hg-ASD link than vaccinations themselves. Kern et al.'s [50] review of 91 papers from 1999 to 2016 found that 74% of these papers identified environmental Hg exposure as a critical risk factor for ASD.

Many animal studies have attempted to determine the neurological mechanisms linking Hg and ASD. Experiments on monkeys show that Hg levels in the brain increase after exposure, and that it is necessary to evaluate the effects of its presence on neurological structures. After administering organic Hg to monkeys, the half-life of Hg in the brain varied considerably in different brain regions. In the thalamus, Hg levels remained the same, and in the pituitary gland, they doubled six months after exposure. Stereologic and autometallographic studies showed that the persistence of Hg in the brain was accompanied by a significant increase in the number of microglia, while the number of astrocytes decreased [51]. An active neuroinflammatory process was detected in the brains of ASD patients, including a marked activation of microglia. Hg-mediated modulation of cytokine production (IL-6, TNF-α) could have an adverse impact on ASD patients, leading to autoimmune brain response, IgG accumulation in brain, and CD4+ T cell infiltration [21]. It is also shown that some cognitive and sensory deficits can be associated with Tryptophan–Kynurenine metabolic system in the human brain [52].

On the other hand, the scientific community's attention has shifted. The focus is not only on how Hg enters the body, but also on the mechanisms of its removal. This shift is particularly vital in the context of ASD children. Numerous investigations have indicated that this sensitive population group exhibits diminished capabilities in eliminating Hg from their bodies [21,49]. Several important factors have been identified, including heightened levels of oxidized glutathione, the far-reaching consequences of oxidative stress, increased use of oral antibiotics (especially during the first year, which disrupts the gut flora and leads to Hg methylation), alterations in cell cycles, epigenetic modifications (such as histone alterations, DNA methylation, and microRNA expression), as well as antagonistic effects on essential trace elements and changes in the expression of metallothioneins, among others. Further in-depth information on these detrimental effects of Hg on multiple biochemical processes can be found in existing literature [48,53].

The present systematic review and comprehensive meta-analysis aim to examine potential aspects of Hg contributing to ASD in children, investigating Hg levels in different biological materials (hair, whole blood, red blood cells, plasma, and urine), and shed light on the role of Hg levels in the context of this neurodevelopmental condition. To achieve that, we categorize, summarize, and discuss the published research papers on this topic.

2. Materials and Methods

The basis for this review and meta-analysis corresponds to the "Preferred Reporting Items for Systematic Reviews and Meta-Analyzes: the PRISMA Statement" [54]. The PRISMA statement was originally proposed in 2009. However, we have utilized the updated PRISMA 2020 statement, which supersedes the 2009 version and incorporates new reporting guidelines that reflect methodological advances in the identification, selection, appraisal, and synthesis of studies.

The main objective of the PRISMA 2020 statement is to ensure that users of review receive a transparent, comprehensive, and accurate account of the rationale for conducting the review, the methodology used, and the findings obtained [55]. It also includes a 27-item checklist, an expanded checklist with detailed reporting recommendations for each item, a PRISMA 2020 abstract checklist, and revised flowcharts for both original and updated reviews.

Prior to commencing the present study, the authors prepared a research protocol.

2.1. Information Sources

First, we searched four databases: SCOPUS, PubMed, ScienceDirect, and Google Scholar. However, as the publications in these databases overlap considerably, we concentrated on two of the most representative databases, SCOPUS and PubMed.

2.2. Search Strategy

Our major objective in this study was to identify all research that examined Hg levels in hair, whole blood, plasma, RBCs, and urine of neurotypical children (controls) and ASD children (cases). We conducted our literature search from 1985 to the present. To do this, we used a comprehensive search strategy with mesh terms such as "autism", "autistic", "child", "preschool", "school", "heavy metals", "toxic metals", "mercury", "Hg", "hair", "blood", "plasma", "red blood cells", and "urine". The authors in our search utilized a total of 1462 ASD-related keywords, with 29 being used most frequently. A graphical representation of these data, illustrating the network visualization and relationships between the observed keywords, can be found in Figure 1A,B (created with VOSviewer 1.6.19 software, copyright (c) 2009–2023 Nees Jan van Eck and Ludo Waltman Centre for Science and Technology Studies of Leiden University, Leiden, The Netherlands).

Additionally, we meticulously reviewed the reference lists of retrieved results. Our inclusion criteria encompassed original, case-control research studies that reported Hg levels in the specified clinical matrices of both cases and controls. Exclusion criteria were studies with adults, studies in which the diagnosis of ASD was not confirmed, studies with cases and controls that were not from the same residence, studies with age- and sex-mismatched cases and controls, studies that reported additional pathologies besides ASD, non-English language studies, studies with insufficient numerical data, and studies with extremely abnormal Hg values. Studies that refer to sufficient numerical data include results where the mean ± standard deviation (SD) or standard error (SE), or some other numerical value from which the SD can be calculated, is accurately reported. In fact, there are many studies that report only the mean without the SD or SE, or studies in which only graphs without numerical values are shown. In our meta-analysis, we set the criterion of using only complete data, i.e., mean values and SDs, that represent sufficient numerical data for us. Further exclusion factors are delineated in Figure 2. For the meta-analysis, we examined original full-length research articles spanning the following timeframes: 1985–2023 for hair (µg/g), 2004–2023 for whole blood (µg/L), 2011–2020 for plasma (µg/L), 2010–2017 for RBCs (μg/L), and 2003–2020 for urine Hg levels (μg/g creatinine). These timeframes were selected to ensure consistency in analytical procedures. Most authors employed inductively coupled plasma mass spectrometry (ICP-MS) to determine Hg concentrations in clinical matrices, while a smaller number utilized atomic absorption spectroscopy (AAS). Two papers used inductively coupled plasma optical plasma spectrometry (ICP-OES), one paper employed the Hg vaporimeter, and one paper utilized atomic fluorescence spectroscopy (AFS).

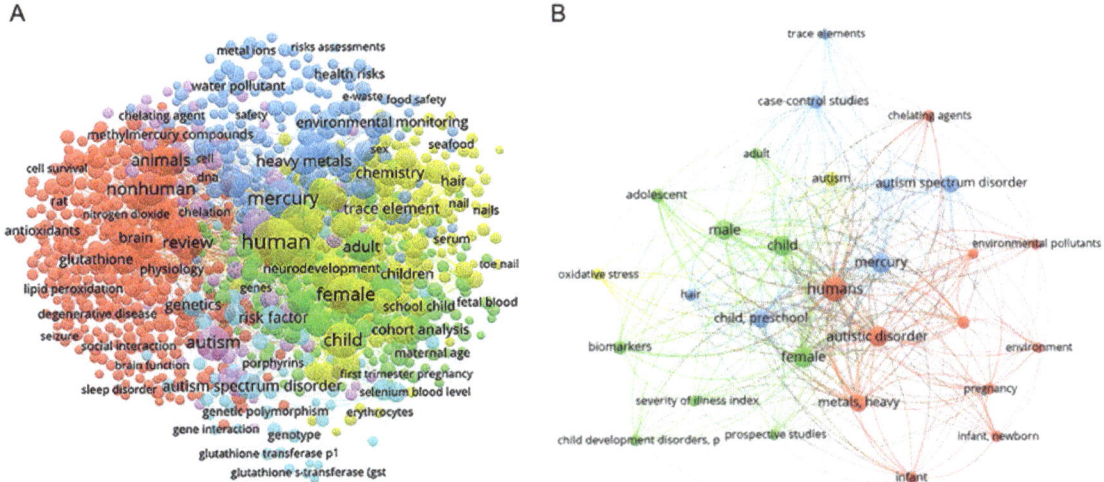

Figure 1. (**A**) Comprehensive network visualization of 1462 ASD-related keywords in scholarly literature; (**B**) focused network visualization of the 29 most commonly used ASD-related keywords in scholarly literature.

2.3. Study Selection and Data Extraction

A graphical representation of the selection process can be found in Figure 2. Two trained researchers (A.S. and S.P.) independently extracted the following data from each study: author(s) and year of publication, country of origin, sample size (controls/cases), age (controls/cases), gender (number of girls/boys in both groups), type of clinical matrices studied, analytical technique used, and Hg level (mean ± SD, given for controls and cases). In cases where results were reported as mean ± SEM, the SEM (standard error of the mean) was converted to SD using the appropriate formula. Similarly, when authors reported results as an interquartile range (IQR), we converted the IQR to SD [56]. Our inclusion criteria only considered papers in which the results were reported as numerical values. After the selection and data extraction process, the final list of studies was compiled through consensus.

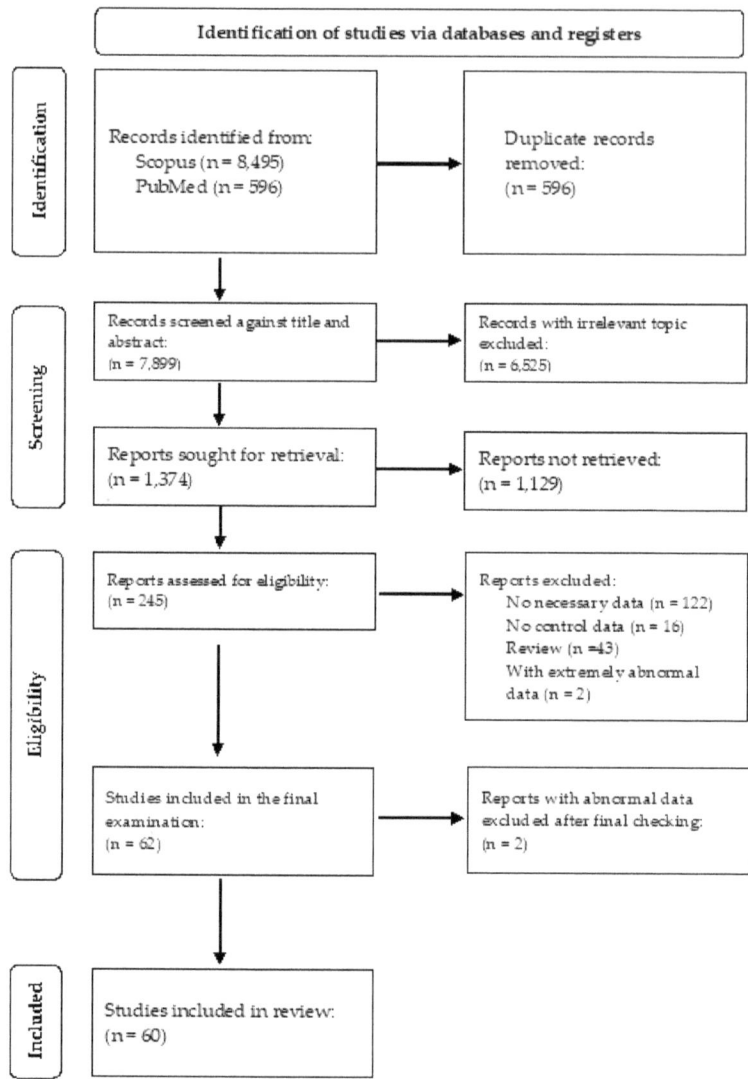

Figure 2. PRISMA flow diagram illustrating the literature search, study identification, inclusion, and exclusion Process. Abbreviation: n (number of studies).

2.4. Quality Assessment

Quality assessment of the enrolled studies was carried out using the Newcastle–Ottawa Scale (NOS) according to [57]. The quality assessment was based on the modified criteria of [58]. The possible scores ranged from 1 to 7, and studies that scored 7 were considered to be of the highest quality, with the lowest risk of bias. Studies that scored less than 7 were considered to be of lower quality, with a higher risk of bias.

We implemented a quality assessment procedure to take account of defects in various parameters. The deficiencies, such as a small sample size, the country of participants' origin, absence of genderi nformation, age data, and method of analysis, were each scored as one "pointless". ICP-MS was deemed the most representative analytical methodology, with all others receiving a score of one "unusable". Finally, the number of points assigned to each study for each clinical matrix was determined, and a mean value for the entire meta-analysis was calculated. A detailed description of the quality assessment procedure can be found.

2.5. Statistical Analysis

The heterogeneity of the selected studies was evaluated using the I-squared (I^2) and the associated Cochran's Q test [59]. An I^2 value exceeding 75% was considered indicative of a high level of heterogeneity, and to account for the limited power of the Q test in detecting heterogeneity, a significance level of $p < 0.1$ was used. In cases where heterogeneity exceeded 70%, pooled estimates were analyzed using the random effects model. We opted for the random effects model for all analyses, as we anticipated that the true effect sizes would vary among studies. Additionally, τ-squared (τ^2), as per [60], was used to assess heterogeneity. A τ^2 value close to 0 suggested low heterogeneity, while a τ^2 value greater than 1 indicated substantial heterogeneity [61].

Effect sizes were calculated as mean differences in Hg levels in clinical materials (hair, whole blood, plasma, RBCs, and urine), and then converted to Hedges's g, with adjustments to account for the influence of small sample sizes [62]. We also calculated 95% confidence intervals (CIs) to measure statistical variance in the pooled effect sizes. In addition, we determined the relative weight of each study to gain insight into the contribution of each study to the overall results of our meta-analysis. This was particularly important for studies categorized as outliers or those with a high risk of bias. The standard residual was also estimated to illustrate the unaccounted-for residual variability between studies. Significance was set at a two-sided p value of less than 0.05.

Statistical analysis was performed using Comprehensive Meta-Analysis software (v. 3.0, Biostat Inc., Frederick, MD, USA). Additionally, as previously mentioned, we employed VOSviewer 1.6.19 software to create network data maps for visualization and exploration.

2.6. Publication Bias

Publication bias is the selective publication of research studies, where studies with positive results are more likely to be published than studies with negative results. To avoid publication bias in the selection of publications for this meta-analysis, we included all studies that met the specified criteria, regardless of whether their outcome was positive or negative. We also performed appropriate statistical tests to mathematically calculate the publication bias. Although combining the data from independent studies using meta-analytical methods can improve statistical precision, it cannot altogether prevent bias.

To assess publication bias, we conducted Egger's regression test [63] and Begg and Mazumdar's rank correlation test [64]. For each type of clinical matrix, publication bias was visually represented using funnel plots. We also utilized the fail-safe method to determine the number of missing studies required to potentially improve the quality of the meta-analysis. However, these results are not presented in this context, given the fact that we did not find a statistically significant publication bias in any of the materials we examined.

3. Results

3.1. Study Selection and Identification

The process of study selection and identification is summarized in Figure 2. Our initial literature search across two primary databases, SCOPUS and PubMed, yielded a total of 9091 records. After removing 596 duplicate records, we further refined the selection based on title and abstract, resulting in the exclusion of 6525 records with irrelevant topics. The remaining 1374 reports were subjected to a detailed search for retrieval. Of these, 1129 reports were not retrievable, and the remaining 245 reports underwent eligibility screening. Within these 245 reports, 122 lacked the necessary data, 16 reports lacked control data, 43 reports were reviews, and 2 reports contained extremely abnormal data, all of which were excluded (total excluded, n = 183 reports). This process led to a final selection of 62 studies for inclusion in the analysis. After a final check, two additional studies with abnormal data were also excluded. Consequently, the meta-analysis included a total of 60 studies. The total number of control participants across all studies was 2991, while the total number of cases was 3892. This resulted in a cumulative total of 6883 participants considered for the meta-analysis.

3.2. Study Characteristics

Table 1 provides an overview of the characteristics of the studies incorporated into the meta-analysis. For the analysis of Hg level in hair, a total of 25 studies were included [65–89], encompassinf various geographic regions. Specifically, there were 7 studies conducted in Europe [70,71,74,76,80,85,88], 5 in North America [73,79,83,86,87], 9 in Asia [65–67,72,77,78,81,82,84], and 4 in Africa [68,69,75,89]. The meta-analysis of Hg levels in whole blood comprised 15 studies [78,86,90–103], with 2 conducted in Europe [85,92], 5 in North America [91,95,96,98,99], 1 in Central America [97], 5 in Asia [77,91,93,100,101], and 2 in Africa [94,102]. For plasma Hg levels, 6 studies were incorporated into the meta-analysis [62,92,103–106], with 2 originating from Europe [92,106], 2 from Asia [62,105], and 2 from Africa [103,104]. In the case of RBCs, the meta-analysis consisted of 5 studies [37,90,107–109], of which 2 were from North America [90,108] and 3 from Asia [37,107,109]. Finally, the analysis of urine Hg values included 9 studies [67,76,78,85,90,110–113], with 3 from Europe [76,85,111], 3 from North America [90,112,113], 2 from Asia [67,78], and 1 from Africa [110]. These studies collectively contributed to our analysis of Hg levels in various clinical matrices and were drawn from diverse geographic regions worldwide.

Table 1. Overview of 60 studies (1985–2023) included in the comprehensive review and meta-analysis of Hg levels in controls and cases as follows: 25 studies (1985–2023) included in the systematic review and meta-analysis of Hg levels in hair (µg/g), 15 studies (2004–2023) included in the systematic review and meta-analysis of Hg levels in whole blood (µg/L), 6 studies (2011–2020) included in the systematic review and meta-analysis of Hg levels in plasma (µg/L), 5 studies (2010–2017) included in the comprehensive review and meta-analysis of Hg levels in red blood cells (RBCs) (µg/L), and 9 studies (2003–2020) included in the comprehensive review and meta-analysis of Hg levels in urine (µg/g creatine).

	Study	Country	Sample Size Controls/Cases	Age Controls/Cases	Gender (Fem/Male) Controls/Cases	Biological Material	Analytical Technique	Mercury Level (Mean ± SD) Controls/Cases
Hair								µg/g
1.	Al-Ayadhi, 2005 [65]	Saudi Arabia	80/65	7.2 ± 0.7/9.0 ± 0.3	not specified; 4/61	Hair	AAS	0.713 ± 0.228/4.204 ± 1.129
2.	Aljumaili et al., 2021 [66]	Iraq	20/75	3–14/3–14	not specified	Hair	AAS	1.25 ± 0.66/3.44 ± 2.93
3.	Blaurock-Bush et al., 2011 [67]	Saudi Arabia	25/25	6.25 ± 2.31/5.29 ± 1.90	6/19; 3/22	Hair	ICP-MS	0.30 ± 0.31/0.47 ± 0.42
4.	Mohamed et al., 2015 [68]	Egypt	100/100	6.80 ± 3.04/6.20 ± 2.40	26/74; 16/84	Hair	AAS	0.25 ± 0.16/0.39 ± 0.37
5.	Ouisselsat et al., 2023 [69]	Morocco	120/107	6.68 ± 2.39/7.14 ± 2.47	36/84; 25/82	Hair	ICP-MS	0.193 ± 0.13/0.200 ± 0.12
6.	Skalny et al., 2017 [70]	Russia	74/74	5.11 ± 2.34/5.12 ± 2.36	not specified	Hair	ICP-MS	0.167 ± 0.077/0.127 ± 0.049
7.	Tinkov et al., 2019 [71]	Russia	30/30	4.8 ± 2.2/4.7 ± 2.1	not specified	Hair	ICP-MS	0.077 ± 0.039/0.229 ± 0.072
8.	Zhai et al., 2019 [72]	China	58/78	4.90 ± 0.97/4.96 ± 1.01	27/31; 22/56	Hair	ICP-MS	0.26 ± 0.13/0.41 ± 0.25
9.	Adams et al., 2006 [73]	USA	40/51	7.5 ± 3.0/7.1 ± 3.0	10/30; 12/39	Hair	ICP-MS	0.29 ± 0.35/0.29 ± 0.41
10.	De Palma et al., 2012 [74]	Italy	61/44	8.4 ± 1.3/9.0 ± 4.0	25/36; 7/37	Hair	AAS	0.25 ± 0.11/0.50 ± 0.14
11.	El-Baz et al., 2010 [75]	Egypt	15/32	5.53 ± 2.75/6.75 ± 3.26	6/9; 10/22	Hair	AAS	0.12 ± 0.019/0.79 ± 0.51
12.	Gil-Hernandez et al., 2020 [76]	Spain	54/54	Not specified	not specified	Hair	AAS	13.00 ± 12.68/8.26 ± 10.57
13.	Ip et al., 2004 [77]	Japan	55/82	7.8 ± 0.4/7.0 ± 0.2	9/46; 9/73	Hair	AAS	1.92 ± 1.58/1.98 ± 1.05
14.	Nabgha-e-Amen et al., 2020 [78]	Pakistan	76/90	3–11/3–11	22/54; 20/70	Hair	ICP-MS	1.0 ± 0.26/1.3 ± 0.4
15.	Wecker et al., 1985 [79]	USA	22/12	4.3 ± 2.6/5.67 ± 0.69	0/22; 0/12	Hair	AAS	15.75 ± 0.35/15.2 ± 0.45
16.	Skalny et al., 2017b [80]	Russia	16/16	5–8/5–8	0/16; 0/16	Hair	ICP-MS	0.151 ± 0.134/0.105 ± 0.09
17.	Hodgson et al., 2014 [81]	Oman	22/22	5.50 ± 1.00/3.5 ± 1.5	6/9; 7/15	Hair	ICP-MS	6.93 ± 0.36/6.03 ± 0.96
18.	Lakshmi and Geetha, 2011 [82]	India	15/50	4–12/4–12	not specified; 20/30	Hair	ICP-MS	0.37 ± 0.04/3.29 ± 0.37
19.	Holmes et al., 2003 [83]	USA	45/94	0.7 ± 0.102/0.7 ± 0.325	11/34; 21/73	Hair	ICP-MS	3.63 ± 3.56/0.47 ± 0.28
20.	Fido and Al-Saad, 2005 [84]	Kuwait	40/40	4.3 ± 2.67/4.2 ± 2.2	0/40; 0/40	Hair	AAS	0.30 ± 0.24/4.50 ± 3.33
21.	Albizzati et al., 2012 [85]	Italy	20/17	10.41 ± 3.05/11.52 ± 3.20	6/14; 2/15	Hair	ICP-MS	0.28 ± 0.08/0.32 ± 0.04
22.	Kern et al., 2007 [86]	USA	45/45	3.0 ± 1.4/3.0 ± 1.4	10/35; 10/35	Hair	AFS	0.16 ± 0.10/0.14 ± 0.11
23.	Adams et al., 2008 [87]	USA	31/78	1.37 ± 0.42/1.38 ± 0.37	11/21; 11/67	Hair	AAS	0.95 ± 0.87/0.87 ± 2.6
24.	Majewska et al., 2010 [88]	Poland	38/55	8.4 ± 0.20/8.1 ± 0.15	19/25; 19/30	Hair	AAS	0.14 ± 0.02/2.1 ± 0.05
25.	Elsheshtawy et al., 2011 [89]	Egypt	32/32	4.0 ± 0.8/4.1 ± 0.8	8/24; 8/24	Hair	ICP-MS	3.2 ± 0.2/0.55 ± 0.06
Whole Blood								µg/L
1.	Adams et al., 2013 [90]	USA	44/55	11.0 ± 3.1/10.0 ± 3.1	5/39; 6/49	Blood	ICP-MS	0.87 ± 0.76/0.75 ± 0.67
2.	Li et al., 2018 [91]	China	184/180	6.12 ± 1.69/5.06 ± 1.37	38/146; 30/150	Blood	AAS	13.47 ± 17.24/55.59 ± 52.56
3.	Macedoni-Lukšič et al., 2015 [92]	Slovenia	22/52	6.6. ± 3.7/6.2 ± 3.0	11/11; 6/46	Blood	AAS	1.55 ± 0.56/1.90 ± 0.97
4.	Zhao et al., 2023 [93]	China	30/30	4.2 ± 1.5/3.8 ± 1.3	15/15; 9/21	Blood	ICP-MS	0.685 ± 0.196/0.796 ± 0.198
5.	Yassa, 2014 [94]	Egypt	45/45	12.40 ± 2.04/11.30 ± 1.02	14/31; 13/32	Blood	ICP-MS	0.00 ± 0.00/4.02 ± 0.54
6.	Stamova et al., 2011 [95]	USA	51/33	2.3–4.7/2.6–4.0	0/51; 0/33	Blood	AAS	0.6 ± 0.82/0.46 ± 0.73
7.	Hertz-Picciotto et al., 2010 [96]	USA	143/249	2–5/2–5	27/116; 28/221	Blood	AAS	0.8 ± 1.3/0.49 ± 1.08
8.	Ip et al., 2004 [77]	Japan	55/82	7.8 ± 0.4/7.0 ± 0.2	9/46; 9/73	Blood	AAS	19.53 ± 5.65/17.68 ± 2.48
9.	Rahbar et al., 2013 [97]	Jamaica	65/65	2–8/2–8	not specified	Blood	ICP-MS	0.98 ± 0.79/0.83 ± 0.67
10.	Yau et al., 2014 [98]	USA, Mexico	78/164	6.6 ± 3.7/6.2 ± 3.0	16/133; 10/68	Blood	ICP-MS	0.32 ± 0.01/0.48 ± 0.13
11.	McKean et al., 2015 [99]	USA	58/164	2–8/2.8	22/36; 149/17	Blood	ICP-MS	4.29 ± 0.84/4.73 ± 0.85
12.	Albizzati et al., 2012 [85]	Italy	20/17	10.41 ± 3.05/11.52 ± 3.20	6/14; 2/15	Blood	ICP-MS	0.57 ± 0.34/0.67 ± 0.31
13.	Mostafa and Al-Ayadhi, 2015 [100]	Saudi Arabia	100/100	8.3 ± 1.6/8.1 ± 1.7	23/77; 22/78	Blood	AAS	0.43 ± 0.14/0.19 ± 0.62
14.	Mostafa et al., 2016 [101]	Saudi Arabia	84/84	7.0 ± 1.8/6.8 ± 1.5	24/60; 22/62	Blood	AAS	0.50 ± 0.14/0.8 ± 0.34
15.	Mostafa and Refai, 2007 [102]	Egypt	40/40	5.25 ± 1.80/5.38 ± 1.85	9/31; 9/31	Blood	AAS	3.9 ± 1.80/19.8 ± 13.9

Table 1. Cont.

	Study	Country	Sample Size Controls/Cases	Age Controls/Cases	Gender (Fem/Male) Controls/Cases	Biological Material	Analytical Technique	Mercury Level (Mean ± SD) Controls/Cases
Plasma								μg/L
1.	Chehbani et al., 2020 [103]	Tunisia	70/89	7.81 ± 3.32/7.52 ± 3.02	29/41; 15/74	Plasma	AAS	0.77 ± 0.53/0.86 ± 1.24
2.	Khaled et al., 2016 [104]	Egypt	40/40	5.23 ± 1.25/4.12 ± 0.94	12/28; 8/32	Plasma	AAS	12.08 ± 4.5/32.9 ± 16.4
3.	Qin et al., 2018 [62]	China	38/34	4.29 ± 1.73/4.10 ± 0.81	17/21; 14/20	Plasma	ICP-OES	1.13 ± 1.05/3.89 ± 0.82
4.	Zhang et al., 2022 [105]	China	30/30	4.21 ± 0.93/4.03 ± 1.12	6/24; 6/24	Plasma	ICP-MS	0.96 ± 0.2/0.81 ± 0.22
5.	Vergani et al., 2011 [106]	Italy	32/28	Not specified /2–6	12/20; 7/21	Plasma	ICP-OES	0.00 ± 0.00/3.21 ± 1.72
6.	Macedoni-Lukšič et al., 2015 [92]	Slovenia	14/42	6.6 ± 3.7/6.2 ± 3.0	7/7; 5/37	Serum	AAS	1.55 ± 0.56/1.90 ± 0.97
RBCs								μg/L
1.	El-Ansary et al., 2017 [37]	Saudi Arabia	30/35	7.2 ± 2.14/7.0 ± 2.34	Not specified	RBCs	AAS	2.71 ± 0.57/3.66 ± 1.13
2.	Alabdali et al., 2014 [107]	Saudi Arabia	32/100	7.2 ± 2.0/7.0 ± 2.34	Not specified; 0/100	RBCs	AAS	5.12 ± 0.83/6.99 ± 0.94
3.	Geier et al., 2010 [108]	USA	89/83	11.4 ± 2.2/7.3 ± 3.7	19/70; 5/58	RBCs	Hg vaporimeter	10.7 ± 4.3/22.2 ± 12.1
4.	Adams et al., 2013 [90]	USA	44/55	11.0 ± 3.1/10.0 ± 3.1	5/39; 6/49	RBCs	ICP-MS	1.3 ± 1.2/1.2 ± 0.81
5.	El-Ansary, 2016 [109]	Saudi Arabia	20/20	7.4/7.4	Not specified	RBCs	AAS	4.64 ± 0.68/6.93 ± 0.94
Urine								μg/g creatinine
1.	Adams et al., 2013 [90]	USA	44/55	11.0 ± 3.1/10.0 ± 3.1	5/39; 6/49	Urine	ICP-MS	2.58 ± 1.10/1.01 ± 3.90
2.	Blaurock-Bush et al., 2011 [67]	Saudi Arabia	25/25	6.25 ± 2.31/5.29 ± 1.90	6/19; 3/22	Urine	ICP-MS	1.10 ± 0.63/2.48 ± 2.34
3.	Metwally et al., 2015 [110]	Egypt	75/55	4.02 ± 4.01	18/57; 16/39	Urine	ICP-MS	2.22 ± 0.35/11.3 ± 6.63
4.	Wright et al., 2012 [111]	UK	28/47	12.6 ± 3.5/9.6 ± 3.6	15/13; 10/37	Urine	ICP-MS	5.4 ± 5.07/4.97 ± 3.04
5.	Woods et al., 2010 [112]	USA	59/59	6.39 ± 3.06/6.01 ± 2.14	0/59; 0/59	Urine	ICP-MS	0.29 ± 0.53/0.36 ± 0.62
6.	Bradstreet et al., 2003 [113]	USA	18/221	8.85/6.25	4/14; 38/183	Urine	ICP-MS	1.29 ± 1.54/4.06 ± 8.59
7.	Albizzati et al., 2012 [85]	Italy	20/17	10.41 ± 3.05/11.52 ± 3.2	6/14; 2/15	Urine	ICP-MS	0.69 ± 0.07/0.70 ± 0.07
8.	Nabgha-e-Amen et al., 2020 [78]	Pakistan	76/90	3–11/3–11	22/54; 20/70	Urine	ICP-MS	1.0 ± 0.31/1.3 ± 0.27
9.	Gil-Hernandez et al., 2020 [76]	Spain	54/54	Not specified	Not specified	Urine	AAS	0.33 ± 0.42/0.54 ± 0.78

Abbreviations: ICP-MS (Inductively Coupled Plasma-Mass Spectrometry); ICP-OES (Inductively Coupled Plasma-Optical Emission Spectrometry); AAS (Atomic Absorption Spectrometry); AFS (Atomic Fluorescence Spectroscopy). Number of controls: 1134 (hair); 1019 (whole blood); 224 (plasma); 215 (RBCs); 399 (urine). Total number of controls: 2991. Number of cases: 1361 (hair); 1345 (whole blood); 263 (plasma); 293 (RBCs); 623 (urine). Total number of cases: 3892. Total number of participants enrolled in the meta-analysis: 6883.

3.3. Quality Assessment

The quality scores assigned to the studies enrolled in the meta-analysis ranged from 1 to 7, with an average score of 6.17. The quality scores differed slightly across the different clinical matrices. Specifically, the quality score for hair studies averaged 6.20, for whole blood studies it was 6.47, for plasma studies it was 6.00, for RBCs studies it was 5.60, and for urine studies it was 6.56 (Table 2). Scores of 5 and 6 were assigned to specific studies, and they generally reflected certain criteria. A score of 5 was typically assigned when participant gender and age were not represented, when numerical data (such as standard deviation or error) were missing, and when ICP-MS was not used as the analytical method. A score of 6 was assigned to studies that did not report either participant gender or age but provided all necessary numerical data required for the meta-analysis. These scores did not imply that the selected studies were of lower quality but rather indicated that they did not fully meet the criteria established for this meta-analysis.

Table 2. Quality assessment of included studies in the meta-analysis: Hg levels in ASD cases (based on the Newcastle–Ottawa Scale).

Study	Selection				Comparability	Outcome		Score	
	Representativeness	Size	Non Respondents	Exposure Determination	Design/ Analysis	Determination of Outcome	Statist. Test	For Sample	Type Average
Hair									
Al-Ayadhi, 2005 [65]	a	a	b	a	a	b	a	5	
Aljumaili et al., 2021 [66]	a	a	b	a	a	b	a	5	
Blaurock-Bush et al., 2011 [67]	a	a	a	a	a	b	a	6	
Mohamed et al., 2015 [68]	a	a	a	a	a	a	a	7	
Ouisselsat et al., 2023 [69]	a	a	a	a	a	a	a	7	
Skalny et al., 2017 [70]	a	a	b	a	a	a	a	6	
Tinkov et al., 2019 [71]	a	a	b	a	a	a	a	6	
Zhai et al., 2019 [72]	a	a	a	a	a	a	a	7	
Adams et al., 2006 [73]	a	a	a	a	a	a	a	7	
De Palma et al., 2012 [74]	a	a	a	a	a	a	a	7	
El-Baz et al., 2010 [75]	a	a	a	a	a	a	a	7	
Gil-Hernandez et al., 2020 [76]	a	a	c	a	a	b	a	4	
Ip et al., 2004 [77]	a	a	a	a	a	b	a	6	
Nabgha-e-Amen et al., 2020 [78]	a	a	a	a	a	b	a	6	
Wecker et al., 1985 [79]	a	a	a	a	a	b	a	6	
Skalny et al., 2017 [80]	a	a	c	a	a	a	a	5	
Hodgson et al., 2014 [81]	a	a	a	a	a	a	a	7	
Lakshmi and Geetha., 2011 [82]	a	a	c	a	a	a	a	5	
Holmes et al., 2003 [83]	a	a	a	a	a	a	a	7	
Fido and Al-Saad, 2005 [84]	a	a	b	a	a	a	a	6	
Albizzati et al., 2012 [85]	a	a	a	a	a	a	a	7	
Kern et al., 2007 [86]	a	a	a	a	a	a	a	7	
Adams et al., 2008 [87]	a	a	a	a	a	b	a	6	
Majewska et al., 2010 [88]	a	a	a	a	a	b	a	6	
Elsheshtawy et al., 2011 [89]	a	a	a	a	a	a	a	7	6.20
Whole blood									
Adams et al., 2013 [90]	a	a	a	a	a	a	a	7	
Li et al., 2018 [91]	a	a	a	a	a	b	a	6	
Macedoni-Lukšić et al., 2015 [92]	a	a	a	a	a	b	a	6	
Zhao et al., 2023 [93]	a	a	a	a	a	a	a	7	
Yassa, 2014 [94]	a	a	a	a	a	a	a	7	
Stamova et al., 2011 [95]	a	a	a	a	a	b	a	6	
Hertz-Picciotto et al., 2010 [96]	a	a	b	a	a	a	a	6	
Ip et al., 2004 [77]	a	a	a	a	a	a	a	7	
Rahbar et al., 2013 [97]	a	a	a	a	a	a	a	7	
Yau et al., 2014 [98]	a	a	b	a	a	a	a	6	
McKean et al., 2015 [99]	a	a	a	a	a	a	a	7	
Albizzati et al., 2012 [85]	a	a	a	a	a	a	a	7	
Mostafa and Al-Ayadhi, 2015 [100]	a	a	a	a	a	b	a	6	
Mostafa et al., 2016 [101]	a	a	a	a	a	b	a	6	
Mostafa and Refai., 2007 [102]	a	a	a	a	a	b	a	6	6.47
Plasma									
Chehbani et al., 2020 [103]	a	a	a	a	a	b	a	6	
Khaled et al., 2016 [104]	a	a	a	a	a	b	a	6	
Qin et al., 2018 [62]	a	a	a	a	a	b	a	6	
Zhang et al., 2022 [105]	a	a	a	a	a	a	a	7	
Vergani et al., 2011 [106]	a	a	b	a	a	a	a	6	
Macedoni-Lukšić et al., 2015 [92]	a	a	a	a	b	b	a	5	6.00

Table 2. Cont.

Study	Selection				Comparability	Outcome		Score
	Representativeness	Size	Non Respondents	Exposure Determination	Design/ Analysis	Determination of Outcome	Statist. Test	For Sample Type Average
RBCs								
El-Ansary et al., 2017 [37]	a	a	b	a	a	b	a	5
Alabdali et al., 2014 [107]	a	a	b	a	a	b	a	5
Geier et al., 2010 [108]	a	a	a	a	a	a	a	7
Adams et al., 2013 [90]	a	a	a	a	a	a	a	7
El-Ansary., 2016 [109]	a	a	c	a	a	b	a	4 5.60
Urine								
Adams et al., 2013 [90]	a	a	a	a	a	a	a	7
Blaurock-Bush et al., 2011 [67]	a	a	a	a	a	a	a	7
Metwally et al., 2015 [110]	a	a	a	a	a	a	a	7
Wright et al., 2012 [111]	a	a	a	a	a	a	a	7
Woods et al., 2010 [112]	a	a	b	a	a	a	a	6
Bradstreet et al., 2003 [113]	a	a	a	a	a	a	a	7
Albizzati et al., 2012 [85]	a	a	a	a	a	a	a	7
Nabgha-e-Amen et al., 2020 [78]	a	a	a	a	a	a	a	7
Gil-Hernandez et al., 2020 [76]	a	a	c	a	a	b	a	4 6.56
								6.17

Selection: (1) Sample representativeness: a, truly representative of the average of the target population; b, reasonably representative of the average of the target population; c, selected group of users. (2) Sample size: a, satisfactory; b, unsatisfactory. (3) Nonrespondents: a, the comparability between the characteristics of the respondents and the nonrespondents is given, and the response rate is satisfactory; b, the response rate is not satisfactory, or the comparability between the respondents and the nonrespondents is not satisfactory; c, no description of response rate or the characteristics of the respondents and the nonrespondents. (4) Exposure determination: a, validated measurement instrument; b, measurement instrument not validated, but the instrument is available or described; c, no description of the measurement instrument. Comparability: (1) Comparability of subjects based on design or analysis: a, the study controls for the main factor; b, the study controls for each additional factor. Outcome: (1) Determination of outcome: a, independent blind assessment; b, record linkage; c, self-report. (2) Statistical test: a, the statistical test used to analyze the data is clearly described and appropriate, and the measure of association is stated, including confidence intervals and probability level (p-value); b, the statistical test is inappropriate, not described, or incomplete. Calculation: a = 1; b = from the maximum 7, 1 is subtracted; c = from the maximum 7, 2 is subtracted. Quality assessment was modified based on criteria as described by [58].

3.4. Meta-Analysis of Hg Levels in Hair

This portion of the analysis included 25 studies with a combined sample size of 1134 controls and 1361 cases. Among these studies, four reported age ranges for controls and cases, one study did not specify age, and the remaining 20 studies had mean ages of 5.64 years for controls and 5.72 years for cases. While four studies did not report the gender of participants, two studies only reported gender for cases, and the other 19 studies provided gender data for both controls and cases. Among these 19 studies, there were 481 girls and 623 boys in the control group, and 222 girls and 626 boys in the case group. Analytical techniques for Hg concentration assessment varied, with 16 studies using ICP-MS, eight studies using AAS, and one study using AFS.

The mean hair Hg levels showed considerable variation, ranging from 0.0077 ± 0.0039 μg/g [71] to 13.00 ± 12.68 μg/g [76] for controls, and from 0.127 ± 0.049 μg/g [70] to 8.26 ± 10.57 μg/g [76] for ASD cases. Out of the 25 studies, nine reported significantly higher Hg levels in the hair of cases compared to controls, eight reported significantly lower levels in cases, and eight reported no significant differences between the two groups.

Pooling of the data using the random effects model revealed no significant differences between cases and controls, with Hedges's g = -0.432 (95% CI: $-0.980, 0.115$) and $p = 0.122$. Individual study effect sizes ranged from -47.909 (95% CI: $-54.806, -41.012, p = 0.000$) in the study by [88] to 1.548 (95% CI: 1.150, 1.945, $p = 0.000$) in the study by [83]. Relative weights and standard residuals for each study are presented in Figure 3. Relative weights ranged from 0.55 [88] to 4.36 [69], and standard residuals ranged from -12.65 [88] to 8.85 [89]. High heterogeneity was observed with $I^2 = 97.170\%$, $Q(24) = 847.959$, and $\tau^2 = 1.772$, $p = 0.000$, indicating substantial variation in the true mean effects between studies.

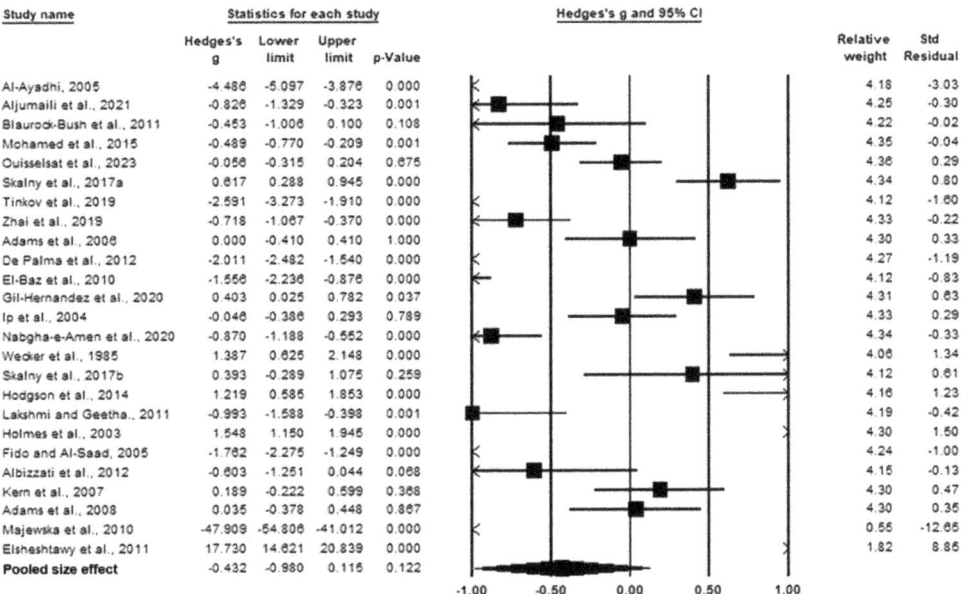

Figure 3. Forest plot for random-effects meta-analysis: variations in hair Hg levels between control children and cases. The size of each square corresponds to the study's weight. The diamond symbol represents the overall pooled effect size for the studies included in the meta-analysis. Abbreviation: CI (Confidence Interval).

Publication bias was assessed using funnel plots, which indicated no significant publication bias. Egger's regression test showed $t_{25} = 1.027$, $p = 0.157$, and Begg and Mazumdar rank correlation demonstrated Kendall's $\tau = -0.120$, $p = 0.200$ (Figure 4).

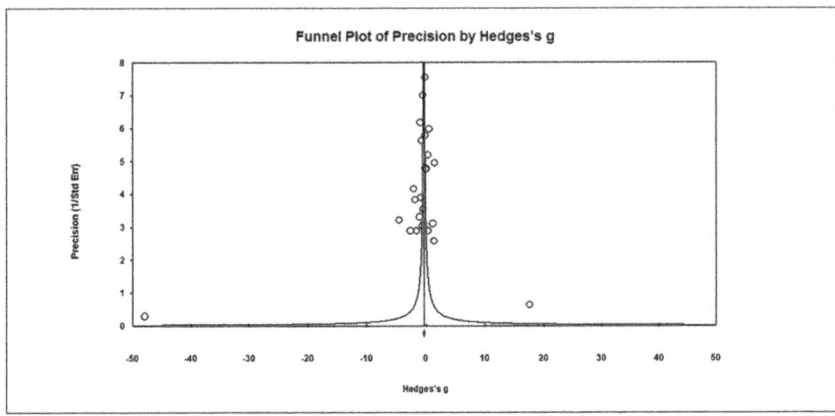

Figure 4. Funnel plots for publication bias assessment in studies comparing hair Hg levels in controls and cases. The plot displays the effect size (Hedges's g) of the studies against their precision (inverse of SE). Observed studies are represented by circles, while the diamond symbol illustrates the overall pooled effect size based on these observed studies. Egger's regression test: $t_{25} = 1.027$; $p = 0.157$; Begg and Mazumdar rank correlation: Kendall's $\tau = -0.120$, $p = 0.200$.

In summary, we did not provide evidence of higher Hg levels in the hair of ASD children compared to neurotypical children ($p = 0.122$).

3.5. Meta-Analysis of Hg Levels in Whole Blood

The meta-analysis of Hg levels in whole blood included 15 studies with a total sample size of 1019 neurotypical children and 1345 ASD children (Table 1). In two studies, age ranges were reported for both controls and cases; in one study, ages ranged from 2 to 5 years in both groups, and in another study, they ranged from 2.3 to 4.7 years for controls and 2.6 to 4.0 years for cases. For the remaining 11 studies, the mean age was 7.15 years for controls and 7.40 years for cases.

One study did not provide information about gender, while the other 14 studies reported that the control group consisted of 219 girls and 806 boys, and the case group included 315 girls and 896 boys. The analytical techniques used varied, with nine studies using ICP-MS and six studies using AAS (Table 1).

The mean Hg levels in whole blood varied markedly. In controls, they ranged from 0.00 ± 0.00 μg/L [94] to 19.53 ± 5.65 μg/L [77]. In cases, the levels ranged from 0.19 ± 0.62 μg/L [100] to 55.59 ± 52.56 μg/L [91]. Seven studies reported significantly higher Hg levels in the whole blood of cases than in controls, three reported levels significantly lower than in controls, while five studies did not find significant differences between the two groups.

The forest plot of pooled data under the random effects model (Figure 5) showed significant differences between cases and controls, with Hedges's $g = -0.813$ (95% CI: $-1.307, -0.318$) and $p = 0.001$. Effect sizes in individual studies ranged from -10.438 (95% CI: $-12.017, -8.859$, $p = 0.000$) in the study by [94] to 0.532 (95% CI: $0.251, 0.813$, $p = 0.000$) in the study by [100]. The relative weights and standard residuals for each study are also displayed in Figure 5. Relative weights ranged from 4.14% [94] to 7.07% [96], and standard residuals ranged from -7.92 [94] to 1.46 [100]. High heterogeneity was observed, with $I^2 = 96.654\%$, $Q(14) = 418.462$, and $\tau^2 = 0.891$, indicating substantial variation in the true mean effects between studies.

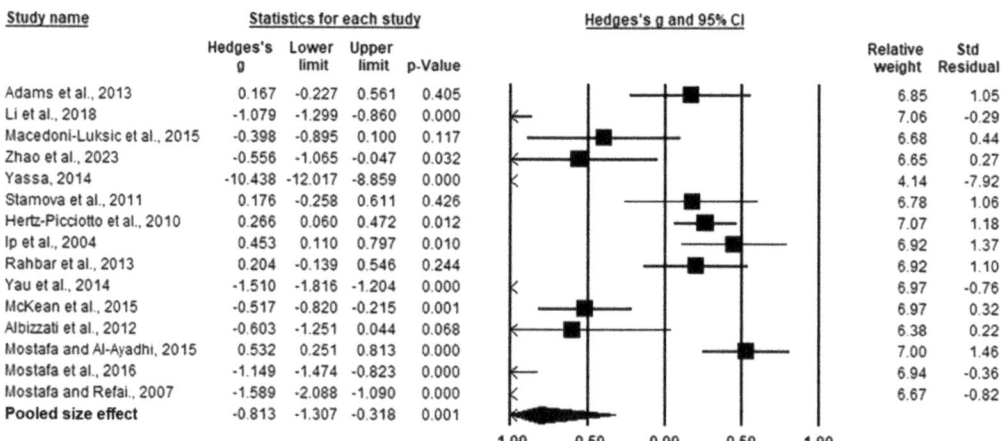

Figure 5. Forest plot for random-effects meta-analysis of differences in whole blood Hg levels between control children and cases. The size of each square corresponds to the study's weight, with the diamond symbol representing the pooled total effect size for the studies included in the meta-analysis. Abbreviation: CI (Confidence Interval).

Publication bias was assessed using funnel plots, which indicated no significant publication bias. Egger's regression test showed $t_{15} = 1.621$, $p = 0.064$, and Begg and Mazumdar rank correlation demonstrated Kendall's $\tau = -0.276$, $p = 0.076$ (Figure 6).

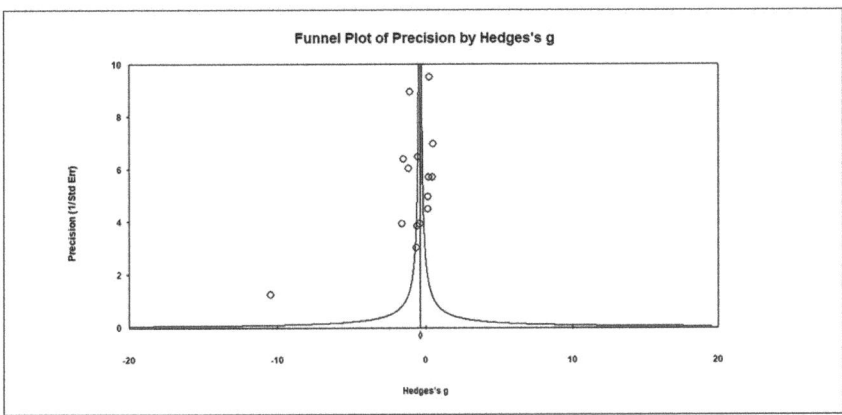

Figure 6. Funnel plots for assessing publication bias in observed studies comparing Hg levels in whole blood between control and case groups. The plot displays the effect size (Hedges's g) of individual studies against their precision (inverse of SE). Observed studies are represented by circles, with the diamond symbol indicating the pooled overall effect size based on these observed studies. Egger's regression test: $t_{15} = 1.621$, $p = 0.064$; Begg and Mazumdar rank correlation: Kendall's $\tau = -0.276$, $p = 0.076$.

In conclusion, the pooled effect size indicates significantly higher Hg levels in whole blood among ASD cases compared to controls ($p = 0.001$).

3.6. Meta-Analysis of Hg Levels in Plasma

The meta-analysis of plasma Hg levels in controls and cases involved six studies with a combined sample size of 224 neurotypical children and 263 ASD children (Table 1). In one study, the mean age was not reported for females and was 2–6 years for males. In the remaining five studies, the mean age was 5.63 years for controls and 5.19 years for cases. The control group consisted of 83 girls and 141 boys, while the case group included 55 girls and 208 boys. Analytical techniques varied across studies, with one study using ICP-MS, two studies using ICP-OES, and three studies using AAS.

The mean Hg levels in plasma ranged from 0.00 ± 0.00 µg/L [106] to 12.08 ± 4.05 µg/L [104] in the control group, and from 0.81 ± 0.22 µg/L [105] to 32.90 ± 16.40 µg/L [104] in the case group. Three studies reported significantly higher plasma Hg levels in cases than in controls, one study found significantly lower levels, and two studies reported no significant differences.

The forest plot of pooled data under the random-effects model is depicted in Figure 7. The results show significant differences between the two groups, with Hedges's g = -1.161 (95% CI: -2.247, -0.075) and $p = 0.036$. Effect sizes in individual studies ranged from -2.878 (95% CI: -3.535, -2.222, $p < 0.001$) in the study by [62] to -0.090 (95% CI: -0.402, 2.222, $p = 0.571$) in the study by [103], indicating high heterogeneity in plasma. The relative weights and standard residuals for each study are also shown in Figure 7. Relative weights ranged from 16.28% [106] to 17.19% [103], and standard residuals ranged from -1.37 [62] to 1.51 [104]. The heterogeneity was $I^2 = 96.256\%$, $Q(5) = 133.562$, and $\tau^2 = 1.761$, $p = 0.000$, indicating high heterogeneity in reporting Hg levels in plasma.

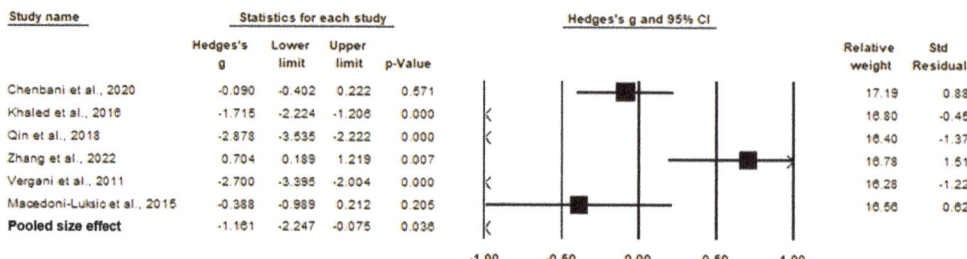

Figure 7. Forest plot for random-effects meta-analysis, depicting variations in plasma Hg levels between control children and cases. The size of each square corresponds to the study's weight, and the diamond symbol represents the pooled total effect size based on the studies included in the meta-analysis. Abbreviation: CI (Confidence Interval).

Funnel plots (Figure 8) were used to assess publication bias, which revealed no significant publication bias. Egger's regression test showed $t_5 = 1.655$, $p = 0.087$, and Begg and Mazumdar rank correlation demonstrated Kendall's $\tau = -0.467$, $p = 0.094$.

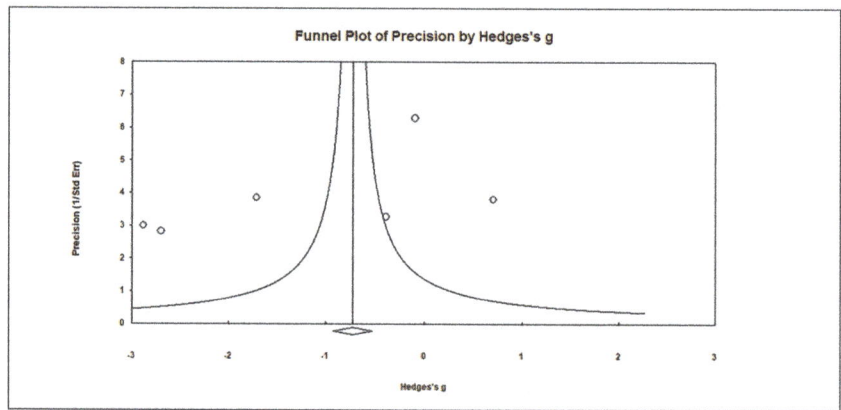

Figure 8. Funnel plots for evaluating publication bias in observed studies comparing Hg levels in the plasma of control and case Groups. The figure illustrates the effect size (Hedges's g) of the studies against their precision (inverse of SE). Observed studies are represented by circles, and the diamond symbol represents the pooled overall effect size based on the observed studies. Egger's regression test: $t_6 = 1.655$, $p = 0.087$; Begg and Mazumdar rank correlation: Kendall's $\tau = -0.467$, $p = 0.094$.

In summary, the pooled effect size indicates significantly higher plasma Hg levels in cases compared to controls ($p = 0.036$).

3.7. Meta-Analysis of Hg Levels in RBCs

The meta-analysis of Hg levels in RBCs involved five studies with a total sample size of 215 neurotypical children and 293 ASD children (Table 1). The mean age in the studies was 8.76 years for controls and 7.74 years for cases. Two studies did not report the gender distribution [37,109], and one study [107] reported the control group's gender, but had an all-boys ASD group. The remaining control group consisted of 24 girls and 119 boys, while the case group included 11 girls and 207 boys. Analytical techniques used included ICP-MS in one study, AAS in three studies, and an Hg vaporimeter in one study.

Mean Hg levels in RBCs varied from 1.30 ± 0.20 µg/L [90] to 10.70 ± 4.30 µg/L [108] in the control group and from 1.20 ± 0.81 µg/L [90] to 22.20 ± 12.10 µg/L [108] in the case group. Four studies reported significantly higher Hg levels in the RBCs of cases compared to controls, while one study did not find significant differences.

The forest plot of pooled data under the random-effects model (Figure 9) indicated significant differences between cases and controls, with Hedges's g = −1.354 (95% CI: −2.197, −0.512) and p = 0.002. Effect sizes in individual studies ranged from −2.736 (95% CI: −3.589, −1.882, p = 0.000) in the study by [37] to −0.099 (95% CI: −0.295, 0.493, p = 0.622) in the study by [90], showing high heterogeneity among RBCs. The relative weights and standard residuals for each study are also displayed in Figure 9. Relative weights ranged from 20.74% [90] to 21.03% [108]. The heterogeneity was high, with I^2 = 93.974%, Q(4) = 66.383, and τ^2 = 0.851, p = 0.000.

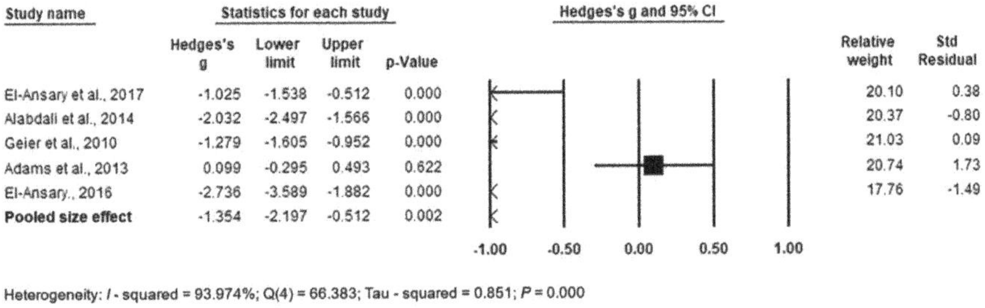

Study name
Statistics for each study
Hedges's g and 95% CI
Hedges's g
Lower limit
Upper limit
p-Value
Relative weight
Std Residual
El-Ansary et al., 2017 -1.025 -1.538 -0.512 0.000 20.10 0.38
Alabdali et al., 2014 -2.032 -2.497 -1.566 0.000 20.37 -0.80
Geier et al., 2010 -1.279 -1.605 -0.952 0.000 21.03 0.09
Adams et al., 2013 0.099 -0.295 0.493 0.622 20.74 1.73
El-Ansary., 2016 -2.736 -3.589 -1.882 0.000 17.76 -1.49
Pooled size effect -1.354 -2.197 -0.512 0.002
-1.00
-0.50
0.00
0.50
1.00
Heterogeneity: I - squared = 93.974%; Q(4) = 66.383; Tau - squared = 0.851; P = 0.000

Figure 9. Forest plot for random-effects meta-analysis, depicting variations in Hg levels in red blood cells (RBCs) between control children and cases. Each square's size corresponds to the study's weight, and the diamond symbol represents the aggregated total effect size for the studies included in the meta-analysis. Abbreviation: CI (Confidence Interval).

Publication bias was assessed using funnel plots, which revealed no significant publication bias. Egger's regression test showed t_5 = 0.901, p = 0.217, and Begg and Mazumdar rank correlation demonstrated Kendall's τ = −0.200, p = 0.312 (Figure 10).

Funnel Plot of Precision by Hedges's g
Precision (1/Std Err)
Hedges's g
0
1
2
3
4
5
6
-3
-2
-1
0
1
2
3

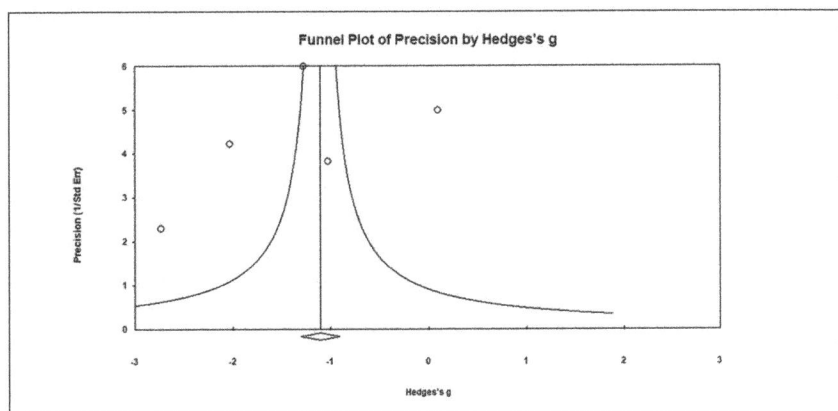

Figure 10. Funnel plots for assessing publication bias in observed studies comparing Hg levels in red blood cells (RBCs) of control and case groups. The figure illustrates the effect size (Hedges's g) of the studies relative to their precision (inverse of SE). Circles represent individual observed studies, while the diamond symbol indicates the overall effect size derived from the observed studies. Egger's regression test: t_5 = 0.901, p = 0.217; Begg and Mazumdar rank correlation: Kendall's τ = −0.200, p = 0.312.

In conclusion, the pooled effect size indicates significantly higher levels of Hg in RBCs in cases compared to controls ($p = 0.002$).

3.8. Meta-Analysis of Hg Levels in Urine

The meta-analysis of urine Hg levels included nine studies with a total sample size of 399 neurotypical children and 623 ASD children (Table 1). In one study [78], the mean age ranged from 3 to 11 years for both groups, while in another study [76], the age was not specified. In the other seven studies, the mean age was 8.50 years for the controls and 7.53 years for the cases. The control group consisted of 76 girls and 233 boys, and the case group included 95 girls and 474 boys. The [112] study used only boys in their experiment, and the gender structure was not specified in the study by [76]. In eight studies, ICP-MS was used, and one study used AAS as the analytical technique.

Mean Hg levels in urine ranged from 0.29 ± 0.53 μg/g creatinine [112] to 5.40 ± 5.07 μg/g creatinine [111] in the control group and from 0.36 ± 0.62 μg/g creatinine [112] to 11.30 ± 6.63 μg/g creatinine [110] in the case group. Four studies reported significantly higher urine Hg levels in cases compared to controls, one study reported significantly lower levels, and four studies did not find significant differences.

The forest plot of pooled data under the random-effects model is depicted in Figure 11. The results showed significant differences between the two groups, with Hedges's $g = -0.471$ (95% CI: -0.981, 0.040) and $p = 0.071$. Effect sizes in individual studies ranged from -0.333 (95% CI: -0.813, 0.147, $p = 0.173$) in the study by [113] to -2.092 (95% CI: -2.521, -1.663, $p = 0.000$) in the study by [110]. The relative weights and standard residuals for each study are shown in Figure 11. Relative weights ranged from 10.26% [85] to 12.61% [78]. Heterogeneity was present, with $I^2 = 92.204\%$, $Q(8) = 102.612$, and $\tau^2 = 0.557$, indicating a high degree of variation among studies. Compared with hair, whole blood, plasma, and RBCs, the least heterogeneity was obtained for studies reporting Hg levels in urine.

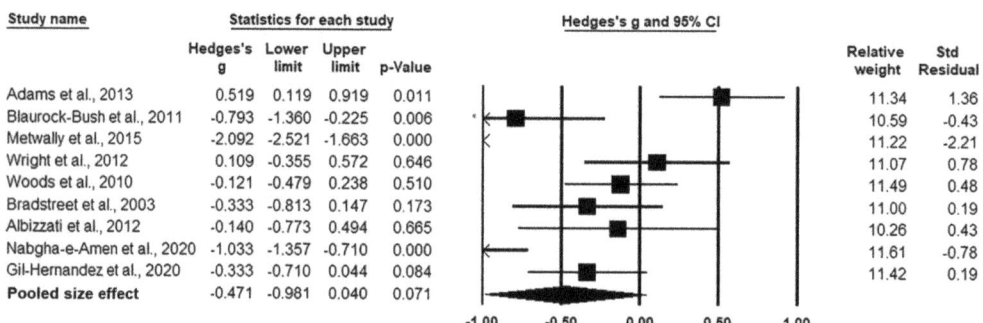

Figure 11. Forest plot for random-effects meta-analysis. Variations in urine Hg levels between control children and cases are presented. The size of each square corresponds to the study's weight, while the diamond symbol represents the combined overall effect size for the studies included in the meta-analysis. Abbreviation: CI (Confidence Interval).

Funnel plots were used to assess publication bias (Figure 12), and they indicated no significant publication bias in urine samples. Egger's regression test showed $t_9 = 0.246$, $p = 0.406$, and Begg and Mazumdar rank correlation demonstrated Kendall's $\tau = 0.000$, $p = 0.500$.

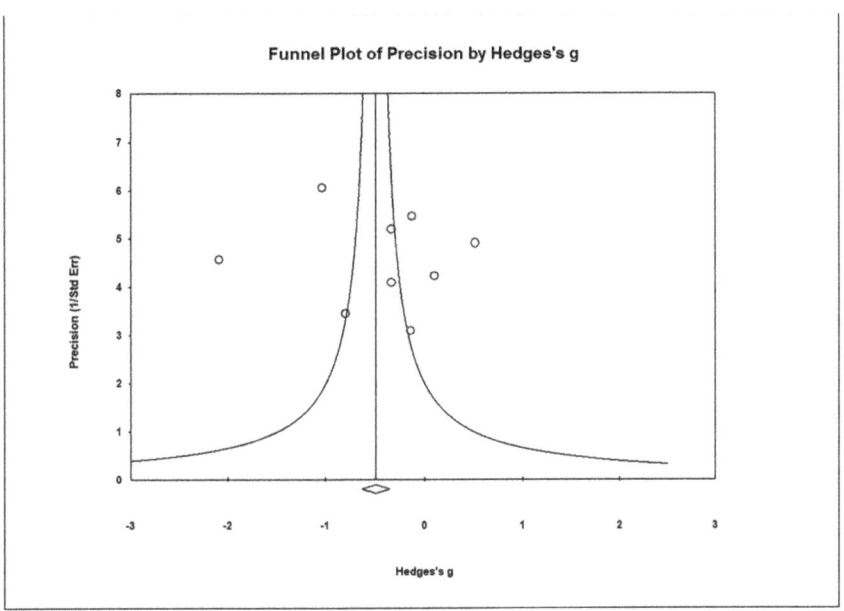

Figure 12. Funnel plots for the evaluation of publication bias in the examined studies, comparing Hg levels in the urine of control and case groups. The figure displays the effect size (Hedges's g) of the individual studies in relation to their precision (inverse of the standard error). Each circle represents an observed study, and the diamond symbol represents the combined overall effect size calculated based on the observed studies. Egger's regression test: $t_9 = 0.246$, $p = 0.406$; Begg and Mazumdar rank correlation: Kendall's $\tau = 0.000$, $p = 0.500$.

In summary, the pooled effect size did not show significantly higher urine Hg levels in cases compared to controls ($p = 0.071$).

Overall, this meta-analysis revealed significantly higher Hg values in cases compared to controls in whole blood, plasma, and RBCs, with high heterogeneity observed. At the same time, no significant differences were found in hair and urine Hg levels between neurotypical children and ASD children. The analysis of publication bias for hair, blood, plasma, RBCs, and urine did not indicate statistically significant publication bias in any of the studies analyzed.

4. Discussion

In this section, we will not provide a detailed discussion of the studies enrolled in the meta-analysis, as presented in Table 1. Studies that provided specific data, such as Hg levels in clinical matrices of cases and controls sorted by gender, age, residence, and other demographic characteristics, will be discussed in more detail.

4.1. Hg in Hair

Scalp hair is considered a suitable sample for assessing Hg levels in ASD children. It is collected noninvasively, reflects long-term Hg exposure, and is a primary sample in evaluating the link between Hg and ASD [78,114]. However, it is important to collect and prepare hair samples appropriately to avoid potential contamination in the pre-analytical phase. Scalp hair grows at a rate of approximately 1.5 cm per month, and can provide insights into Hg exposure over time [115].

The 1999–2000 NHANES study reported a mean hair Hg value of 0.12 µg/g for healthy neurotypical USA children (n = 838, aged 1 to 5 years) [116]. Their study also highlighted that hair can contain significantly higher Hg levels compared to blood, making it a suitable sample for environmental science. When assessing hair from children with ASD, it is essential to consider the age of the children, as younger children with ASD could exhibit different Hg levels than older children with ASD. Majewska et al. [88] pointed out that younger children with ASD had lower Hg levels than older children with ASD. This discrepancy might be attributed to increased Hg exposure or variations in detoxification mechanisms over time. Nevertheless, it is crucial to explore these variables' dynamics as children with ASD grow, depending on their Hg exposure and detoxification mechanisms.

Several studies reported significantly lower Hg levels in the hair of ASD cases compared to controls, and the specifics can be found in Table 1. A meta-analysis conducted by Saghazadeh and Rezaei [117], involving 1092 cases and 973 controls, did not establish a link between Hg and ASD in hair samples. However, it reported substantially higher hair Hg levels in ASD cases from developing countries compared to those from developed countries. These findings of unaltered levels of Hg in hair were consistent with the data we obtained in this meta-analysis of 1361 cases and 1134 controls. It is important to note that studies with exceptionally high Hg levels in hair, such as the one by Fido and Al-Saad [84], were excluded from our analysis.

To date, limited research has explored differences in hair Hg levels in ASD cases and neurotypical controls based on demographic and clinical factors. Adams et al. [73] found no significant differences in hair Hg levels for age groups 3–15 years and 3–6 years in the USA. In contrast, Zhai et al. [72] found significantly different hair Hg levels between female cases and female controls, but not between male cases and male controls in China. Geier et al. [53] reported a significant correlation between increasing ASD severity and higher hair Hg levels. However, research findings vary, as Lakshmi Priya and Geetha [82] did not find a significant association between ASD symptom severity and hair Hg levels. Fiore et al. [118] also reported no significant correlation between hair Hg levels and ASD symptom severity in participants from Catania, Southern Italy. Given these discrepancies, further extensive research is needed to better understand Hg levels in ASD children from different countries, accounting for demographic and clinical factors.

4.2. Hg in Whole Blood and Its Parts (Plasma/Serum and RBCs)

Whole blood and RBCs provide long-term information on Hg levels, particularly RBCs, which have a lifespan of approximately 120 days [31]. In contrast, plasma offers only short-term information on Hg exposure, making it less crucial as a clinical matrix in ASD [119]. Therefore, it is imperative to conduct comprehensive studies on the Hg status in the blood, hair, and urine of pregnant women, lactating women, and young children to gain in-depth insights into prenatal and early postnatal Hg exposure, potentially during the period when ASD begins to develop [41]. For instance, a study by Ryu et al. [120] found a connection between prenatal and early childhood Hg exposure and ASD behavior at age 5 by analyzing Hg levels from early pregnancy to age 3 in a longitudinal cohort study of 458 mother–child pairs.

Most studies have reported higher Hg values in whole blood, plasma, and RBCs of ASD cases compared to matched controls, particularly in children older than 3 years. For instance, Baj et al. [48] indicated higher serum Hg levels in 78.3% of children with ASD. Geier et al. [108] reported a twofold increase in Hg levels in RBCs of cases compared to gender- and age-matched controls. Nevertheless, a few studies have reported the opposite pattern, where Hg levels were lower in cases compared to controls (Table 1).

In addition to quantifying total Hg and Hg-species in whole blood and its derivatives, it is crucial to assess essential trace elements, primarily zinc (Zn) and selenium (Se). Some studies have indicated a deficiency of these two elements in ASD cases with elevated Hg profiles. For instance, Babaknejad et al. [121] reported a deficiency of Zn in ASD cases compared to controls, while El-Ansary et al. [37] found protective effects of Se in ASD cases with high Hg levels in RBCs. It is interesting to note that an occupational study by Chen et al. [122] with participants from an Hg-contaminated region reported significantly higher serum and urine Hg levels in the exposed population. McDowell et al. [116] found higher Hg levels in older women, women who consumed more seafood, and women of different ethnicities.

While a previous meta-analysis by Jafari et al. [35] reported significantly lower Hg levels in hair for cases compared to controls, they also reported higher Hg levels in whole blood and RBCs for ASD cases compared to controls. Shiani et al. [123] reported significantly higher Hg levels in 952 cases compared to 650 controls in their meta-analysis, which included 13 studies. These results corroborate previous findings of higher Hg levels in ASD cases compared to controls, but the current meta-analysis enrolled a substantially larger number of participants and samples, including plasma samples.

4.3. Hg in Urine

Urine reflects the short-term status of Hg exposure, and is easily accessible without invasive procedures [31,114,124]. Urine Hg excretion is particularly important in ASD cases receiving chelation therapy, such as dimercaptosuccinic acid (DMSA), which has been reported to lead to increased urine Hg excretion [113,125].

To date, three meta-analyses of urine Hg levels between cases and controls have been conducted. Jafari et al. [35] included eight studies (491 cases and 417 controls) and reported no significant differences in urine Hg levels between cases and controls. They also found no significant difference in urine Hg levels between cases in the US and certain other continents. Saghazadeh and Rezaei [117] similarly reported no significant differences between ASD cases and controls in terms of urine Hg levels. In contrast, Shiani et al. [122] conducted a meta-analysis involving seven studies (466 cases and 325 controls), and reported that children with ASD had significantly lower urine Hg levels compared to controls. Our meta-analysis observed no variations in urine Hg levels between cases and controls, consistent with the findings of Jafari et al. [35] and Saghazadeh and Rezaei [117], but on a larger sample.

As with hair and blood, there is limited knowledge about urine Hg levels in cases and controls concerning age, gender, and other demographic factors. We identified only one study that reported significantly lower urine Hg levels in children aged 2 to 4 years (n = 16, median value of 0.77 µg/L) compared to age-matched controls (n = 16, median value of 0.97 µg/L) [105]. In the comparison of urine Hg levels between children aged 4 to 6 years, no statistically significant differences in Hg levels were observed. This scarcity of data highlights the need for additional research in this direction to better understand the variations in urine Hg levels among different demographic groups.

In addition to measuring Hg levels in urine, several studies have focused on quantifying porphyrins in urine (pre-coproporphyrin, coproporphyrin, etc.), which could serve as specific biomarkers for Hg profiles in the body [38]. Porphyrins are heterocyclic compounds required for heme formation, an essential component of hemoglobin [48]. Many studies have reported significant increases in urine porphyrin levels in ASD cases compared to controls [35,77,104,112,126–129]. For instance, Geier and Geier [125] noted that children with ASD had 83% higher levels of urine coproporphyrin. Additionally, Geier et al. [130] established a link between high urinary porphyrin levels and ASD severity, although one study did not support this relationship [131]. This area warrants further research to enhance our understanding of urinary Hg and porphyrin levels in relation to ASD. In our meta-analysis, we did not include studies of children with ASD who underwent chelation therapy and subsequently had urinary Hg levels measured, which is actually evidence of the presence of a toxic metal in the organs.

4.4. Are Hg Levels in the Teeth a Promising Link to ASD?

Compared to other biological materials, deciduous teeth are perhaps the most promising clinical matrices for examining the link between Hg and ASD. Unfortunately, only two studies have been published on this topic to date, making it impossible to conduct a meta-analysis [41,112]. For a comprehensive understanding of the role of Hg in ASD, it is important to analyze tooth enamel rather than the entire tooth or dentin, because deciduous teeth's enamel begins to develop in utero, and concludes between 3 months and 1 year after birth. This provides insight into prenatal and early postnatal exposure, a critical period when ASD begins to develop [112]. Of note, the Hg levels recorded by Adams et al. [41] for neurotypical children corresponded to levels found in brain tissue from monkeys subjected to thimerosal, simulating the US childhood vaccination schedule, emphasizing the importance of deciduous teeth, particularly enamel, in understanding the role of Hg in ASD. Hg levels ranging from 260 to over 600 ng/g have been reported in Minamata disease [41]. Further research in this area is needed to explore the potential relationship between Hg exposure through deciduous teeth and ASD.

4.5. Advantages and Limitations of Study Design and Further Directions

Although systematic review can provide useful overviews of the current state of knowledge on a topic if they are conducted with rigorous and clear methods, meta-analysis has some limitations. Although strict criteria were used to appropriately include individuals and exclude papers with very high levels of Hg in clinical matrices, the current study also had some limitations. We were unable to separate participants by gender, age, or residence, as the dimensionality required for reliable meta-analysis was lost. We have generalized results despite differences in primary research, combined different types of studies, and the summary effect may ignore important differences between studies, including the temporal relationship between exposure and outcome. In addition, it is possible that older children with ASD show more mouth behavior than healthy controls, leading to increased Hg levels in their biological tissues. There are not enough studies for nails and teeth, disease severity, and geographical region for ASD, and the measurement of total Hg but not inorganic or organic forms separately.

One of the primary challenges in elucidating the etiological role of Hg in ASD is the lack of access to the most authoritative clinical matrices to either confirm or refute a causal relationship. This primarily pertains to the inability to collect brain tissue from children with ASD due to the impracticality of surgical or biopsy procedures. The situation is further complicated by the fact that the exact timing of ASD onset remains unknown; symptoms emerge at varying ages.

For all the positive and negative aspects of the meta-analysis, we did our best to strictly follow all the rules of the PRISMA protocol to generate an appropriate study design to avoid heterogeneity, bias, and subjectivity. We are aware that this is not completely possible, but we hope that with this study, we have contributed to a better understanding of the relationship between Hg and ASD.

To address these limitations and further advance our understanding of the potential link between Hg and ASD, future investigations should consider the following:

Comprehensive Hg Analysis: Future studies should focus on detailed Hg analysis, including speciation and quantification (MeHg, EtHg, etc.), across a substantial number of participants diagnosed with ASD. These studies should ensure that participants are rigorously matched by factors such as gender, age, residence, diet, socio-economic status, and other uniform characteristics with neurotypical children.

Non-Invasive Clinical Matrices: To overcome the challenges of collecting brain tissue, researchers should emphasize non-invasive clinical matrices, such as hair, urine, and deciduous teeth, or less invasive clinical matrices (whole blood).

5. Conclusions

The present study provides valuable insights into Hg exposure and its potential link to ASD. Patients with ASD had higher whole blood, RBCs, and plasma levels of Hg, while Hg levels in hair and urine were unchanged. The findings support the hypothesis about the role of Hg as an environmental factor in the etiology of ASD. In addition, the findings of this study suggest that ASD children could have impaired excretory mechanisms for removing Hg from their bodies. Our results suggest that we must consider alternative explanations, such as different environmental exposure and increased deposition of Hg in other body tissues, which could lead to decreased excretion. We stress the promising avenue of investigating Hg levels in offering timely insights into MeHg and other Hg species' impact on ASD. Furthermore, we emphasize the urgency of international collaboration to curtail environmental Hg exposure, amenable to non-invasive collection, offering timely insights into MeHg and other Hg species' impact on ASD, highlighting the vital role of human–environment interaction in shaping future generations' health. Through ongoing research and exploration, we aspire to unveil the intricate connection, if any, between Hg exposure and ASD.

Finally, we strongly recommended future research studies to examine the level of Hg in other biological materials, such as nail and deciduous teeth enamel, amenable to non-invasive collection, offering timely insights into MeHg and other Hg species' impact on ASD.

Additional research is needed to shed light on the reliable reduction of Hg levels in the bodies of children with ASD and, thereby, reduce or prevent harmful effects.

Author Contributions: A.S. designed the research, conducted the comprehensive review, participated in the statistical analysis, and drafted the initial and final versions of the paper; N.L. contributed important information regarding ASD and participated in the paper's composition; S.P. was involved in the comprehensive review, conducted the complete meta-analysis, and contributed to the writing of the paper. All authors made critical contributions to the paper's development and provided final approval for its publication. All authors have read and agreed to the published version of the manuscript.

Funding: This research was financially supported by the Ministry of Science, Technological Development, and Innovation of the Republic of Serbia, Contract Numbers 451-03-47/2023-01/200161 and 451-03-47/2023-01/200007.

Institutional Review Board Statement: Not applicable.

Informed Consent Statement: Not applicable.

Data Availability Statement: The authors declare that all data supporting the findings of this study are available from the corresponding author upon reasonable request.

Conflicts of Interest: The authors declare no conflict of interest.

References

1. Veselinović, A.; Petrović, S.; Žikić, V.; Subotić, M.; Jakovljević, V.; Jeremić, N.; Vučić, V. Neuroinflammation in autism and supplementation based on omega-3 polyunsaturated fatty acids: A narrative review. *Medicina* **2021**, *57*, 893. [CrossRef]
2. Awadh, S.M.; Yaseen, Z.M.; Al-Suwaiyan, M.S. The role of environmental trace element toxicants on autism: A medical biogeochemistry perspective. *Ecotoxicol. Environ. Saf.* **2023**, *251*, 114561. [CrossRef] [PubMed]
3. WHO. World Health Organization. 2022. Available online: https://www.who.int/standards/classifications/classification-of-diseases (accessed on 18 May 2023).
4. EAIS. European Autism Information System. 2023. Available online: https://ec.europa.eu/health (accessed on 16 August 2023).
5. Basu, S.; Parry, P. The autism spectrum disorder 'epidemic': Need for biopsychosocial formulation. *Aust. N. Z. J. Psychiatry* **2013**, *7*, 1116–1118. [CrossRef] [PubMed]
6. WHO. World Health Organization. 2023. Available online: https://www.who.int/news-room/factsheets/detail/autismspectrumdisorders#:~:text=About%201%20in%20100%20children,and%20can%20evolve%20over%20time (accessed on 30 June 2023).
7. CDC. Centers for Disease Control and Prevention. 2023. Available online: https://www.cdc.gov/ncbddd/autism/data.html (accessed on 7 September 2023).

8. Arora, M.; Reichenberg, A.; Willfors, C.; Austin, C.; Gennings, C.; Berggren, S.; Lichtenstein, P.; Anckarsäter, H.; Tammimies, K.; Bölte, S. Fetal and postnatal metal dysregulation in autism. *Nat. Commun.* **2017**, *8*, 15493. [CrossRef] [PubMed]
9. Behl, S.; Mehtam, S.; Pandey, M.K. Abnormal levels of metal micronutrients and autism spectrum disorder: A perspective review. *Front. Mol. Neurosci.* **2020**, *13*, 586209. [CrossRef] [PubMed]
10. Maenner, M.J.; Warren, Z.; Williams, A.R.; Amoakohene, E.; Bakian, A.V.; Bilder, D.A.; Durkin, M.S.; Fitzgerald, R.T.; Furnier, S.M.; Hughes, M.M.; et al. Prevalence and characteristics of autism spectrum disorder among children aged 8 years—Autism and developmental disabilities monitoring network, 11 sites, United States. *MMWR Surveill. Summ.* **2020**, *72*, 1–14. [CrossRef] [PubMed]
11. Lord, C.; Brugha, T.S.; Charman, T.; Cusack, J.; Dumas, G.; Frazier, T.; Jones, E.J.H.; Jones, R.M.; Pickles, A.; State, M.W.; et al. Autism spectrum disorder. *Nat. Rev. Dis. Primers* **2020**, *6*, 5. [CrossRef] [PubMed]
12. Hirota, T.; King, B.H. Autism spectrum disorder: A review. *JAMA* **2023**, *329*, 157–168. [CrossRef]
13. LeClerc, S.; Easley, D. Pharmacological therapies for autism spectrum disorder: A review. *PT* **2015**, *40*, 389–397.
14. DeFilippis, M.; Wagnerm, K.D. Treatment of autism spectrum disorder in children and adolescents. *Psychopharmacol. Bull.* **2016**, *46*, 18–41.
15. Siafis, S.; Çıray, O.; Wu, H.; Schneider-Thoma, J.; Bighelli, I.; Krause, M.; Rodolico, A.; Ceraso, A.; Deste, G.; Huhn, M.; et al. Pharmacological and dietary-supplement treatments for autism spectrum disorder: A systematic review and network meta-analysis. *Mol. Autism* **2022**, *13*, 10. [CrossRef] [PubMed]
16. Dong, H.Y.; Feng, J.Y.; Li, H.H.; Yue, X.J.; Jia, F.Y. Non-parental caregivers, low maternal education, gastrointestinal problems and high blood lead level: Predictors related to the severity of autism spectrum disorder in Northeast China. *BMC Pediatr.* **2022**, *22*, 11. [CrossRef] [PubMed]
17. Sauer, A.K.; Stanton, J.E.; Hans, S.; Grabrucker, A.M. Autism spectrum disorders: Etiology and pathology. In *Autism Spectrum Disorders [Internet]*; Grabrucker, A.M., Ed.; Exon Publications: Brisbane, Australia, 2021; Chapter 1.
18. Dickerson, A.S.; Rotem, R.S.; Christian, M.A.; Nguyen, V.T.; Specht, A.J. Potential sex differences relative to autism spectrum disorder and metals. *Curr. Environ. Health Rep.* **2017**, *4*, 405–414. [CrossRef] [PubMed]
19. Marquès, M.; Correig, E.; Capdevila, E.; Gargallo, E.; González, N.; Nadal, M.; Domingo, J.L. Essential and Non-essential Trace Elements in Milks and Plant-Based Drinks. *Biol. Trace Elem. Res.* **2022**, *200*, 4524–4533. [CrossRef] [PubMed]
20. Jagodić, J.; Pavlović, S.; Borković-Mitić, S.; Perović, M.; Miković, Ž.; Đurđić, S.; Manojlović, D.; Stojsavljević, A. Examination of trace metals and their potential transplacental transfer in pregnancy. *Int. J. Mol. Sci.* **2022**, *23*, 8078. [CrossRef] [PubMed]
21. Kaur, I.; Behl, T.; Aleya, L.; Rahman, M.H.; Kumar, A.; Arora, S.; Akter, R. Role of metallic pollutants in neurodegeneration: Effects of aluminum, lead, mercury, and arsenic in mediating brain impairment events and autism spectrum disorder. *Environ. Sci. Pollut. Res. Int.* **2021**, *28*, 8989–9001. [CrossRef] [PubMed]
22. Skogheim, T.S.; Weyde, K.V.F.; Engel, S.M.; Aase, H.; Surén, P.; Øie, M.G.; Biele, G.; Reichborn-Kjennerud, T.; Caspersen, I.H.; Hornig, M.; et al. Metal and essential element concentrations during pregnancy and associations with autism spectrum disorder and attention-deficit/hyperactivity disorder in children. *Environ. Int.* **2021**, *152*, 106468. [CrossRef]
23. McCaulley, M.E. Autism spectrum disorder and mercury toxicity: Use of genomic and epigenetic methods to solve the etiologic puzzle. *Acta Neurobiol. Exp.* **2019**, *79*, 113–125. [CrossRef]
24. Grabrucker, A.M. Environmental factors in autism. *Front. Psychiatry* **2013**, *3*, 118. [CrossRef]
25. Santos-Sacramento, L.; Arrifano, G.P.; Lopes-Araújo, A.; Augusto-Oliveira, M.; Albuquerque-Santos, R.; Takeda, P.Y.; Souza-Monteiro, J.R.; Macchi, M.; do Nascimento, J.L.M.; Lima, R.R.; et al. Human neurotoxicity of mercury in the Amazon: A scoping review with insights and critical considerations. *Ecotoxicol. Environ. Saf.* **2021**, *208*, 111686. [CrossRef]
26. Rice, K.M.; Walker, E.M., Jr.; Wu, M.; Gillette, C.; Blough, E.R. Environmental mercury and its toxic effects. *J. Prev. Med. Public Health* **2014**, *47*, 74–83. [CrossRef]
27. Bjørklund, G.; Skalny, A.V.; Rahman, M.M.; Dadar, M.; Yassa, H.A.; Aaseth, J.; Chirumbolo, S.; Skalnaya, M.G.; Tinkov, A.A. Toxic metal(loid)-based pollutants and their possible role in autism spectrum disorder. *Environ. Res.* **2018**, *166*, 234–250. [CrossRef]
28. Bernhoft, R.A. Mercury toxicity and treatment: A review of the literature. *J. Environ. Public Health* **2012**, *2012*, 460508. [CrossRef] [PubMed]
29. Magos, L.; Clarkson, T.W. Overview of the clinical toxicity of mercury. *Ann. Clin. Biochem.* **2006**, *43*, 257–268. [CrossRef]
30. Sweet, L.I.; Zelikoff, J.T. Toxicology And Immunotoxicology Of Mercury: A Comparative Review In Fish And Humans. *J. Toxicol. Environ. Health B* **2001**, *4*, 161–205. [CrossRef]
31. Burtis, C.A.; Ashwood, E.R.; Bruns, D.E.; Tietz, N.W. *Textbook of Clinical Chemistry and Molecular Diagnostics*, 5th ed.; Elsevier: Amsterdam, The Netherlands, 2012.
32. Ijomone, O.M.; Olung, N.F.; Akingbade, G.T.; Okoh, C.O.A.; Aschner, M. Environmental influence on neurodevelopmental disorders: Potential association of heavy metal exposure and autism. *J. Trace Elem. Med. Biol.* **2020**, *62*, 126638. [CrossRef]
33. Hsueh, Y.-M.; Lee, C.-Y.; Chien, S.-N.; Chen, W.-J.; Shiue, H.-S.; Huang, S.-R.; Lin, M.-I.; Mu, S.-C.; Hsieh, R.-L. Association of blood heavy metals with developmental delays and health status in children. *Sci. Rep.* **2017**, *7*, 43608. [CrossRef]
34. Osman, M.A.; Yang, F.; Massey, I.V.Y. Exposure routes and health effects of heavy metals on children. *BioMetals* **2019**, *32*, 563–573. [CrossRef]
35. Jafari, T.; Rostampour, N.; Fallah, A.A.; Hesami, A. The association between mercury levels and autism spectrum disorders: A systematic review and metaanalysis. *J. Trace Elem. Med. Biol.* **2017**, *44*, 289–297. [CrossRef]

36. Amadi, C.N.; Orish, C.N.; Frazzoli, C.; Orisakwe, O.E. Association of autism with toxic metals: A systematic review of case-control studies. *Pharmacol. Biochem. Behav.* **2022**, *212*, 173313. [CrossRef]
37. El-Ansary, A.; Bjørklund, G.; Tinkov, A.A.; Skalny, A.V.; Al Dera, H. Relationship between selenium, lead, and mercury in red blood cells of Saudi autistic children. *Metab. Brain Dis.* **2017**, *32*, 1073–1080. [CrossRef]
38. Błażewicz, A.; Grabrucker, A.M. Metal profiles in autism spectrum disorders: A crosstalk between toxic and essential metals. *Int. J. Mol. Sci.* **2022**, *24*, 308. [CrossRef] [PubMed]
39. Shandley, K.; Austin, D.W. Ancestry of pink disease (infantile acrodynia) identified as a risk factor for autism spectrum disorders. *J. Toxicol. Environ. Health A* **2011**, *74*, 1185–1194. [CrossRef]
40. Lai, O.; Parsi, K.K.; Wu, D.; Konia, T.H.; Younts, A.; Sinha, N.; McNelis, A.; Sharon, V.R. Mercury toxicity presenting as acrodynia and a papulovesicular eruption in a 5-year-old girl. *Dermatol. Online J.* **2016**, *22*, 13030/qt6444r7nc. [CrossRef]
41. Adams, J.B.; Romdalvik, J.; Ramanujam, V.M.; Legator, M.S. Mercury, lead, and zinc in baby teeth of children with autism versus controls. *J. Toxicol. Environ. Health A* **2007**, *70*, 1046–1051. [CrossRef]
42. Dadar, M.; Peyghan, R.; Memari, H.R. Evaluation of the bioaccumulation of heavy metals in white shrimp (Litopenaeus vannamei) along the Persian Gulf coast. *Bull. Environ. Contam. Toxicol.* **2014**, *93*, 339–343. [CrossRef] [PubMed]
43. Jinadasa, B.K.K.K.; Jayasinghe, G.D.T.M.; Pohl, P.; Fowler, S.W. Mitigating the impact of mercury contaminants in fish and other seafood-A review. *Mar. Pollut. Bull.* **2021**, *171*, 112710. [CrossRef]
44. FDA. The Food and Drug Administration. 2023. Available online: https://www.fda.gov/food/consumers/advice-about-eating-fish (accessed on 5 October 2023).
45. Windham, G.C.; Zhang, L.; Gunier, R.; Croen, L.A.; Grether, J.K. Autism spectrum disorders in relation to distribution of hazardous air pollutants in the San Francisco bay area. *Environ. Health Perspect.* **2006**, *114*, 1438–1444. [CrossRef]
46. Palmer, R.F.; Blanchard, S.; Wood, R. Proximity to point sources of environmental mercury release as a predictor of autism prevalence. *Health Place* **2009**, *15*, 18–24. [CrossRef]
47. Gorini, F.; Muratori, F.; Morales, M.A. The role of heavy metal pollution in neurobehavioral disorders: A focus on autism. *Rev. J. Autism Dev. Disord.* **2014**, *1*, 354–372. [CrossRef]
48. Baj, J.; Flieger, W.; Flieger, M.; Forma, A.; Sitarz, E.; Skórzyńska-Dziduszko, K.; Grochowski, C.; Maciejewski, R.; Karakuła-Juchnowicz, H. Autism spectrum disorder: Trace elements imbalances and the pathogenesis and severity of autistic symptoms. *Neurosci. Biobehav. Rev.* **2021**, *129*, 117–132. [CrossRef]
49. Ye, B.S.; Leung, A.O.W.; Wong, M.H. The association of environmental toxicants and autism spectrum disorders in children. *Environ. Pollut.* **2017**, *227*, 234–242. [CrossRef]
50. Kern, J.K.; Geier, D.A.; Sykes, L.K.; Haley, B.E.; Geier, M.R. The relationship between mercury and autism: A comprehensive review and discussion. *J. Trace Elem. Med. Biol.* **2016**, *37*, 8–24. [CrossRef] [PubMed]
51. Geier, D.A.; King, P.G.-; Sykes, L.K.; Geier, M.R. A comprehensive review of mercury provoked autism. *Indian J. Med. Res.* **2008**, *128*, 383–411.
52. Battaglia, M.R.; Di Fazio, C.; Battaglia, S. Activated Tryptophan-Kynureninemetabolic system in the human brain is associated with learned fear. *Frontiers Mol. Neurisci.* **2023**, *16*, 1217090. [CrossRef]
53. Geier, D.A.; Kern, J.K.; King, P.G.; Sykes, L.K.; Geier, M.R. Hair toxic metal concentrations and autism spectrum disorder severity in young children. *Int. J. Environ. Res. Public Health* **2012**, *9*, 4486–4497. [CrossRef] [PubMed]
54. Moher, D.; Liberati, A.; Tetzlaff, J.; Altman, D.G. PRISMA Group. Preferred reporting items for systematic reviews and meta-analyses: The PRISMA statement. *PLoS Med.* **2009**, *21*, e1000097. [CrossRef]
55. Page, M.J.; McKenzie, J.E.; Bossuyt, P.M.; Boutron, I.; Hoffmann, T.C.; Mulrow, C.D.; Shamseer, L.; Tetzlaff, J.M.; Akl, E.A.; Brennan, S.E.; et al. The PRISMA 2020 statement: An updated guideline for reporting systematic reviews. *BMJ* **2021**, *372*, n71. [CrossRef] [PubMed]
56. Zar, J.H. *Biostatistical Analysis*, 4th ed.; Prentice Hall International Inc.: New Jersey, NJ, USA, 1999.
57. Wells, G.; Shea, B.; O'Connell, D.; Peterson, J.; Welch, V.; Losos, M.; Tugwell, P. *The Newcastle–Ottawa Scale (NOS) for Assessing the Quality of Nonrandomized Studies in Meta-Analyses*; Ottawa Hospital Research Institute: Ottawa, ON, Canada, 2009.
58. Nakhaee, S.; Amirabadizadeh, A.; Farnia, V.; Ali Azadi, N.; Mansouri, B.; Radmehr, F. Association between biological lead concentrations and autism spectrum disorder (ASD) in children: A systematic review and meta-analysis. *Biol. Trace Elem. Res.* **2023**, *201*, 1567–1581. [CrossRef]
59. Higgins, J.P.T.; Green, S. Cochrane Handbook for Systematic Reviews of Interventions. The Cochrane Collaboration Version 5.1.0. 2011. (Updated March 2011). The Cochrane Collaboration. Available online: www.cochrane-handbook.org (accessed on 13 September 2013).
60. Mata, D.A.; Ramos, M.A.; Bansal, N.; Khan, R.; Guille, C.; Di Angelantonio, E.; Sen, S. Prevalence of depression and depressive symptoms among resident physicians: A systematic review and meta-analysis. *JAMA* **2015**, *314*, 2373–2383. [CrossRef]
61. Peeters, W.; Van den Brande, R.; Polinder, S.; Brazinova, A.; Steyerberg, E.W.; Lingsma, H.F.; Maas, A.I. Epidemiology of traumatic brain injury in Europe. *Acta Neurochir.* **2015**, *157*, 1683–1696. [CrossRef]
62. Qin, Y.Y.; Jian, B.; Wu, C.; Jiang, C.Z.; Kang, Y.; Zhou, J.X.; Yang, F.; Liang, Y. A comparison of blood metal levels in autism spectrum disorder and unaffected children in Shenzhen of China and factors involved in bioaccumulation of metals. *Environ. Sci. Pollut. Res. Int.* **2018**, *25*, 17950–17956. [CrossRef] [PubMed]

63. Egger, M.; Smith, G.D.; Minder, C. Bias in meta-analysis detected by a simple, graphical test. *BMJ* **1997**, *315*, 629–634. [CrossRef] [PubMed]
64. Begg, C.B.; Mazumdar, M. Operating characteristics of a rank correlation test for publication bias. *Biometrics* **1994**, *50*, 1088–1101. [CrossRef] [PubMed]
65. Al-Ayadhi, L.Y. Heavy metals and trace elements in hair samples of autistic children in central Saudi Arabia. *Neurosciences* **2005**, *10*, 213–218. [PubMed]
66. Aljumaili, O.I.; Ewais, E.E.D.A.; El-Waseif, A.A.; AbdulJabbar Suleiman, A. Determination of hair lead, iron, and cadmium in a sample of autistic Iraqi children: Environmental risk factors of heavy metals in autism. *Mater. Today Proc.* **2021**, *80*, 2712–2715. [CrossRef]
67. Blaurock-Busch, E.; Amin, O.R.; Rabah, T. Heavy metals and trace elements in hair and urine of a sample of Arab children with autistic spectrum disorder. *Maedica* **2011**, *6*, 247–257.
68. Mohamed Fel, B.; Zaky, E.A.; El-Sayed, A.B.; Elhossieny, R.M.; Zahra, S.S.; Salah Eldin, W.; Youssef, W.Y.; Khaled, R.A.; Youssef, A.M. Assessment of hair aluminum, lead, and mercury in a sample of autistic Egyptian children: Environmental risk factors of heavy metals in autism. *Behav. Neurol.* **2015**, *2015*, 545674. [CrossRef]
69. Ouisselsat, M.; Maidoumi, S.; Elmaouaki, A.; Lekouch, N.; Pineau, A.; Sedki, A. Hair trace elements and mineral content in Moroccan children with autism spectrum disorder: A case-control study. *Biol. Trace Elem. Res.* **2023**, *201*, 2701–2710. [CrossRef]
70. Skalny, A.V.; Simashkova, N.V.; Klyushnik, T.P.; Grabeklis, A.R.; Bjørklund, G.; Skalnaya, M.G.; Nikonorov, A.A.; Tinkov, A.A. Hair toxic and essential trace elements in children with autism spectrum disorder. *Metab. Brain Dis.* **2017**, *32*, 195–202. [CrossRef]
71. Tinkov, A.A.; Skalnaya, M.G.; Simashkova, N.V.; Klyushnik, T.P.; Skalnaya, A.A.; Bjørklund, G.; Notova, S.V.; Kiyaeva, E.V.; Skalny, A.V. Association between catatonia and levels of hair and serum trace elements and minerals in autism spectrum disorder. *Biomed. Pharmacother.* **2019**, *109*, 174–180. [CrossRef] [PubMed]
72. Zhai, Q.; Cen, S.; Jiang, J.; Zhao, J.; Zhang, H.; Chen, W. Disturbance of trace element and gut microbiota profiles as indicators of autism spectrum disorder: A pilot study of Chinese children. *Environ. Res.* **2019**, *171*, 501–509. [CrossRef]
73. Adams, J.B.; Holloway, C.E.; George, F.; Quig, D. Analyses of toxic metals and essential minerals in the hair of Arizona children with autism and associated conditions, and their mothers. *Biol. Trace Elem. Res.* **2006**, *110*, 193–209. [CrossRef] [PubMed]
74. De Palma, G.; Catalani, S.; Franco, A.; Brighenti, M.; Apostoli, P. Lack of correlation between metallic elements analyzed in hair by ICP-MS and autism. *J. Autism. Dev. Disord.* **2012**, *42*, 342–353. [CrossRef]
75. El-Baz, F.; Elhossiny, R.M.; Elsayed, A.B.; Gaber, G.M. Hair mercury measurement in Egyptian autistic children. *Egypt. J. Med. Hum. Gen.* **2010**, *11*, 135–141. [CrossRef]
76. Gil-Hernández, F.; Gómez-Fernández, A.R.; de la Torre-Aguilar, M.J.; Pérez-Navero, J.L.; Flores-Rojas, K.; Martín-Borreguero, P.; Gil-Campos, M. Neurotoxicity by mercury is not associated with autism spectrum disorders in Spanish children. *Ital. J. Pediatr.* **2020**, *46*, 19. [CrossRef] [PubMed]
77. Ip, P.; Wong, V.; Ho, M.; Lee, J.; Wong, W. Mercury exposure in children with autistic spectrum disorder: Case-control study. *J. Child Neurol.* **2004**, *19*, 431–434, Erratum in: *J. Child. Neurol.* **2004**, *22*, 1324. [CrossRef]
78. Nabgha-e-Amen Eqani, S.A.M.A.S.; Khuram, F.; Alamdar, A.; Tahir, A.; Shah, S.T.A.; Nasir, A.; Javed, S.; Bibi, N.; Hussain, A.; Rasheed, H.; et al. Environmental exposure pathway analysis of trace elements and autism risk in Pakistani children population. *Sci. Total Environ.* **2020**, *712*, 136471. [CrossRef]
79. Wecker, L.; Miller, S.B.; Cochran, S.R.; Dugger, D.L.; Johnson, W.D. Trace element concentrations in hair from autistic children. *J. Intellect. Disabil. Res.* **1985**, *29*, 15–22. [CrossRef]
80. Skalny, A.V.; Simashkova, N.V.; Klyushnik, T.P.; Grabeklis, A.R.; Radysh, I.V.; Skalnaya, M.G.; Tinkov, A.A. Analysis of hair trace elements in children with autism spectrum disorders and communication disorders. *Biol. Trace Elem. Res.* **2017**, *107*, 215–223. [CrossRef]
81. Hodgson, N.W.; Waly, M.I.; Al-Farsi, Y.M.; Al-Sharbati, M.M.; Al-Farsi, O.; Ali, A.; Ouhtit, A.; Zang, T.; Zhou, Z.S.; Deth, R.C. Decreased glutathione and elevated hair mercury levels are associated with nutritional deficiency-based autism in Oman. *Exp. Biol. Med.* **2014**, *239*, 697–706. [CrossRef]
82. Lakshmi Priya, M.D.; Geetha, A. Level of trace elements (copper, zinc, magnesium and selenium) and toxic elements (lead and mercury) in the hair and nail of children with autism. *Biol. Trace Elem. Res.* **2011**, *142*, 148–158. [CrossRef] [PubMed]
83. Holmes, A.S.; Blaxill, M.F.; Haley, B.E. Reduced levels of mercury in first baby haircuts of autistic children. *Int. J. Toxicol.* **2003**, *22*, 277–285. [CrossRef] [PubMed]
84. Fido, A.; Al-Saad, S. Toxic trace elements in the hair of children with autism. *Autism* **2005**, *9*, 290–298. [CrossRef] [PubMed]
85. Albizzati, A.; Morè, L.; Di Candia, D.; Saccani, M.; Lenti, C. Normal concentrations of heavy metals in autistic spectrum disorders. *Minerva Pediatr.* **2012**, *64*, 27–31. [PubMed]
86. Kern, J.K.; Grannemann, B.D.; Trivedi, M.H.; Adams, J.B. Sulfhydryl-reactive metals in autism. *J. Toxicol. Environ. Health A* **2007**, *70*, 715–721. [CrossRef] [PubMed]
87. Adams, J.B.; Romdalvik, J.; Levine, K.E.; Hu, L.W. Mercury in first-cut baby hair of children with autism versus typically-developing children. *Toxicol. Environ. Chem.* **2008**, *90*, 739–753. [CrossRef]
88. Majewska, M.D.; Urbanowicz, E.; Rok-Bujko, P.; Namyslowska, I.; Mierzejewski, P. Age-dependent lower or higher levels of hair mercury in autistic children than in healthy controls. *Acta Neurobiol. Exp.* **2010**, *70*, 196–208.

89. Elsheshtawy, E.; Tobar, S.; Sherra, K.; Atallah, S.; Elkasaby, R. Study of some biomarkers in hair of children with autism. *MECP* **2011**, *18*, 6–10. [CrossRef]
90. Li, H.; Li, H.; Li, Y.; Liu, Y.; Zhao, Z. Blood mercury, arsenic, cadmium, and lead in children with autism spectrum disorder. *Biol. Trace Elem. Res.* **2018**, *181*, 31–37. [CrossRef]
91. Adams, J.B.; Audhya, T.; McDonough-Means, S.; Rubin, R.A.; Quig, D.; Geis, E.; Gehn, E.; Loresto, M.; Mitchell, J.; Atwood, S.; et al. Toxicological status of children with autism vs. neurotypical children and the association with autism severity. *Biol. Trace Elem. Res.* **2013**, *151*, 171–180. [CrossRef] [PubMed]
92. Macedoni-Lukšič, M.; Gosar, D.; Bjørklund, G.; Oražem, J.; Kodrič, J.; Lešnik-Musek, P.; Zupančič, M.; France-Štiglic, A.; Sešek-Briški, A.; Neubauer, D.; et al. Levels of metals in the blood and specific porphyrins in the urine in children with autism spectrum disorders. *Biol. Trace Elem. Res.* **2015**, *163*, 2–10. [CrossRef]
93. Zhao, G.; Liu, S.J.; Gan, X.Y.; Li, J.R.; Wu, X.X.; Liu, S.Y.; Jin, Y.S.; Zhang, K.R.; Wu, H.M. Analysis of whole blood and urine trace elements in children with autism spectrum disorders and autistic behaviors. *Biol. Trace Elem. Res.* **2023**, *201*, 627–635. [CrossRef]
94. Yassa, H.A. Autism: A form of lead and mercury toxicity. *Environ. Toxicol. Pharmacol.* **2014**, *38*, 1016–1024. [CrossRef]
95. Stamova, B.; Green, P.G.; Tian, Y.; Hertz-Picciotto, I.; Pessah, I.N.; Hansen, R.; Yang, X.; Teng, J.; Gregg, J.P.; Ashwood, P.; et al. Correlations between gene expression and mercury levels in blood of boys with and without autism. *Neurotox. Res.* **2011**, *19*, 31–48. [CrossRef] [PubMed]
96. Hertz-Picciotto, I.; Green, P.G.; Delwiche, L.; Hansen, R.; Walker, C.; Pessah, I.N. Blood mercury concentrations in CHARGE Study children with and without autism. *Environ. Health Perspect.* **2020**, *118*, 161–166. [CrossRef] [PubMed]
97. Rahbar, M.H.; Samms-Vaughan, M.; Loveland, K.A.; Ardjomand-Hessabi, M.; Chen, Z.; Bressler, J.; Shakespeare-Pellington, S.; Grove, M.L.; Bloom, K.; Pearson DALalor, G.C.; et al. Seafood consumption and blood mercury concentrations in Jamaican children with and without autism spectrum disorders. *Neurotox. Res.* **2013**, *23*, 22–38. [CrossRef]
98. Yau, V.M.; Green, P.G.; Alaimo, C.P.; Yoshida, C.K.; Lutsky, M.; Windham, G.C.; Delorenze, G.; Kharrazi, M.; Grether, J.K.; Croen, L.A. Prenatal and neonatal peripheral blood mercury levels and autism spectrum disorders. *Environ. Res.* **2014**, *133*, 294–303. [CrossRef]
99. McKean, S.J.; Bartell, S.M.; Hansen, R.L.; Barfod, G.H.; Green, P.G.; Hertz-Picciotto, I. Prenatal mercury exposure, autism, and developmental delay, using pharmacokinetic combination of newborn blood concentrations and questionnaire data: A case control study. *Environ. Health* **2015**, *14*, 62. [CrossRef]
100. Mostafa, G.A.; Al-Ayadhi, L.Y. The possible association between elevated levels of blood mercury and the increased frequency of serum anti-myelin basic protein autoantibodies in autistic children. *J. Clin. Cell Immunol.* **2015**, *310*, 6. [CrossRef]
101. Mostafa, G.A.; Bjørklund, G.; Urbina, M.A.; Al-Ayadhi, L.Y. The levels of blood mercury and inflammatory-related neuropeptides in the serum are correlated in children with autism spectrum disorder. *Metab. Brain Dis.* **2016**, *31*, 593–599. [CrossRef]
102. Mostafa, G.A.; Refai, T.M. Antineuronal antibodies in autistic children: Relation to blood mercury. *Egypt J. Pediatr. Allergy Immunol.* **2007**, *5*, 21–30.
103. Chehbani, F.; Gallello, G.; Brahim, T.; Ouanes, S.; Douki, W.; Gaddour, N.; Cervera Sanz, M.L. The status of chemical elements in the blood plasma of children with autism spectrum disorder in Tunisia: A case-control study. *Environ. Sci. Pollut. Res. Int.* **2020**, *27*, 35738–35749. [CrossRef] [PubMed]
104. Khaled, E.M.; Meguid, N.A.; Bjørklund, G.; Gouda, A.; Bahary, M.H.; Hashish, A.; Sallam, N.M.; Chirumbolo, S.; El-Bana, M.A. Altered urinary porphyrins and mercury exposure as biomarkers for autism severity in Egyptian children with autism spectrum disorder. *Metab. Brain Dis.* **2016**, *31*, 1419–1426. [CrossRef]
105. Zhang, J.; Lin, J.; Zhao, X.; Yao, F.; Feng, C.; He, Z.; Cao, X.; Gao, Y.; Khan, N.U.; Chen, M.; et al. Trace element changes in the plasma of autism spectrum disorder children and the positive correlation between chromium and vanadium. *Biol. Trace Elem. Res.* **2022**, *200*, 4924–4935. [CrossRef] [PubMed]
106. Vergani, L.; Cristina, L.; Paola, R.; Luisa, A.M.; Shyti, G.; Edvige, V.; Giuseppe, M.; Elena, G.; Laura, C.; Adriana, V. Metals, metallothioneins and oxidative stress in blood of autistic children. *Res. Autism Spectr. Disord.* **2011**, *5*, 286–293. [CrossRef]
107. Alabdali, A.; Al-Ayadhi, L.; El-Ansary, A. A key role for an impaired detoxification mechanism in the etiology and severity of autism spectrum disorders. *Behav. Brain Funct.* **2014**, *10*, 14. [CrossRef] [PubMed]
108. Geier, D.A.; Audhya, T.; Kern, J.K.; Geier, M.R. Blood mercury levels in autism spectrum disorder: Is there a threshold level? *Acta Neurobiol. Exp.* **2010**, *70*, 177–186.
109. El-Ansary, A. Data of multiple regressions analysis between selected biomarkers related to glutamate excitotoxicity and oxidative stress in Saudi autistic patients. *Data Brief.* **2016**, *7*, 111–116. [CrossRef]
110. Metwally, F.M.; Abdelraoof, E.R.; Rashad, H.; Hasheesh, A.; Elsedfy, Z.B.; Gebril, O.; Meguid, N.A. Toxic effect of some heavy metals in Egyptian autistic children. *Int. J. Pharm. Clin. Res.* **2015**, *7*, 206–211.
111. Wright, B.; Pearce, H.; Allgar, V.; Miles, J.; Whitton, C.; Leon, I.; Jardine, J.; McCaffrey, N.; Smith, R.; Holbrook, I.; et al. A comparison of urinary mercury between children with autism spectrum disorders and control children. *PLoS ONE* **2012**, *7*, e29547. [CrossRef] [PubMed]
112. Woods, J.S.; Armel, S.E.; Fulton, D.I.; Allen, J.; Wessels, K.; Simmonds, P.L.; Granpeesheh, D.; Mumper, E.; Bradstreet, J.J.; Echeverria, D.; et al. Urinary porphyrin excretion in neurotypical and autistic children. *Environ. Health Perspect.* **2010**, *118*, 1450–1457. [CrossRef]

113. Bradstreet, J.; Geier, D.A.; Kartzinel, J.J.; Adams, J.B.; Geier, M.R. A case–control study of mercury burden in children with autistic spectrum disorders. *J. Am. Phys. Surg.* **2003**, *8*, 76–79.
114. Abdullah, M.M.; Ly, A.R.; Goldberg, W.A.; Clarke-Stewart, K.A.; Dudgeon, J.V.; Mull, C.G.; Chan, T.J.; Kent, E.E.; Mason, A.Z.; Ericson, J.E. Heavy metal in children's tooth enamel: Related to autism and disruptive behaviors? *J. Autism Dev. Disord.* **2012**, *42*, 929–936. [CrossRef] [PubMed]
115. Ambeskovic, M.; Laplante, D.P.; Kenney, T.; Elgbeili, G.; Beaumier, P.; Azat, N.; Simcock, G.; Kildea, S.; King, S.; Metz, G.A.S. Elemental Analysis of hair provides biomarkers of maternal hardship linked to adverse behavioral outcomes in 4-year-old children: The QF2011 Queensland Flood Study. *J. Trace Elem. Med. Biol.* **2022**, *73*, 127036. [CrossRef]
116. McDowell, M.A.; Dillon, C.F.; Osterloh, J.; Bolger, P.M.; Pellizzari, E.; Fernando, R.; Montes de Oca, R.; Schober, S.E.; Sinks, T.; Jones, R.L.; et al. Hair mercury levels in U.S. children and women of childbearing age: Reference range data from NHANES 1999–2000. *Environ. Health Perspect.* **2004**, *112*, 1165–1171. [CrossRef] [PubMed]
117. Saghazadeh, A.; Rezaei, N. Systematic review and meta-analysis links autism and toxic metals and highlights the impact of country development status: Higher blood and erythrocyte levels for mercury and lead, and higher hair antimony, cadmium, lead, and mercury. *Prog. Neuropsychopharmacol. Biol. Psychiatry B* **2017**, *79*, 340–368. [CrossRef]
118. Fiore, M.; Barone, R.; Copat, C.; Grasso, A.; Cristaldi, A.; Rizzo, R.; Ferrante, M. Metal and essential element levels in hair and association with autism severity. *J. Trace Elem. Med. Biol.* **2020**, *57*, 126409. [CrossRef]
119. Bridle, T.G.; Kumarathasan, P.; Gailer, J. Toxic Metal Species and 'Endogenous' Metalloproteins at the Blood–Organ Interface: Analytical and Bioinorganic Aspects. *Molecules* **2021**, *26*, 3408. [CrossRef]
120. Ryu, J.; Ha, E.H.; Kim, B.N.; Ha, M.; Kim, Y.; Park, H.; Hong, Y.C.; Kim, K.N. Associations of prenatal and early childhood mercury exposure with autistic behaviors at 5years of age: The Mothers and Children's Environmental Health (MOCEH) study. *Sci. Total Environ.* **2017**, *15*, 251–257. [CrossRef]
121. Babaknejad, N.; Sayehmiri, F.; Sayehmiri, K.; Mohamadkhani, A.; Bahrami, S. The relationship between zinc levels and autism: A systematic review and meta-analysis. *Iran J. Child. Neurol.* **2016**, *10*, 1–9.
122. Chen, C.; Yu, H.; Zhao, J.; Li, B.; Qu, L.; Liu, S.; Zhang, P.; Chai, Z. The roles of serum selenium and selenoproteins on mercury toxicity in environmental and occupational exposure. *Environ. Health Perspect.* **2006**, *114*, 297–301. [CrossRef]
123. Shiani, A.; Sharafi, K.; Omer, A.K.; Kiani, A.; Karamimatin, B.; Massahi, T.; Ebrahimzadeh, G. A systematic literature review on the association between exposures to toxic elements and an autism spectrum disorder. *Sci. Total Environ.* **2023**, *857*, 59246. [CrossRef]
124. Stojsavljević, A.; Lakićević, N.; Pavlović, S. Does lead have a connection to autism? a systematic review and meta-analysis. *Toxics* **2023**, *11*, 753. [CrossRef]
125. Soden, S.E.; Lowry, J.A.; Garrison, C.B.; Wasserman, G.S. 24-hour provoked urine excretion test for heavy metals in children with autism and typically developing controls, a pilot study. *Clin. Toxicol.* **2007**, *45*, 476–481. [CrossRef] [PubMed]
126. Nataf, R.; Skorupka, C.; Amet, L.; Lam, A.; Springbett, A.; Lathe, R. Porphyrinuria in childhood autistic disorder: Implications for environmental toxicity. *Toxicol. Appl. Pharmacol.* **2006**, *14*, 99–108. [CrossRef] [PubMed]
127. Geier, D.A.; Geier, M.R. A prospective assessment of porphyrins in autistic disorders: A potential marker for heavy metal exposure. *Neurotox. Res.* **2006**, *10*, 57–64. [CrossRef] [PubMed]
128. Kern, J.K.; Geier, D.A.; Adams, J.B.; Geier, M.R. A biomarker of mercury body burden correlated with diagnostic domain specific clinical symptoms of autistic disorders. *Biometals* **2010**, *23*, 1043–1051. [CrossRef] [PubMed]
129. Heyer, N.J.; Echeverria, D.; Woods, J.S. Disordered porphyrin metabolism: A potential biological marker for autism risk assessment. *Autism Res.* **2012**, *5*, 84–92. [CrossRef]
130. Geier, D.A.; Kern, J.K.; Geier, M.R. A prospective blinded evaluation of urinary porphyrins verses the clinical severity of autism spectrum disorders. *J. Toxicol. Environ. Health A* **2009**, *72*, 1585–1591. [CrossRef] [PubMed]
131. Shandley, K.; Austin, D.W.; Bhowmik, J.L. Are urinary porphyrins a valid diagnostic biomarker of autism spectrum disorder? *Autism Res.* **2014**, *7*, 535–542. [CrossRef] [PubMed]

Disclaimer/Publisher's Note: The statements, opinions and data contained in all publications are solely those of the individual author(s) and contributor(s) and not of MDPI and/or the editor(s). MDPI and/or the editor(s) disclaim responsibility for any injury to people or property resulting from any ideas, methods, instructions or products referred to in the content.

MDPI
St. Alban-Anlage 66
4052 Basel
Switzerland
www.mdpi.com

Biomedicines Editorial Office
E-mail: biomedicines@mdpi.com
www.mdpi.com/journal/biomedicines

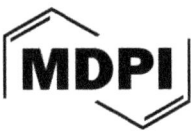

Disclaimer/Publisher's Note: The statements, opinions and data contained in all publications are solely those of the individual author(s) and contributor(s) and not of MDPI and/or the editor(s). MDPI and/or the editor(s) disclaim responsibility for any injury to people or property resulting from any ideas, methods, instructions or products referred to in the content.